T0383029

Medical Devices

This book provides an overview of the wide variety of medical devices that are an integral part of clinical practice. This practical book includes descriptions of medical devices by both clinical specialty and purpose, thus ensuring that a wide variety of devices are included, covering important elements such as body contact, duration of contact, the mechanism of each device, its intended use, single and/or multiple use, benefits and any side/adverse/toxicological effects to the patient, and how to avoid user error. Authored by clinicians, researchers, and educators who are experienced in medical device use, regulation, and research, the content will be of benefit to postgraduate clinicians and employees of medical device companies.

Medical Devices

A Practical Guide

Edited by
Prakash Srinivasan Timiri Shanmugam

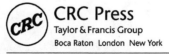

CRC Press is an imprint of the
Taylor & Francis Group, an **informa** business

First edition published 2023
by CRC Press
6000 Broken Sound Parkway NW, Suite 300, Boca Raton, FL 33487-2742

and by CRC Press
4 Park Square, Milton Park, Abingdon, Oxon, OX14 4RN

CRC Press is an imprint of Taylor & Francis Group, LLC

Library of Congress Cataloging-in-Publication Data

Names: Shanmugam, Prakash Srinivasan Timiri, editor.
Title: Medical devices : a practical guide / [edited by] Prakash Srinivasan Timiri Shanmugam.
Other titles: Medical devices (Shanmugam)
Description: First edition. | Boca Raton : CRC Press, 2023. | Includes bibliographical references and index. | Summary: "An overview of the wide variety of medical devices that are an integral part of clinical practice. This practical book includes descriptions of medical devices by both clinical specialty and purpose, thus ensuring that a wide variety of devices are included"-- Provided by publisher.
Identifiers: LCCN 2022017833 (print) | LCCN 2022017834 (ebook) | ISBN 9781032062525 (hardback) | ISBN 9781032116051 (paperback) | ISBN 9781003220671 (ebook)
Subjects: MESH: Equipment and Supplies | Prostheses and Implants
Classification: LCC R857.M3 (print) | LCC R857.M3 (ebook) | NLM W 26 | DDC 610.28/4--dc23/eng/20220701
LC record available at https://lccn.loc.gov/2022017833
LC ebook record available at https://lccn.loc.gov/2022017834

ISBN: 9781032062525 (hbk)
ISBN: 9781032116051 (pbk)
ISBN: 9781003220671 (ebk)

DOI: 10.1201/9781003220671

Typeset in Times
by Deanta Global Publishing Services, Chennai, India

Contents

Contributor List

K. P. G. Uma Anitha
Vellore Institute of Technology
Chennai, India

Sayan Kumar Das
Department of Pharmacology,
Manipal-TATA Medical College, Jamshedpur,
Manipal Academy of Higher Education,
    Manipal, India

T. Y. Sri Hari
Consultant Critical Care
Omni Hospital
Hyderabad, Telangana, India

Indumathy Jagadeeswaran
Department of Biological Sciences
Southern Methodist University
University Park, Texas, USA

B. Karthika
Tamil Nadu Dr. MGR Medical University
Chennai, India

Sameer Khasbage
Department of Pharmacology
All India Institute of Medical Sciences
Bhopal, India

Z. Naveen Kumar
Department of Physiology
Santhiram Medical College
Nandyal, India

Basanta Manjari Naik
Department of Physiology
Jawaharlal Institute of Postgraduate Medical
    Education and Research
Pondicherry, India

Shamsul Nisa
Bharati Vidyapeeth
Pune, India

Shalini Pattabiraman
School of Health Professions
Rutgers, The State University of New Jersey
New Brunswick, New Jersey, USA

M. Pavani
Tamil Nadu Dr. MGR Medical University
Chennai, India

Thamizharasan S
Department of Pharmacology and
    Toxicology
Saveetha Medical College and Hospital
SIMATS
Chennai, India

K. S. B. S. Krishna Sasanka
Department of ENT
All India Institute of Medical Sciences
Deoghar, India

Mythili Sathiavelu
Vellore Institute of Technology
Chennai, India

Gayathri Segaran
Vellore Institute of Technology
Chennai, India

**Prakash Srinivasan Timiri
    Shanmugam**
Global Product Safety and Toxicology
Avanos Medical Inc
Alpharetta, Georgia, USA

Surjit Singh
Additional Professor
Department of Pharmacology
AIIMS
Jodhpur, India.

Harini Sriram
Covabind Joint Research Private Limited
Hosur, India

Sandhiya Thamizharasan
Saasha Smile Clinic
Saasha Garden
Chennai, India

Sree Sudha T. Y.
Department of Pharmacology
All India Institute of Medical
   Sciences
Deoghar, India

Pugazhenthan Thangaraju
Department of Pharmacology
All India Institute of Medical Sciences
Raipur, India

Krithaksha V
Georgian National University SEU
Tbilisi, Georgia

Yakaiah Vangoori
Department of Pharmacology
Santhiram Medical College
Nandyal, India

Anjaly Mary Varghese
Department of Pharmacology
Santhiram Medical College
Nandyal, India

Shobhan Babu Varthya
Department of Pharmacology
All India Institute of Medical Sciences
Jodhpur, India

Hemasri Velmurugan
Department of Pharmacology
All India Institute of Medical Sciences
Raipur, India

Introduction

1

Thamizharasan S, Sandhiya Thamizharasan,
Krithaksha V, and Prakash Srinivasan
Timiri Shanmugam

Medical devices play an important role in the delivery of many health care services. "Medical device" means any instrument, apparatus, implement, machine, appliance, implant, in vitro reagent or calibrator, software, material or other similar or related article, intended by the manufacturer to be used, alone or in combination, for human beings for one or more of the specific purposes of:

- diagnosis, prevention, monitoring, prediction, prognosis, treatment or alleviation of disease
- diagnosis, monitoring, treatment, alleviation of or compensation for an injury or disability
- investigation, replacement or modification of the anatomy or of a physiological or pathological process or state
- providing information by means of in vitro examination of specimens derived from the human body, including organ, blood and tissue donations
- and which does not achieve its principal intended action by pharmacological, immunological or metabolic means, in or on the human body, but which may be assisted in its function by such means (1)

The following products shall also be deemed to be medical devices:

- devices for the control or support of conception
- products specifically intended for the cleaning, disinfection or sterilization of devices

The term applies to everything from common medical supplies such as latex gloves and syringes to advanced imaging equipment and implantable devices such as cardiac defibrillators. The medical device industry is thus an important component of the larger health care system and plays an essential role by developing new medical technologies that can improve the ability to diagnose and treat illness. Some types of medical devices include:

- single-use devices (i.e. syringes, catheters)
- implantable (i.e. hip prothesis, pacemakers)
- imaging (i.e. ultrasound and CT scanners)
- medical equipment (i.e. anesthesia machines, patient monitors, hemodialysis machines)
- software (i.e. computer aided diagnostics)
- in vitro diagnostics (i.e. glucometer, HIV tests)

DOI: 10.1201/9781003220671-1

- personal protective equipment (i.e. mask, gowns, gloves)
- surgical and laboratory instruments

BACKGROUND

As early as 2000 to 5000 years ago, many ancient civilizations used tools such as forceps, knives, scalpels, saws, lancets, needles, trocars, cauteries and knives for several medical procedures. Scalpels were used to make big incisions across the abdomen, and clean, precise incisions on the arms, neck and legs. Punctures in various parts of the body were made using needles. Hooks held up blood vessels and skin, and lifted and moved tissue during a medical procedure. Hand drills were used to remove parts of the skull to access the brain, to either cut out portions in a lobotomy or to remove dead tissue from the body. Forceps, an extremely versatile tool during surgery, were used to grasp or position tissues, immobilize blood flow and hold skin together while adding or removing stitches. Suturing techniques used crude forms of needle and thread. Early procedures included tracheotomy, amputations, bloodletting, cataract surgery, bone surgeries, removal of bladder stones, trepanation (making a hole in the skull), organ removal, etc. The earliest instruments used in these procedures were made of stone, flint or obsidian, and later on from metals like silver, gold and bronze.

From about the 1st century CE to the 17th century, most medical procedures involved the treatment of injuries of soldiers at war on the battlefields, or the ailments of the very rich. Devices were used to treat battleground wounds received from arrows, knives, sabers, guns and cannons. With the formalization of the scientific method in the 17th century such devices became more prevalent. Many medical devices were manufactured by doctors or small companies and sold directly to the public with no government standards or oversight for safety or effectiveness. Hospitals were created as a place where soldiers and patients could be treated by doctors with access to specialized equipment and care. Universities began teaching science, medicine, anatomy and medical-related topics. Medical knowledge and know-how continued to expand and evolve. Advances were made in the areas like ophthalmology, optometry, prostheses, catheterization with devices like syringes for the removal of cataracts, eyeglasses, metallic or wooden artificial limbs and metallic catheters respectively.

Discovery of what would be considered a medical device by modern standards dates as far back as c. 7000 BC in Baluchistan where Neolithic dentists used flint-tipped drills and bowstrings. The study of archeology and Roman medical literature also indicates that many types of medical devices were in widespread use during the time of ancient Rome. In the United States it wasn't until the Federal Food, Drug, and Cosmetic Act (FD&C Act) in 1938 that medical devices were regulated. Later, in 1976, the Medical Device Amendments to the FD&C Act established medical device regulation and oversight as we know it today (2).

The road to modern medicine has been a long one, and doctors have come up with a variety of tools along the way. But some of the early iterations were, shall we say, a little crude. Here are some of the more cringe-inducing instruments from medicine's past.

Artificial leeches: When in the 1800s live leeches were unavailable, or perhaps too gross, this metal cylinder with blades performed the same function. Its rotating blades cut into the skin, while the tube suctioned the blood out. A similar tool, called a scarificator, used up to ten spring-loaded blades. They quickly sliced into the skin and then the device was heated to create a vacuum.

Hernia tool: Recognizing that the human body could often patch things up better than they could, doctors in the 1850s had a tool specifically for hernias. Once doctors repaired the tear in the muscle or tissue, they would insert the hernia tool into the area. This thing would be in place for about a week while scar tissue formed on it to help seal your repaired hernia.

Amputation saw: Medicine also has a long history of doctors lopping off problems they didn't yet know how to fix, such as infections. From the pre-antibiotic bacteria of old to the antibiotic-resistant bacteria of today, infection has always been a major reason for amputations. But doctors often took pride in the instruments used for this grisly purpose. Saws like this had decorative swirls, grooves and other designs that were, ironically, probably also a place for germs to breed.

Ecraseur: Used in the 19th century, this instrument strangled uterine and ovarian tumors as well as hemorrhoids. Its wire loop or chain was placed around the base of the unwanted growth and gradually tightened. That would eventually either cut through the base of the growth or cut off its blood supply until it gave up and dropped off. Doing this was painful, particularly with hemorrhoids, but experts of the day argued that the pain was short-lived compared with cutting.

Arrow remover: When a patient in the 1500s sported a protruding arrow, the medical professionals didn't just yank it out. Instead, they held the shaft of the arrow in the center barrel of a scissor-like arrow remover. But unlike scissors, the sharp edges of the blades faced away from the center. So, as if having an arrow stuck in you wasn't bad enough, the blades cut the skin so that the arrow's head could be removed without much further injury.

Speculum: Long before the speculum was actually called that, there were tools for getting an intimate look at a woman's reproductive organs. In the 1600s, it was a rather frilly-looking sort of inverted salad tongs. Once the leading end was inserted into the entry of the vagina or other orifice, the user would turn the crank at the other end to widen the opening for a better view.

Syringe: Syringes are still in use today, but this simple piston syringe was special. With its long, thin tube and pump, it was way bigger than the hypodermics we use today. It was used in the 1500s to inject mercury as a treatment for syphilis, often contracted by amorous sailors on the high seas. With such a huge syringe, the good news is that you didn't get stabbed with it. The bad news is that it was a urethral syringe, so the injection went directly into the penis through its natural opening. Worse yet, mercury often killed people long before syphilis complications (3).

The 1800s was a groundbreaking era for medical devices, therapeutic and medical inventions and the development of modern medicine. In 1867, Joseph Lister published his "Antiseptic Principle of the Practice of Surgery". This was one of the most seminal and pivotal moments in medical science that would ultimately lead to cleaner operating theatres, more successful outcomes and higher survival rates of patients. Louis Pasteur and Robert Koch identified "germs" as the cause of many diseases around the world (4). In the 19th century, devices such as the stethoscope, the hypodermic syringe, the ophthalmoscope, the electrocardiogram, hearing aids, the kymograph and nitrous oxide as an anesthetic were brought to market. In addition, drugs such as quinine, aspirin and cholera vaccines were also discovered, significantly changing the health outcomes of the public. The design of devices such as forceps, knives, scalpels, saws, lancets, needles, trocars, cauteries and knives continued to evolve with the use of materials like steel. The 20th century saw an explosion of medical devices and procedures that included the cardio defibrillator, hip and knee replacements, heart surgeries, laparoscopes, dialysis machines, infusion pumps, insulin pumps, balloon catheters, disposable catheters, disposables, the iron lung, heart lung machines, inhalers, prostheses, cardiovascular devices, respirators, ventilators and implants such as stents and pacemakers. The growth of medical devices has been exponential in the last 100 years.

TERMS AND DEFINITIONS

"**Accessory to a medical device**" means an article which, while not being itself a medical device, is intended by its manufacturer to be used together with one or several particular medical device(s) to specifically enable the medical device(s) to be used in accordance with its/their intended purpose(s) or to specifically and directly assist the medical functionality of the medical device(s) in terms of its/their intended purpose(s).

"**Active medical device**" means any device, the operation of which depends on a source of energy other than that generated by the human body for that purpose, or by gravity, and which acts by changing the density of or converting that energy. Devices intended to transmit energy, substances or other elements between an active device and the patient, without any significant change, shall not be deemed to be active devices.

"**Active therapeutic device**" means any active device used, whether alone or in combination with other devices, to support, modify, replace or restore biological functions or structures with a view to treatment or alleviation of an illness, injury or disability.

"**Active device intended for diagnosis and monitoring**" means any active device used, whether alone or in combination with other devices, to supply information for detecting, diagnosing, monitoring or treating physiological conditions, states of health, illnesses or congenital deformities.

"**Adverse event**" means any untoward medical occurrence, unintended disease or injury or any untoward clinical signs, including an abnormal laboratory finding, in subjects, users or other persons, in the context of a clinical investigation, whether or not related to the investigational device.

"**Biomaterial**" is a material brought into contact with living tissue for the treatment of medical and dental conditions.

"**Calibrator**" means a measurement reference material used in the calibration of a device.

"**Companion diagnostic**" means a device which is essential for the safe and effective use of a corresponding medicinal product to identify, before and/or during treatment, patients who are most likely to benefit from the corresponding medicinal product; or identify, before and/or during treatment, patients likely to be at increased risk of serious adverse reactions as a result of treatment with the corresponding medicinal product.

"**Common specifications**" (**CS**) means a set of technical and/or clinical requirements, other than a standard, that provides a means of complying with the legal obligations applicable to a device, process or system.

"**Clinical performance**" means the ability of a device, resulting from any direct or indirect medical effects which stem from its technical or functional characteristics, including diagnostic characteristics, to achieve its intended purpose as claimed by the manufacturer, thereby leading to a clinical benefit for patients, when used as intended by the manufacturer.

"**Compatibility**" is the ability of a device, including software, when used together with one or more other devices in accordance with its intended purpose, to perform without losing or compromising the ability to perform as intended, and/or integrate and/or operate without the need for modification or adaption of any part of the combined devices, and/or be used together without conflict/interference or adverse reaction.

"**Conformity assessment**" means the process of demonstrating whether the requirements of a regulation relating to a device have been fulfilled.

"**Corrective action**" means action taken to eliminate the cause of a potential or actual non-conformity or other undesirable situation.

"**Custom-made device**" means any device specifically made in accordance with a written prescription of any person authorized by national law by virtue of that person's professional qualifications which gives, under that person's responsibility, specific design characteristics, and is intended for the sole use of a particular patient exclusively to meet their individual conditions and needs. However, mass-produced devices which need to be adapted to meet the specific requirements of any professional user and devices which are mass-produced by means of industrial manufacturing processes in accordance with the written prescriptions of any authorized person shall not be considered to be custom-made devices.

"**Device deficiency**" means any inadequacy in the identity, quality, durability, reliability, safety or performance of an investigational device, including malfunction, use errors or inadequacy in information supplied by the manufacturer.

"**Falsified device**" means any device with a false presentation of its identity and/or its source and/or its Conformitè Europëenne (CE) marking certificates or documents relating to CE marking procedures. This definition does not include unintentional non-compliance and is without prejudice to infringements of intellectual property rights.

"**Harmonized standard**" means a European standard as defined in point (1)(c) of Article 2 of Regulation (EU) No 1025/2012.

"**Implantable device**" means any device, including those that are partially or wholly absorbed, which is intended to be totally introduced into the human body, or to replace an epithelial surface or the surface of the eye, by clinical intervention, and which is intended to remain in place after the procedure. Any device intended to be partially introduced into the human body by clinical intervention and intended to remain in place after the procedure for at least 30 days shall also be deemed to be an implantable device.

"**In vitro diagnostic medical device**" means any medical device which is a reagent, reagent product, calibrator, control material, kit, instrument, apparatus, piece of equipment, software or system, whether used alone or in combination, intended by the manufacturer to be used in vitro for the examination of specimens, including blood and tissue donations, derived from the human body, solely or principally for the purpose of providing information on one or more of the following:

- concerning a physiological or pathological process or state
- concerning congenital physical or mental impairments
- concerning the predisposition to a medical condition or a disease
- to determine the safety and compatibility with potential recipients
- to predict treatment response or reactions
- to define or monitor therapeutic measures
- specimen receptacles shall also be deemed to be in vitro diagnostic medical devices

"**Invasive device**" means any device which, in whole or in part, penetrates inside the body, either through a body orifice or through the surface of the body.

"**Investigational device**" means a device that is assessed in a clinical investigation.

"**Legacy devices**" are considered to include all devices previously CE marked under the European Medical Devices Directive 93/42/EEC (MDD) or Active Implantable Medical Devices Directive 90/385/EEC (AIMDD).

"**Life cycle**" means a series of all phases in the life of a medical device, from the initial conception to final decommissioning and disposal.

"**Nanomaterial**" means a natural, incidental or manufactured material containing particles in an unbound state or as an aggregate or as an agglomerate and where, for 50% or more of the particles in the number size distribution, one or more external dimensions is in the size range 1–100 nm; fullerenes, graphene flakes and single-wall carbon nanotubes with one or more external dimensions below 1 nm shall also be deemed to be nanomaterials.

"**Non-viable**" means having no potential for metabolism or multiplication.

"**Notified body**" means a conformity assessment body designated in accordance with this Regulation.

"**Performance evaluation**" means an assessment and analysis of data to establish or verify the scientific validity and the analytical and, where applicable, the clinical performance of a device.

"**Recall**" means any measure aimed at achieving the return of a device that has already been made available to the end user.

"**Risk**" means the combination of the probability of occurrence of harm and the severity of that harm.

"**Risk management**" means the systematic application of management policies, procedures and practices to the tasks of analyzing, evaluating, controlling and monitoring risk.

"**Serious adverse event**" means any adverse event that leads to any of the following:

- a patient management decision resulting in death or an imminent life-threatening situation for the individual being tested, or in the death of the individual's offspring
- death
- serious deterioration in the health of the individual being tested or the recipient of tested donations or materials that results in any of the following:
  - life-threatening illness or injury
  - permanent impairment of a body structure or a body function
  - hospitalization or prolongation of patient hospitalization
  - medical or surgical intervention to prevent life-threatening illness or injury or permanent impairment to a body structure or a body function
  - chronic disease
  - fetal distress, fetal death or a congenital physical or mental impairment or birth defect

"**Single-use device**" means a device that is intended to be used on one individual during a single procedure.

"**System**" means a combination of products, either packaged together or not, which are intended to be inter-connected or combined to achieve a specific medical purpose.

"**Unique device identifier**" ("**UDI**") means a series of numeric or alphanumeric characters that are created through internationally accepted device identification and coding standards and that allows unambiguous identification of specific devices on the market.

"**Withdrawal**" means any measure aimed at preventing a device in the supply chain from being further made available on the market.

CLASSIFICATION OF MEDICAL DEVICES

The Food and Drug Administration (FDA) has established classifications for approximately 1700 different generic types of devices and grouped them into 16 medical specialties referred to as panels. Each of these generic types of devices is assigned to one of three regulatory classes based on the level of control necessary to assure the safety and effectiveness of the device.

Class 1 – Low Risk

There are currently approximately 780 Class I devices on the market. General controls include Adulteration/Misbranding, Electronic Establishment, Registration, Electronic Device Listing, Premarket Notification, Quality Systems, Labeling and Medical Device Reporting (MDR).

Examples: Corrective glasses and frames, manual wheelchairs.
Type of certification: Self-certification/self-declaration.

Class 1s – Low Risk (Sterile)

Examples: Personal protection kits, sterile urine bags, etc.
Type of certification: Notified body.

Class 1m – Low Risk (Measuring Body Attributes)

Examples: Stethoscopes, weighing balance.
Type of certification: Notified body.

Class 1r – Low Risk (Reused Device)

Examples: Surgical forceps (all types of SS/Tit surgical equipment sterilized and reused by hospitals).
Type of certification: Notified body.

Class IIa – Medium Risk

Examples: Orthodontic wires, surgical gloves, lancets.
Type of certification: Notified body.

Class IIb – Medium to High Risk

Most devices are classified as Class II, an intermediate-risk device that is subject to "special controls" to assure safety. The majority of Class II devices are subject to premarket review and clearance by FDA through the 510 (k)-premarket notification process and may have rigorous review requirements in line with a Class III device. There are currently over 800 Class II devices on the market.

Examples: Orthopedic nails and plates, intra-ocular lenses, pregnancy test kits, incubators for babies.
Type of certification: Notified body.

Class III – High Risk

These devices are subject to the most rigorous review process that includes general controls, special controls and premarket approval. There are fewer than 120 Class III devices currently on the market.

Examples: Pacemakers, prosthetic heart valves, cardiovascular sutures, brain spatulas, drug-device combination products.
Type of certification: Notified body.

Medical Device Classification: 21 CFR 862–892

Most medical devices can be classified by finding the matching description of the device in Title 21 of the Code of Federal Regulations (CFR), Parts 862–892. FDA has classified and described over 1,700 distinct types of devices and organized them in the CFR into 16 medical specialty panels such as cardiovascular devices or in vitro diagnostics.

862 = Chemistry/Toxicology
864 = Hematology/Pathology
866 = Immunology/Microbiology
868 = Anesthesiology
870 = Cardiovascular
872 = Dental
874 = Ear, Nose and Throat
876 = Gastro/Urology
878 = General Plastic Surgery
880 = General Hospital
882 = Neurological
884 = Obstetrical/Gynecological
886 = Ophthalmic
888 = Orthopedic
890 = Physical Medicine
892 = Radiology Regulations

For each of the devices classified by the FDA, the CFR gives a general description including the intended use, the class to which the device belongs (i.e. Class I, II or III) and information about marketing requirements. Your device should meet the definition in a classification regulation contained in 21 CFR 862–892.

MATERIALS USED IN MEDICAL DEVICES

The most common classes of materials used in the devices are metals, polymers, ceramics and composite (Table 1.1). These four classes are used singly and in combination to form most of the implantation devices available today. Metals are particularly inert, ceramics may be inert, active or resorbable and polymers may be inert or resorbable in nature. Biomaterials must be nontoxic, noncarcinogenic, chemically inert, stable and mechanically strong enough to withstand the repeated forces of a lifetime (5).

In the development of medical devices, selecting appropriate material for each part is a vital step, one which demands an understanding of issues ranging from physical performance and manufacturing constraints to fund limitations and supply chain logistics. There are few "trivial" components in a medical device, and identifying materials for all but the most direct demands a robust decision process to check that appropriate options are assessed. In device design, several essential factors need to be considered when deciding whether a material, and its specific grade, are appropriate for use on a component. Biomaterial used in the devices and implants should have some important properties in order for long-term usage in the body without rejection.

Materials testing: Materials are tested to determine the properties of biomaterials used in various devices. The data thus obtained can be used in specifying the suitability of materials for various applications like medical devices and implants. The materials chosen must be able to support the device's function. Safety is the most important reason material testing is done, and it also prevents the failure of devices. Standard test methods have been established by such national and international bodies as the International Organization for Standardization (ISO), with headquarters in Geneva, and the American Society for Testing and Materials (ASTM), Philadelphia.

Biocompatibility

Biocompatibility is a key demand for several medical devices, especially newer drug delivery devices which must be made of materials suitable for contact with both the drug and the user. Materials that are biocompatible are called biomaterials, and biocompatibility is a descriptive term which indicates the ability of a material to perform with an appropriate or specific host response, in a device application. For new materials not already approved, extensive material test programs could be required to check extractables and leachables, toxicity or irritation, depending on the application and risk. For considerations such as long-term implantation or primary drug packaging, where permeability to substances including moisture or oxygen can also be a vital property, these issues can be the dominant factor driving material/material grade selection. It should not adversely affect the local and systemic host environment of interaction (bone, soft tissues, ionic composition of plasma, as well as intra- and extracellular fluids). Biocompatibility refers

TABLE 1.1 Classification of Materials Used in Medical Devices

MATERIALS CLASSIFICATION	
MATERIALS	*SUBCATEGORIES*
Metals	Gold, tantalum, Ti6A14V, stainless steel, Co-Cr alloys, titanium, nitinol
Polymers	Ultra-high molecular weight polyethylene (UHMWPE), polyurethane (PE), polyurethane (PU), polytetrafluoroethylene (PTFE), polyacetal (PA), polymethylmethacrylate (PMMA), polyethylene terephthalate (PET), silicone rubber (SR), polyetheretherketone (PEEK), poly (lactic acid) (PLA), polysulfone (PS)
Ceramics	Alumina, zirconia, carbon, titania, bioglass, hydroxyapatite (HA)
Composites	Silica/SR, CF/UHMWPE, CF/PTFE, HA/PE, CF/epoxy, CF/PEEK, CF/C, Al2O3/PTFE

to a set of properties that a material must have to be used safely in a biological organism. A biocompatible material must be noncarcinogenic, non-pyrogenic, nontoxic, non-allergenic, blood compatible and noninflammatory. The operational definition of biocompatible is "The patient is alive so the material must be biocompatible".

Bio Functionality

Bio functionality fulfills a specific function in physical and mechanical terms. The material must satisfy its design requirements in service:

- load transmission and stress distribution (e.g. bone replacement)
- articulation to allow movement (e.g. artificial knee joint)
- control of blood and fluid flow (e.g. artificial heart)
- space filling (e.g. cosmetic surgery)
- electrical stimuli (e.g. pacemaker)
- light transmission (e.g. implanted lenses)
- sound transmission (e.g. cochlear implant)

Toxicology

A biomaterial should not be toxic to the human, unless it is specifically engineered for such requirements (for example a "smart bomb" drug delivery system that targets cancer cells and destroys them). Toxicology for biomaterials deals with the substances that migrate or are released out of the biomaterials. It is reasonable to say that a biomaterial should not give off anything from its mass unless it is specifically designed to do so.

BIOLOGICAL EVALUATION OF MEDICAL DEVICES

Biological safety evaluation and hazard testing of medical devices shall be performed in compliance with ISO 10993 "Biological Evaluation of Medical Devices" series as the international standard. Based on the framework and principles of ISO 10993-1 "Evaluation and Testing", the necessary evaluation items can be selected corresponding to the nature and duration of exposure of individual medical devices to the human body. The test method guidelines in the ISO 10993 series generally include lists of multiple test methods for each evaluation item. ISO 10993-3 specifies strategies for risk estimation, selection of hazard identification tests and risk management, with respect to the possibility of the following potentially irreversible biological effects arising as a result of exposure to medical devices:

- acute toxicity
- chronic toxicity
- irritation (eye, skin, mucosal surfaces)
- hypersensitivity
- genotoxicity
- carcinogenicity
- reproductive and developmental toxicity

The international standards have been continuously revised according to the development of science and technology. Accordingly, an appropriate test method must be selected, considering the most current international standards at the time when testing is conducted.

MEDICAL DEVICES REGULATIONS

In the United States, medical devices are regulated by the FDA with an aim of ensuring the safety and effectiveness of the devices. The FDA's Center for Devices and Radiological Health (CDRH) is responsible for regulating firms who manufacture, repackage, relabel and/or import medical devices sold in the United States. In addition, CDRH regulates radiation-emitting electronic products (medical and non-medical) such as lasers, X-ray systems and ultrasound equipment (6). The basic regulatory requirements that manufacturers of medical devices distributed in the United States must comply with are:

Establishment Registration and Medical Device Listing – 21 CFR Part 807

Owners or operators of establishments that are involved in the production and distribution of medical devices intended for use in the United States are required to register annually with the FDA. This process is known as establishment registration.

Manufacturers must list their devices with the FDA. Establishments required to list their devices include:

manufacturers
contract manufacturers
contract sterilizers
repackagers and relabelers
specification developers
reprocessors of single-use devices
remanufacturers
manufacturers of accessories and components sold directly to the end user
US manufacturers of "export only" devices

Premarket Notification 510(k) – 21 CFR Part 807 Subpart E

A company that wants to market a Class I, II or III device intended for human use in the United States, for which a Premarket Approval (PMA) application is not required, must submit a 510(k) to FDA unless the device is exempt from the 510(k) requirements of the FD&C Act. There is no 510(k) form; however, 21 CFR 807 Subpart E describes the requirements for a 510(k) submission. Before marketing a device, each submitter must receive an order, in the form of a letter, from the FDA which finds the device to be substantially equivalent (SE) and states that the device can be marketed in the United States. This order "clears" the device for commercial distribution (7).

Premarket Approval (PMA) – 21 CFR Part 814

Products requiring PMAs are Class III devices which are high risk devices that pose a significant risk of illness or injury, or devices found not substantially equivalent to Class I and II predicates through the 510(k) process. The PMA process is more involved and includes the submission of clinical data to support claims made for the device.

Investigational Device Exemption (IDE) for Clinical Studies – 21CFR Part 812

An investigational device exemption (IDE) allows the investigational device to be used in a clinical study in order to collect the safety and effectiveness data required to support a PMA application or a Premarket Notification 510(k) submission to FDA. Clinical studies with devices of significant risk must be approved by the FDA and by an Institutional Review Board (IRB) before the study can begin. Studies with devices of nonsignificant risk must be approved by the IRB only before the study can begin.

Quality System (QS) Regulation 21 CFR Part 820

The quality system regulation includes requirements related to the methods used in and the facilities and controls used for the designing, purchasing, manufacturing, packaging, labeling, storing, installing and servicing of medical devices. Manufacturing facilities undergo FDA inspections to assure compliance with the QS requirements.

Labeling Requirements – 21 CFR Part 801

The US FDA develops and administers regulations under authority granted by laws passed by Congress that apply to food, drugs, cosmetics, biologics, radiation-emitting electronic products and medical devices. Labeling regulations pertaining to medical devices are found in the following Parts of Title 21 of the CFR.

Medical Device Reporting (MDR) – 21 CFR Part 803

Incidents in which a device may have caused or contributed to a death or serious injury must be reported to the FDA under the Medical Device Reporting program. In addition, certain malfunctions must also be reported. The MDR regulation is a mechanism for the FDA and manufacturers to identify and monitor significant adverse events involving medical devices. The goals of the regulation are to detect and correct problems in a timely manner.

EU Regulation

EU Regulation of Restriction of Hazardous Substances (RoHS): European Union directives have restricted the use of certain hazardous substances in medical devices and implants. Hazardous substances are categorized per EU Regulation 1272/2008 (Classification, Labelling and Packaging of Substances/ Mixtures and Substances Identified in EU Regulation 1907/2006) (REACH: Registration, Evaluation, Authorization, and Restriction of Chemicals). EU 1272/2008 REACH contains a list of all hazardous chemicals. A substance of very high concern (SVHC) contains carcinogenic, mutagenic, reproductive toxic (CMR) substances like N, N-dimethylanilinium tetrakis borate, dibutylin hydrogen borate, perboric acid and restricted substances of endocrine disruptives (EDs), persistent, bioaccumulative and toxic (PBT) and very persistent and very bioaccumulative (vPvB). Chemicals that are substances of very high concern are to be phased out and replaced with safer alternative chemicals (8). In addition to CMR, EDs, PBTs and vPvB, the list extends to flammable gases, flammable aerosols, oxidizing gases, gases under pressure, flammable liquids, flammable solids, self-reactive substances or mixtures, chemicals capable of causing skin corrosion, irritation, serious eye irritation, respiratory/skin sensitization, germ cell mutagenicity or specific target organ toxicity and chemicals hazardous to the aquatic environment or ozone layer. RoHS specifies maximum levels by weight for the following ten restricted materials. The first six were included in the original RoHS while the last four phthalates were added under RoHS III. The expanded list for RoHS 3 is thus as follows:

- lead (0.1%)
- mercury (0.1%)
- cadmium (0.01%)
- hexavalent chromium (0.1%)
- polybrominated biphenyls (PBB) (0.1%)
- polybrominated diphenyl ethers (PBDE) (0.1%)
- **bis (2-ethylhexyl) phthalate (DEHP) (0.1%)**
- **butyl benzyl phthalate (BBP) (0.1%)**
- **dibutyl phthalate (DBP) (0.1%)**
- **diisobutyl phthalate (DIBP) (0.1%)**

As per RoHS guidelines, device designers are required to replace these chemicals in their products with less hazardous alternatives. The hazardous substances present in any medical device or implant should be less than 0.1 W/W of the device. Acceptable justification must be given if the CMR or endocrine-disrupting substances (for example, lead compounds, other heavy metals, phenols) are present above 0.1% by weight in these device types. The restriction of DEHP, BBP, DBP and DIBP shall apply to medical devices, including in vitro medical devices, and monitoring and control instruments, including industrial monitoring and control instruments, from 22 July 2021. Medical device manufacturers are advised to thoroughly review the conformity assessment procedures applicable to their device to avoid delays in the product review and approval process. In addition to the requirements of RoHS III (EU Directive 2015/863), medical device manufacturers may be subject to other EU directives and regulations addressing the use of hazardous substances and the control of electrical and electronic waste. These include EU Directive 2012/19/EC on Waste Electrical and Electronic Equipment (II), and EU Regulation (1907/2006), as well as EU directives on the disposal of batteries, and on product packaging and packaging waste. According to EU Directive (2011/65/EU) medical devices have to follow the restrictions regarding the use of hazardous substances.

PHASES IN THE LIFE SPAN OF A MEDICAL DEVICE

It is important to recognize that any of these phases can affect the safety and performance of a medical device. Examples of how each phase can create health hazards are described below (9):

Conception and development: The scientific principles upon which a device is based are fundamental to its safety and performance. For example, a cardiac pacemaker should deliver a minute electrical impulse of a certain size and shape that simulates the natural functioning of the heart. Significant deviation from this may compromise safety and performance. The more complex the device, the higher the risk of user error. Soundness of concept and adequacy of design, construction and testing (including verification, validation and clinical trials) require the scrutiny of scientific experts to ensure that design parameters and performance characteristics do not impose unwarranted risks (10).

Manufacture: Functional medical devices are produced when the manufacturing process is adequately managed. However, poor manufacturing management can produce inconsistency in the quality of products, such that non-conforming devices can filter through the production line to the market, even when the original prototype has been well-designed. This consideration has led to the development of good manufacturing practice (GMP) for drugs, biological products and medical devices. Now, GMP is more commonly referred to as "quality systems in manufacturing", and these are addressed later in this guide.

Packaging and labeling: Properly packaged medical devices pose little risk to individuals handling them, even if the medical device is biohazardous. This highlights the importance of well-designed packaging systems in delivering clean, sterile and protected medical devices to the point of use. Shipping is one of the hazards a medical device and its packaging must survive. Subtle damage can result during transportation and handling unless the total packaging system is designed robustly and can withstand various stresses. Well-sealed packaging is essential for those medical devices that must be kept sterile. Labeling is crucial in identifying the medical device and specifying instructions for its proper use. As with drugs, the mislabeling of medical devices can result in serious consequences for the user. Hazard warnings or cautions and clear instructions for use are very important.

Advertising: Advertisement has the potential to create expectations and powerfully influence the belief in a medical device's capabilities. It is important, therefore, that medical device marketing and advertising are regulated to prevent misrepresentation of a medical device and its performance. Misleading or fraudulent advertising of medical devices may increase sales. However, from the buyer's perspective, the purchase of an inappropriate medical device is a waste of money that may deprive the patient of more appropriate treatment and could lead to patient or user injury.

Sale: The sale of medical devices by the vendor is a critical stage that leads to the device being put into actual use. If the vendor is not subject to regulation, then there is a higher risk of exposing the public to low-quality or ineffective devices.

Use: Users of medical devices can have a profound effect on their safety and effective performance. Unfamiliarity with a certain technology or operating procedure, and the use of products for clinical indications outside the scope of those specified in the labeling, can cause device failure even in the absence of any inherent design or manufacturing defects. Within the clinical engineering community, it is widely believed that user error underlies at least half of all medical device-related injuries and deaths. The re-use of disposable devices contrary to the manufacturer's instructions, and without proper control or precautions for minimizing associated risks, can be dangerous. The lack of, or inappropriate, calibration and maintenance of medical devices can seriously jeopardize their safety and performance. These issues are often overlooked or underestimated (11).

Disposal: Disposal of certain types of devices should follow specific and stringent safety rules. For example, devices that are contaminated after use (e.g. syringes) or devices that contain toxic chemicals, can present hazards to people or the environment and must be disposed of properly.

It is people who manage each phase in the life span of a medical device, and these people should be identified and called on to participate in ensuring medical device safety.

MEDICAL DEVICE SAFETY AND RISK MANAGEMENT

The optimum assurance of medical device safety has several essential elements:

- absolute safety cannot be guaranteed
- it is a risk management issue
- it is closely aligned with device effectiveness/performance
- it must be considered throughout the life span of the device
- it requires shared responsibility among the stakeholders

All devices carry a certain degree of risk and could cause problems in specific circumstances. Many medical device problems cannot be detected until extensive market experience is gained. For example, an implantable device may fail in a manner that was not predictable at the time of implantation; the failure may reflect conditions unique to certain patients. For other devices, component failure can also be unpredictable or random. The current approach to device safety is to estimate the potential of a device becoming a hazard that could result in safety problems and harm. This estimate is often referred to as the risk assessment. Hazard is the potential for an adverse event, a source of danger. Risk is a measure of the combination of (1) the hazard; (2) the likelihood of occurrence of the adverse event; (3) the severity or overall impact. Risk assessment begins with risk analysis to identify all possible hazards, followed by risk evaluation to estimate the risk of each hazard. In general, risk assessment is based on experience, evidence, computation or even guesswork. Risk assessment is complex, as it can be influenced by personal perception and other factors such as cultural background, economic conditions and political climates.

References

1. *Medical Device Regulations: Global Overview and Guiding Principles.* WHO, https://www.who.int/medical_devices/publications/en/MD_Regulations.pdf
2. Leah Samuel. Most gruesome medical devices in history, June 17, 2016, https://www.statnews.com/2016/06/17/medical-devices-history
3. https://bio.libretexts.org/Bookshelves/Biotechnology/Quality_Assurance_and_Regulatory_Affairs_for_the_Biosciences/08%3A_Medical_Device_and_Combination_Products/8.01%3A_Section_1-.
4. https://www.johner-institute.com/articles/regulatory-affairs/glossary-for-medical-device-manufacturers.
5. Thamizharasan Sampath, Sandhiya Thamizharasan, Monisha Saravanan, Prakash Srinivasan Timiri Shanmugam. (2020) *Material Testing, Trends in Development of Medical Devices.* Elsevier.
6. *A History of Medical Device Regulation & Oversight in the United States.* U.S. Food & Drug Administration. 2018-11-03. Retrieved 16 March 2019. https://www.fda.gov/medical-devices/overview-device-regulation/history-medical-device-regulation-oversight-united-states.
7. *A Textbook of Materials and Materials Testing.* Ch-10, 184–195.
8. Chris Hurlstone. Selecting materials for medical devices. https://www.team-consulting.com/insights/selecting-materials-for-medical-devices.
9. Amit Aherwar, Amit Kumar Singh, Amar Patnaik. (2016) Cobalt based alloy: A better choice biomaterial for hip implants. *Society for Biomaterials and Artificial Organs*, vol 30(1), 34–39.
10. International Organisation for Standardization. (2006) ISO 10993-2:2006, Biological evaluation of medical devices - Part 2: Animal welfare requirements, https://www.iso.org/standard/36405.html
11. https://www.fda.gov/medical-devices/overview-device-regulation/classify-your-medical-device.

Cosmetic Devices

2

Thamizharasan S, Sandhiya Thamizharasan, Krithaksha V, and Prakash Srinivasan Timiri Shanmugam

---

ABBREVIATIONS

EU	European Union
FDA	Food and Drug Administration
GMP	good manufacturing practice
RF	radiofrequency
LED	light-emitting diode
HA	hyaluronic acid
HIFU	high-intensity focused ultrasound
MDA	microdermabrasion

INTRODUCTION

Medical aesthetic devices refer to all medical devices that are used for various cosmetic procedures, which include plastic surgery, unwanted hair removal, excess fat removal, anti-aging, aesthetic implants, skin tightening, etc., that are used for beautification, correction, and improvement of the body. Aesthetic procedures include both surgical and non-surgical procedures. The surgical procedures include liposuction, breast implants, facelifts, radiofrequency, and other related procedures. The non-surgical procedures include chemical peels, non-surgical liposuction, and skin-tightening procedures, among others. Medical aesthetic devices are classified based on types of devices (energy-based aesthetic devices and non-energy-based aesthetic devices) and application (skin resurfacing and tightening, body contouring and cellulite reduction, hair removal, facial aesthetic procedures, breast augmentation, and other applications) (1).

The beauty industry can thank the consumer for continually driving innovation forward due to their insatiable appetite for products that improve the aesthetics of the human body. Some of the developments involve biologically active cosmetics, others more invasive chemical and surgical techniques. An increasing number involve beauty devices, which are oftentimes used in combination with cosmetic products. Device technology can provide the consumer with superior results during their beauty routines, and results that are not always achievable by the use of cosmetics alone.

DOI: 10.1201/9781003220671-2

Medical aesthetic technology has advanced rapidly over the past two decades in various countries, especially in the United States. The factors that are expected to impact market growth positively include technological advancement in devices, increasing awareness regarding aesthetic procedures, rising adoption of minimally invasive devices, and an increasingly obese population in the region. According to the American Society of Plastic Surgeons, 18.1 million cosmetic procedures were recorded in 2019, an increase of 2% from 2018, which included around 1.8 million cosmetic surgical and 16.3 million cosmetic minimally invasive procedures. The global market for medical aesthetic devices is expected to surpass $8.2 billion by 2024. These devices look to revitalize and tighten skin, soften or reduce wrinkles, and deliver a more youthful appearance. These products are approved by the FDA. The FDA recognizes them as Class II devices if they are electrosurgical, cutting or coagulation devices, or accessories. These products are noninvasive and perform non-surgical tightening of the skin.

Devices that massage, irradiate, or manipulate the skin to alter its structure or function, or underlying tissue, fall into the medical device category. For cosmetic companies venturing into this space, there is a completely different quality paradigm that governs medical devices. Instead of GMP/ISO 22716 for cosmetic products, medical devices adhere to strict ISO 13489 requirements. While there are similarities in these quality systems, there are also substantial differences. The quality management system for medical devices is much more extensive, given the design complexity and risk of these products. Production facilities used for the manufacture of consumer products or cosmetics will be in for a shock should they be required to meet ISO 13489 standards. Even the design of the product will be governed by these strict ISO standards, and the documentation required is enormous.

But before the regulatory and quality system is outlined, a product must first be defined as a drug, medical device, or cosmetic product. Although this may appear simple, it can be challenging as new innovative technologies are created. Cleansing brushes have been popular for many years now. Clarisonic's Mia, for example, claims to lift dirt and oil by oscillating at 300 movements a second to work with the natural elasticity of the skin to remove the impurities. It is classified as a Class I medical device. If a device is to be used in contact with the human body, but its primary function is aesthetic in nature, does that make it a medical device? Something as simple as topical gel is a great example. If the gel is used as a moisturizer, it is considered a cosmetic. However, once it is used for scar reduction, or in an ultrasound procedure, it becomes a medical device. There is a legal distinction between cosmetics and medical devices, and in cases such as this, a highly trained eye is necessary in order to correctly classify and manage newly emerging technologies.

TYPES OF AESTHETIC DEVICES

1. Energy-based aesthetic devices
    i.   Laser-based aesthetic devices
    ii. Radiofrequency (RF)-based aesthetic devices
    iii. Light-based aesthetic devices
    iv. Ultrasound aesthetic devices
2. Non-energy-based aesthetic devices
    i.   Botulinum toxin
    ii. Dermal fillers and aesthetic threads
    iii. Microdermabrasion
    iv. Implants
        – Facial implants
        – Breast implants
        – Other implants
3. Other aesthetic devices

Dermal Fillers

Aesthetic medicine has advanced greatly in the past decade in terms of our understanding of facial anatomy; the cumulative effects of the aging process; and how dermal fillers may be used to repair, reduce, and even reverse these changes. The four major structural components of the face are skin, fat, muscle, and bone. A reduction in volume in these regions leads to aging. Age-related bone loss in the face can lead to retraction of the jawline, descent of the nose, and loss of high cheekbones. The facial muscles also decrease in volume and elasticity, and the deflation and movement of facial fat further accentuate the signs of aging. Finally, the skin stretches and loses elasticity compounded by the loss of scaffolding provided by fat, muscle, and bone; this leads to wrinkles, sagging skin, and other familiar signs of aging. Dermal fillers help to reduce these sights (2).

Dermal fillers are soft, gel-like substances that are injected under the skin. The areas where dermal fillers are injected are the temporal hollows, cheeks, sub-malar, nose, nasolabial folds, marionette lines, mental crease and lines, oral commissure, and jawline. Most dermal fillers today consist of hyaluronic acid, a naturally occurring polysaccharide that is present in skin and cartilage. Some people may need more than one injection to achieve the wrinkle-smoothing effect. The effect lasts for about six months or longer. Successful results depend on the health of the skin, skill of the health care provider, and type of filler used. Regardless of material (whether synthetic or organic) filler duration is highly dependent on the amount of activity in the region where it is injected. Exercise and high-intensity activities such as manual labor can stimulate blood flow and shorten the lifespan of fillers (3).

Materials used: Fillers are made of sugar molecules or composed of hyaluronic acids, collagens which may come from pigs, cows, cadavers, or the person's own transplanted fat may be generated in a laboratory and biosynthetic polymers. Examples: Calciumhydroxylapatite, polycaprolactone, polymethylmethacrylate, and polylactic acid.

Injection Techniques

A certain amount of practice and experience is required to inject dermal fillers. It is essential to choose the filling agent best suited to each patient and anatomical site, and to determine the appropriate amount of filler to be injected. Another crucial aspect in achieving a good outcome with dermal fillers is the depth at which the material is implanted. Most dermal fillers are injected into the deep dermis or the fatty tissue. A number of different injection techniques are

- Linear threading or tunneling
- Serial puncture
- Radial fanning
- Crosshatching

The filler should be injected deeply. The most common complications are overcorrection and the appearance of lumps, bruises, and localized edema. Only experienced practitioners should undertake this procedure because this is one of the most complicated and delicate treatment areas. Isolated cases of blindness following treatment have been reported, probably caused by poor technique. The likelihood of such a complication can be minimized by administering nerve block anesthesia with epinephrine, which produces vasoconstriction. The recommended technique is to use 30-gauge needles to slowly inject small amounts of filler (4).

Less Common Indications for Dermal Fillers

Scarring

Although no studies in the literature have demonstrated any long-term benefits associated with the treatment of scars with dermal fillers, the injection of HA can improve the patient's appearance, especially in the case of atrophic acne scars. Small amounts of filler should be injected over a number of sessions. Good long-term results have also been reported with poly-L-lactic acid, and porcine collagen has also been used.

Chin Shaping in Patients with Implants

In patients with chin implants, contouring with HA can improve the transition between the implant and the adjacent soft tissue. To obtain the best results, these treatments are usually combined with botulinum toxin treatment.

Earlobe Treatment

With age, the earlobes tend to sag and create folds, and the injection of fillers such as HA can improve their appearance. The effects of treatment last longer in the earlobes than elsewhere, probably because it is metabolically inactive tissue that moves very little.

Hand Rejuvenation

Hands can also be improved with dermal fillers, although this application is not very widespread. Stabilized HA fillers are a good choice. Other fillers that have been used in the hand include calcium hydroxylapatite and bovine collagen (5).

Temporary Dermal Fillers

Autologous fat: Subcutaneous fat is distributed across independent compartments separated by fibrous septa. In the youthful face, the transition between these subcutaneous fat compartments is subtle, but aging gives rise to abrupt changes of contour between these spaces, whether due to loss of volume or fat misplacement. One example is orbital fat, which tends to herniate and create bags around the eyes. The use of the patient's own fat as a filler is a safe and natural method (6). One drawback of this technique is that it must be performed in an operating theater environment with local anesthesia and sedation; specific instruments and materials are also required. Fat is extracted from areas such as the thighs or abdomen using special cannulas. The harvested fat is then purified by centrifugation. Using a different type of cannula, the processed fat is then injected into the treatment areas depending on the needs of the patient (forehead, brow, cheeks, suborbital region, perioral areas, jawline, etc.). Fat is injected at different depths (subdermal, intramuscular, and subperiosteal) and in different quantities depending on the patient and the anatomical area treated. The longevity of injected autologous fat ranges from eight months to several years.

   Hyaluronic acid: Under normal circumstances, HA is present in the human body as a component of the extracellular matrix. It is a polysaccharide (a glycosaminoglycan disaccharide composed of an alternating and repeating unit of D-glucuronic acid and N-acetyl-D-glucosamine) with hydrophilic properties (a very high affinity for attracting and binding water molecules). Owing to their hydrophilic properties, HA filler materials can achieve substantial soft tissue augmentation after injection. The initial filling effect is directly related to the volume of the exogenous HA injected, but it has been shown that HA also has an indirect effect in that, once deposited in the dermis, it activates the dermal fibroblasts. HA is a temporary injectable filler. However, unlike collagen fillers, which only remain in tissue for a few weeks or months, HA can last for as long as six to nine months or sometimes longer, depending on the type of HA filler used. When an appropriate volume is correctly placed, this material cannot be detected either visually or by palpation. Most of the HA products on the market are synthetic, sourced from stabilized nonanimal HA. This makes pretreatment skin testing unnecessary since there is no possibility of an allergic reaction. To further its longevity in tissue, the HA is manipulated using a process called crosslinking that involves the use of substances such as divinyl sulfone, 1,2,7,8-diepoxyoctane, and butanediol-diglycidyl-ether (7). The differences between the types of HA on the market are due in part to the degree of crosslinking and the agent used in this process. Crosslinking modifies the solubility of HA, and the degree of crosslinking is directly related to the viscosity of the gel. Any allergic reaction produced by such products is thought to be caused by the agent used in the crosslinking process.

Collagen Fillers

Collagen makes up 70% to 80% of the dermis. With age, dermal collagen is lost and becomes fragmented, as the transformation from new and complete collagen (type I) to fibrotic collagen (type III) gives rise to the appearance of rhytides and folds. Collagen fillers can be bovine, human, or porcine in origin. One of the advantages of collagen fillers over HA is that they are less viscous and can be more useful for the correction of fine lines and wrinkles because they are less likely to produce irregularities when injected superficially.

Bovine Collagen

The two bovine collagen products most used are Zyderm® and Zyplast®. Bovine collagen, a temporary and biodegradable filler, was the first collagen to be sold as a filler. Pretreatment skin testing is necessary. Some authors even recommend administering two skin tests separated by an interval of two to four weeks. The incidence of local hypersensitivity reactions in patients tested prior to treatment is estimated to be between 3% and 5%. Zyderm® is indicated for superficial rhytides and Zyplast® for deeper rhytides or defects. Zyplast® should never be used in the glabellar region because cases of local cutaneous necrosis caused by intra-arterial injection of the product have been reported. A shorter duration of effect in the treatment of nasolabial folds than that obtained with HA fillers has been reported. These products remain in tissue for between two and six months (8).

Human Collagen

Human collagen is produced from human dermal fibroblast cell lines using bioengineering techniques. No pretreatment skin test is required. The two most frequently used dermal filling products are Cosmoderm® and Cosmoplast®. Both products are biodegradable and therefore temporary and have a duration of effect from three to seven months. Cosmoderm® is indicated for superficial and Cosmoplast® for deep rhytides or defects, and both contain the anesthetic agent lidocaine. Collagen can also be obtained from the tissue of human cadavers. Products that contain collagen of human origin include Fascian®.

Porcine Collagen

Porcine collagen is also temporary and biodegradable and has a duration in tissue of around 12 months. A number of products on the market contain porcine collagen, including Evolence® and Evolence Breeze®. The porcine collagen in these products is cross-linked using natural sugar, a technology called Glymatrix®. Collagen extracted from porcine tendons is broken down using enzymes, and the crosslinking is then reconstituted using the Glymatrix® system. Since this proprietary technology does not involve the use of chemical crosslinking agents, it eliminates all potentially antigenic compounds that might induce allergic reactions. No pretreatment skin test is required. The particles are incorporated into the recipient tissue, and neovascularization occurs. The product is broken down over time by enzymatic mechanisms. Another advantage of this type of filler is the low incidence of edema and hematomas following injection because of the hemostatic properties of collagen. Other porcine collagen products on the market include Fibroquel® and Permacol®. Evolence® is indicated for moderate to deep lines, wrinkles, and folds, and for the correction of contour defects. It is not used on the lips because of the possibility of nodule formation. Evolence Breeze® is used to fill fine lines and for lip enhancement (9).

Poly-L-lactic Acid

Poly-L-lactic acid is a temporary dermal filler composed of a biocompatible and biodegradable synthetic polymer. No pretreatment skin test is required. The only commercially available product of this type is marketed in the United States under the brand name Sculptra® and in Europe as New Fill®. Poly L-lactic acid belongs to the category of fillers that produce their effect by stimulating new collagen formation through fibroblast activation. As a result, the volume increases in the treated area over time. This effect has been studied in a murine model and has been described in isolated cases in humans in a series reported in the literature. The amount of collagen present has been found to continue to increase on follow-up at 3 and 6 months; after a longer interval, between 8 and 30 months, breakdown of the poly-L-lactic acid is observed but type I collagen continues to increase. The poly-L-lactic acid continues to break down 9 to 24 months after its introduction. Degradation is not enzymatic but rather involves metabolism into water and carbon dioxide. The de novo collagen may, however, remain in tissue, and its presence has been detected up to 24 months after treatment (10).

Calcium Hydroxylapatite

The calcium hydroxylapatite filler is Radiesse®, a product formerly marketed under the brand name Radiance FN®. Although Radiesse is a temporary filler, it has a longer duration of effect than either HA or collagen fillers, leading some authors to classify it as semipermanent. Radiesse is composed of microspheres of synthetic calcium hydroxylapatite (a chemical composition identical to that found in teeth and bone) suspended in a water-based carboxymethyl cellulose gel carrier. The microspheres are very smooth and vary in size from 25 to 45 μm. As the product is totally biocompatible, no pretreatment skin test is required. In addition to the direct volumizing effect produced by the presence of the filler itself, this product also stimulates endogenous collagen production, an effect that can be observed months after treatment as a consequence of the attempts of macrophages to break down the calcium hydroxylapatite; macrophages have been observed to engulf the calcium hydroxylapatite microspheres. This filler remains in tissue for as long as 1 year or even 18 months in some studies, exceeding the longevity of HA (11). It is indicated for the correction of moderate to severe facial wrinkles and oral and maxillofacial defects and for the treatment of HIV-associated facial lipoatrophy. Radiesse is also used for radiographic tissue marking and vocal cord augmentation. The incidence of associated complications is low, and there are no reports of calcification or osteogenesis at injection sites.

Permanent Dermal Fillers

Polymethyl Methacrylate Microspheres

Polymethyl methacrylate microspheres can be suspended in either bovine collagen (Artecoll® and Artefill®) or HA (Dermalive® and Dermadeep®). The characteristics of each of these two types of dermal fillers are detailed below. The two most widely known fillers in this group are Artecoll®, a second-generation product, and, more recently Artefill®, a third-generation product. Arteplast®, the original polymethyl methacrylate filler, is no longer in use. The bovine collagen, in addition to being the carrier of the polymethyl methacrylate microspheres, prevents the needle from becoming obstructed during injection and has the effect of stimulating the growth of tissue in which it is deposited. This product is mainly used as a filler for nasolabial folds (12).

Hydroxyethyl Methacrylate in Hyaluronic Acid

The products based on a combination of hydroxyethyl methacrylate and HA are Dermalive® and Dermadeep®. Dermalive® is a mixture of 60% cross-linked HA fluid produced by fermentation in bacterial culture and 40% hydroxyethyl methacrylate and ethyl methacrylate particles. The particles have an irregular surface and vary in size from 45 to 65 μm. This filler must be implanted in the deep dermis and is not indicated for the treatment of superficial rhytides. Dermadeep® must be implanted even more deeply, in the hypodermis or periosteum. The use of these materials is not very widespread because of the high incidence of associated adverse effects (13).

Polyacrylamide Gel

The two most widely known polyacrylamide gel products are Bio-Alcamid® and Aquamid®. Bio-Alcamid® is composed of 96% water and 4% polyalkylimide. It is generally used for the treatment of deep defects. Aquamid® is a hydrogel, composed of 2.5% polyacrylamide and 97.5% water that is not absorbed. This product is also used to correct deep defects. Since Aquamid has a high complication rate and its use is often associated with the formation of granulomas, its use is increasingly rare (14).

Silicone

Injectable liquid silicone was one of the permanent fillers most used in the past. There are various products on the market, including Adato SIL-OL 5000®, Silikon 1000®, and SilSkin 1000®. There is also a product, marketed under the brand name Bioplastique®, that consists of solid silicone particles suspended in a polyvinylpyrrolidone carrier. All these materials must be implanted in the deep dermis or on the dermis-panniculus adiposus plane. As well as affording an immediate effect due to the volume of the injected silicone, these products also induce the formation of fibroplasia in the long term. However, since complications are frequent, these products are now rarely used for facial rejuvenation (15).

Risks: An improper injection technique leads to severe side effects like swelling and lumpiness. In many cases, if the filler gets accidentally injected into the blood vessels instead of skin, it may affect the blood flow by blocking it which leads to skin loss or wounds and also causes skin necrosis (death of tissue). In the long term, damage includes wrinkling of the lip and disturbance of the attachment of the facial pads and irregularity.

Microneedling Devices

Microneedling devices are instruments with technological features, such as many small needles, tips, or pins on the surface, which are repeatedly inserted into and removed from the skin. The devices create many small puncture holes in the skin by moving over the skin repeatedly. Some microneedling devices are manual, meaning the needles always project from the surface, and they enter the skin when the device is rolled or stamped on the surface. Other devices use a motor to move needles in and out of the device surface. In some motorized devices, the health care practitioner can adjust and control the depth and speed of penetration of needles into the skin.

Microneedling may help address many skin-related complaints, including wrinkles, scarring, acne, alopecia, skin pigmentation issues, stretch marks, rosacea, and loose skin, such as after weight loss or liposuction, and it also helps in rejuvenating the skin. Some professionals also use microneedling to fill medication, such as topical tretinoin or vitamin C, deeper into the skin. This can boost the treatment of many issues including acne scarring. It also increases the amount of collagen in the skin as the collagen keeps the skin looking youthful, wrinkle free, smooth, and firm. The microneedling procedure is not a quick fix as it involves the growth of new skin, and it may take some months for the person to see the full result (16).

There are three types of microneedling procedures:

Mechanical microneedling: This technique uses a motorized pen with tiny slender needles to create thousands of channels that are up to 2.5 mm deep. These channels disrupt photo-aging, wrinkles, or scar tissues to allow for the growth of new skin to occur. This type of microneedling creates the most channels per square inch of skin. Because of this, patients do experience a mild amount of bleeding and redness. This is the most popular type of microneedling because it is both relatively economical and it is an excellent maintenance treatment for delaying the aging process. Examples: SkinPen Precision, MDpen, Pen Stylus.

Fractional radiofrequency microneedling: Frictional radiofrequency microneedling uses thicker needles to transmit heat deep into the skin. The basis of this therapy is thermal coagulation of tissue to stimulate collagen denaturation and renewal. The main goal of RF is to lift the skin and thicken the collagen, whereas mechanical microneedling plays an important role in resurfacing the upper layers of skin. Examples: There are a handful of RF devices on the market including Endymed Intensif, Secret RF, Vivace, Virtue RF, and Morpheus.

Mesotherapy: Mesotherapy is the least invasive of all the needling options. This minimally invasive option only affects the very topmost layer of skin, about 600 micrometers deep, which is very superficial. Mesotherapy increases the permeability of the stratum corneum, allowing skincare ingredients to penetrate a little bit deeper. Typical skincare products applied during mesotherapy include hyaluronic acid, vitamin C, or Botox. Examples: Aquagold, stamps, dermarollers (17).

Risks in microneedling: Skin damage is a risk that commonly occurs with microneedling devices. The damage may include bleeding, bruising, redness, tightness, itching, and peeling, and these typically go away without any treatment after a few days or weeks. Less common risks include stinging or itching when cosmetics or other skincare products such as moisturizers and sunscreen are applied, dark or light spots on the skin, lines on the face, a flareup of cold sores, swollen lymph nodes, and infection.

Indications of Mesotherapy

Mesotherapy, like corticosteroids, is claimed to have a wide array of applications especially in the field of cosmetic dermatology. However, only the current and widely practiced indications in the field of dermatology along with the drugs used in them are discussed below.

1. Body – cellulite, lipodissolve, body contouring (not very effective)
2. Skin – rejuvenation/glow, lift, pigmentation
3. Hair – telogen effluvium, androgenetic alopecia

Various Mixtures and Protocols in Mesotherapy

Materials used in mesotherapy can be broadly classified into two categories:

i. Principal (P)/major
ii. Complementary (C)/minor

A cocktail or mixture should contain at least two to three principal agents for it to be effective.

1. Mesolift
   Hyaluronic acid (P)
   Silorgamine = silorg + DMAE (P) + taurinox (C) + Puretinol/vitamin A (P)
2. Mesoglow
   Hyaluronic acid (P)
   Silorg (P)
   Purascorbol/vitamin C (P) + xadenal (C)
3. Mesolighten
   Kojic acid (P)
   Azelaic acid (P) + either tretinoin (C) or glycolic acid (C)
   Vitamin C (P)
4. Localized fat dissolve
   Phosphatidylcholine (P) and deoxycholic acid (P) +/– vitamin complex +/– taurine +/– L-carnitine +/– alfa lipoic acid +/– organic silicium +/– aminophylline amino acids +/– pantothenic acid

5. Meso cellulite: principal agents L-carnitine
   Aminophylline pentoxiphylline DMAE
   Vitamin C procaine
6. Mesostretch: principal agents Silorgamine = silorg + DMAE or
   Idebe = idebenone + DMAE or
   Centella asiatica, fibronectin, vegetal proteins
7. Telogen effluvium
   Biotin (P) + multivitamins, trace elements (C)
   Dexenol (P)
8. Androgenetic alopecia
   Minoxidil (P)
   Dutasteride (P) + zinc, azelaic acid (C) + biotin (P)
   Dexenol (P)

Equipment Needed

Classical Injection Method

- Needles 27G, 30G, 32G
- Syringes – slip tip, luer lock 5 mL, 10 mL, 20 mL linear multiple injector
- Circular multiple injectors
- Multi injector plates – three, five, and seven connectors

Meso Gun

The benefits of the meso gun include faster injections, precise dose delivery, consistent depth of penetration, and more comfort for the physician and patient. It has different modes, for example continuous, dosimetric, nappage, and mesoperfusion modes (18).

Skin and Scalp Rollers

These are available in 48 and 96 needle configurations with 4 needles in each row with a gap of 5 mm in between. They stimulate comparatively deeper layers of skin and are used mainly in the management of acne, stretch marks, and alopecia.

Facial Care Devices

Microdermabrasion

Microdermabrasion is sometimes referred to as "microderm," lunchtime peel, Parisian Peel, or Diamond Peel. Micro-dermabrasion is a procedure used to renew overall skin tone and texture. It is a simple, quick, and painless cosmetic treatment with no downtime and minimal risk. It improves the appearance of sun damage, wrinkles, fine lines, age spots, acne scarring, melisma, and other skin-related concerns and conditions. Microdermabrasion uses fine crystals or minute diamond-studded tips to abrade the skin and vacuum suction to remove dead skin cells. It has low risk and rapid recovery; it is painless and requires no needles or anesthesia. Skin may become noticeably smoother even after one treatment and may better absorb moisturizers. It is an affordable professional treatment with a fairly low cost. Most often, microdermabrasion may be repeated every three to four weeks for optimal results. Microdermabrasion is not a laser-based treatment. Microdermabrasion works by removing a few of the top layers of the skin called the stratum corneum. Much like brushing your teeth, microderm helps to gently remove "plaque" and skin debris. Since human skin typically regenerates at approximately 30-day intervals, skin improvement with microdermabrasion is temporary and needs to be repeated at average intervals of 2 to 4 weeks for continued improvement. Multiple treatments in combination with sunscreen, sun avoidance, and other skincare creams yield the best results. Several at-home microdermabrasion creams and home machines are now available.

Microdermabrasion is useful for people with dull or sallow skin, mild acne, acne discoloration, pock marks, and very superficial acne scars. Microdermabrasion may be a good treatment option for patients with superficial skin problems and busy lifestyles who are looking for minimal benefits with virtually no side effects or downtime. Individuals with deeper acne scars may expect a much longer series of treatments or likely benefit from physician-performed surgical dermabrasion, chemical peeling, or laser resurfacing.

Mechanism: The crystal microdermabrasion system contains a pump, a connecting tube, a hand piece, and a vacuum. While the pump creates a high-pressure stream of inert crystals, such as aluminum oxide, magnesium oxide, sodium chloride, or sodium bicarbonate, to abrade the skin, the vacuum removes the crystals and exfoliated skin cells. Alternatively, the inert crystals can be replaced by a tip with a roughened surface in the diamond microdermabrasion system.

Unlike the crystal microdermabrasion system, the diamond microdermabrasion machine does not produce particles from crystals that may be inhaled into a patient's nose or blown into the eyes. Hence, diamond microdermabrasion is safer for use on areas around the eyes and lips. Generally, the slower the movement of the hand piece against the skin and the more passes over the skin, the deeper the treatment.

Applications

- Improves age spots and blackheads
- Improves hyperpigmentation (patches of darkened skin)
- Exfoliates your skin, resulting in a refreshed appearance
- Lessens the appearance of stretch marks
- Reduces fine lines and wrinkles
- Reduces or eliminates enlarged pores
- Treats acne and the scars left by acne

Microdermabrasion helps to thicken your collagen, which results in a younger looking complexion. Collagen is a protein in your skin which is abundant when you're a child and makes skin appear taut and smooth. Collagen production declines as we age, resulting in looser, uneven skin (19).

CONTRAINDICATIONS

Microdermabrasion is contraindicated in areas of active cutaneous infection, such as herpes simplex virus, varicella-zoster virus, human papillomavirus, and impetigo. In individuals with contact allergies to the abrasive crystals (i.e., aluminum allergy), a different crystal or a crystal-free system should be used. MDA should be used cautiously in individuals with a known history of hypertrophic scarring (keloids). Rosacea and telangiectasias are considered relative contraindications.

Microdermabrasion Devices

Microdermabrasion devices are categorized as either crystal or crystal-free systems. The crystal-based system propels abrasive crystals at the skin at a predetermined flow rate. The most common crystal used is aluminum oxide. Sodium chloride, magnesium oxide, and sodium bicarbonate crystals are less commonly employed. With the crystal-free systems, diamonds embedded in the handpiece provide the abrasive stimulus. The following equipment is needed to perform the procedure:

- Microdermabrasion handpiece
- Disposable handpiece tips or autoclave-safe handpiece tips
- Fresh abrasion crystals (for crystal-based systems)
- Filters (for machines with a closed-loop vacuum system)
- Gentle skin cleanser
- Protective equipment (eyewear, gloves, mask)

Technique

The area of desired treatment should be cleaned with a mild cleanser prior to the start of the procedure. Moist gauze is placed over the eyes to prevent contact with the abrasive crystals. Contact is made between the skin and the device tip. Using negative pressure, the device pulls the skin into the handpiece. The device then releases the abrasive crystals at a controlled flow rate. Surface debris and the stratum corneum layer of cells are removed, and the particles collect in a reservoir. The device is then passed over the skin to target the desired surface area. A single treatment usually requires three passes over the treated area. The remaining crystals and debris are wiped away with a washcloth, and a gentle moisturizer is applied. The entire procedure typically takes 30–60 minutes. Patients often require four to six weekly treatments to achieve the desired results. The degree of stratum corneum removal is dependent on the crystal flow rate and procedure exposure time. The pressure generated by the vacuum device has little effect on stratum corneum removal (20).

Complications

Side effects of microdermabrasion are minimal, and most patients experience no adverse events. Common complications include tenderness, swelling, redness, petechiae, and bruising. Eye irritation can occur if the crystals come in contact with the conjunctiva. There is an increased risk of autoinoculation of viral cutaneous lesions (e.g., molluscum contagiosum) and reactivation of latent herpes simplex virus in an affected dermatome. Since stratum corneum removal occurs during MDA, the skin is more sensitive to photodamage for a few days after the treatment.

Clinical Significance

The primary clinical significance of microdermabrasion lies in cosmetic and aesthetic benefits. It is a minimally invasive procedure that can offer evened skin tone, bright complexion, and reduced appearance of dark spots and wrinkles, with cleaned-out pores and improved smoothness of the skin. Microdermabrasion has also been shown to enhance transdermal drug delivery by allowing the drug to diffuse more freely in the viable epidermis. The theoretical benefits of this are thought to include improved transdermal insulin delivery, transdermal vitamin C delivery, transdermal lidocaine delivery, and transdermal 5-fluorouracil delivery. Although there are several ongoing clinical trials with promising results, the feasibility of using microdermabrasion in a clinical setting to enhance transdermal drug delivery is still unknown.

There are no specific age or sex restrictions; typically children over age 12 up to adults aged 65 can get microdermabrasion. While there is no age maximum, mature skin over age 70 may have slightly higher risks of bruising and skin abrasions. Individuals younger than age 12 may sometimes also receive treatment under the care of a dermatologist or plastic surgeon.

Vacuum's role in microdermabrasion: It gently pulls and lifts a small section of skin for micro abrasion. It can spray a stream of crystals across the targeted skin area. It focally stimulates blood circulation and creates mild swelling in the skin. It collects the used crystals and dead skin in a receptacle for easy disposal.

Microdermabrasion with scars: Useful for people with active acne, mild acne discoloration, pock marks, and very superficial or raised acne scars. Dermatologists use microdermabrasion to help unclog pores and clear acne. Often used in combination with gentle glycolic peels and medical acne extractions, microderm can help speed up acne clearing. Individuals with deeper acne scars might be candidates for surgical dermabrasion or laser resurfacing (21).

Microdermabrasion with melasma: Microderm can be helpful in treating melasma and other types of hyperpigmentation. Optimal melasma treatment might typically include biweekly or monthly microderm combined with glycolic acid peels, fading creams like hydroquinone 4%, and daily sunscreens. Multiple treatments in combination with sunscreen and sun avoidance and other creams help yield the best results, although permanent improvement is not to be expected.

Side Effects and Risks

People who have taken the acne medicine isotretinoin in the past six months may need to wait before having microdermabrasion. They have an increased risk of complications such as scarring. Excessive bleeding, growth, or changing on any spot or scar can indicate skin cancer.

For a few days after microdermabrasion, a person may notice:

- Skin swelling
- Skin redness, similar to sunburn
- Bruising
- A burning or stinging sensation

Many home microdermabrasion kits are available in stores or online. Spas and salons also offer the procedure. The American Academy of Dermatologist (AAD) advise people to speak to a dermatologist before undergoing the procedure outside a clinical setting. This is to ensure that the person's skin is suitable for microdermabrasion and that they are not likely to experience complications.

Cosmetic lymphatic drainage device: The lymphatic system is a crucial part of your immune system. Through a network of hundreds of lymph nodes, it drains fluid called lymph to be transported back into your bloodstream. It also removes bodily waste and carries white blood cells that help prevent infection. When there's any kind of obstruction in your lymphatic system, fluid can start to build up. That's where lymphatic drainage, a specialized type of massage therapy, comes in.

It's been used to treat lymphedema, a condition marked by chronic swelling that can occur after lymph node removal. But in recent years, some have started incorporating facial lymphatic drainage into their beauty regimen as a weapon against puffy, dull complexion and skin irritation. This increasingly popular procedure can be performed to target areas from head to toe, and can be done at home with a few key tools, or experienced in a professional setting depending on your budget and personal preference (22).

The technique stimulates and encourages the accumulated fluid between the cells to return to the vessels and move towards the bloodstream. The blood will bring nutrition and oxygen to the cell. After cell metabolism, some debris is absorbed by the bloodstream through small capillaries while excessive fluid and larger molecules are drained by the lymphatic system. This manual technique ultimately will increase the lymph flow and the process of filtration through lymph nodes. Lymphatic drainage, historically performed on the body (below the neck), is the application of one or more noninvasive techniques to enhance the movement of lymphatic fluids into lymph nodes for the clearance of waste and toxins from the body. More recently, aspects of lymphatic drainage have been incorporated into aesthetic facials. This type of massage encourages the movement of lymph fluids around the body. The lymph system is what works to eliminate waste and toxins in our body, so this massage can help flush out what we don't need to support our natural lymph function. The process also helps reduce bodily swelling and water retention and supports blood circulation. Lymphatic drainage massage can benefit people who suffer from a number of ailments, including lymphedema, fibromyalgia, edema, fatigue, insomnia, stress, digestive problems, and migraine. Also, studies have proven that lymphatic drainage can help with cellulite.

Radiofrequency Device

Radiofrequency (RF) devices are commonly used in aesthetic practices. RF devices are used for skin tightening, collagen production, body contouring by heating up and destroying fat cells, and facial rejuvenation. A larger area, such as the abdomen or flank, can be treated in a shorter period of time. The procedure involves using energy waves to heat the deep layer of your skin known as your dermis. This heat stimulates the production of collagen. Collagen is the most common protein in your body. It creates the framework of your skin and gives your skin its firmness. As you age, your cells produce less collagen, which leads to sagging skin and wrinkles. Skin laxity occurs around age 35 to 40 when the quantity and quality of your collagen begin to decline. RF therapy has been used since 2001 to fight against sagging skin and signs of aging. These skin-bypassing technologies can be effective with a wide range of patients, including those with darker color skin that may experience discoloration with a laser (23).

Mechanism: Radiofrequency energy consists of an alternating wavelength current that is delivered by a specialized electrode(s). As the energy travels across the tissue, the polarity or electrical charge of the skin tissue is changed. The friction of the movement of the energy current creates heat in the epidermis and/or dermis. Radiofrequency devices can be designed to be "monopolar" thus using a dispersive electrode that is worn by the client during the procedure. Since RF energy travels the path of least resistance or impedance in the skin, the RF energy travels across the body and returns back to the device via the dispersive pad. Some RF devices are "bipolar" and travel more superficially across the tissue. The current travels from the positively charged electrode to the negatively charged electrode that is contained in the tip of the device or handpiece. No dispersive electrode needs to be worn during the procedure. RF energy can be used alone or in combination with lasers or with intense pulsed light. Thermalift was the first type of RF available for skin tightening. Each type of technology works the same way. RF waves heat the deep layer of your skin to between 122 and 167°F (50–75°C). Maintaining a temperature over 115°F (46°C) for over 3 minutes causes your body to release heat-shock proteins. These proteins stimulate your body to create new collagen fibers.

Radiofrequency Delivery

There are two major electrode configurations available in current RF devices: Monopolar and bipolar.

Monopolar RF energy has been successfully used to accomplish noninvasive skin tightening of the face, periorbita, abdomen, and extremities. The first monopolar RF device was the ThermaCool device, which was introduced in 2001 and approved by the FDA for the noninvasive treatment of periorbital rhytids and wrinkles in 2002, for full-face treatment in 2004, and for body contouring in 2006. By three months posttreatment, there was a statistically significant average elevation of 4.3 mm of the mid-brow and 2.4 mm of the lateral brow with a 1.9 mm increase at the level of the palpebral crease. Skin tightening improved from 35% to 40% at the end of treatment to 70% to 75% at three months following treatment (24).

Monopolar devices typically have mild and self-limited adverse effects mainly limited to transient erythema and edema. Weiss et al. published a thorough review of adverse effects following ThermaCool consistent with mild side effects. There were rare cases of superficial crusting, slight contour deformities, subcutaneous erythematous papules, and neck tenderness. The overall rate of adverse side effects was 2.7%, but none of these side effects were experienced when using a lower energy multiple-pass treatment algorithm.

Bipolar devices differ from monopolar because they pass electrical current only between two positioned electrodes. The tissue to be heated and tightened is between these two electrodes, and the depth of penetration is approximately half the distance between the electrodes. Thus, bipolar radiofrequency devices offer a shallower depth of penetration when compared with monopolar. However, this configuration does provide a more controlled or localized distribution of energy and less discomfort. No grounding pad is necessary with these systems because the current does not flow through the rest of the body. Although this heat is targeted between the two electrodes, monopolar devices are believed to lead to a more uniform volumetric heating. The clinical skin contraction obtained was reported at 40% improved. Minor complications included erythema, prolonged swelling past two months, and subdermal banding.

Applications: Sun damage is among the most frequent reasons patients visit aesthetic practitioners. With sun damage, UV light radiation increases the production of free radicals in the skin. This causes damage to the DNA, as well as inflammation of the collagen and other proteins that provide elasticity and tone to skin. Excessive sun exposure leads to the appearance of premature aging in the form of lines, wrinkles, brown or red spots, broken capillaries, and leathery, dry, and rough skin. Some people may even develop pre-cancerous lesions or melanoma. A 2011 study found that three months of RF treatment led to clinically significant improvements in a small group of people with mild to moderate signs of sun damage.

Body Contouring

RF devices such as ThermaCool TC offer a nonablative and noninvasive treatment option for unwanted skin concerns of the head, neck, and body. By manipulating skin cooling and delivering radiofrequency energy to precise skin depths, these treatments are highly effective in reducing fat pockets. RF thermal stimulation happens regardless of skin color type, so it is a powerful treatment for patients of every ethnicity. Body contouring or body sculpting can eliminate fat, shape areas of the body, and tighten skin. Lipolysis is a non-surgical option that uses cold, heat, lasers, and other methods. It aims to get rid of extra skin, eliminate excess fat, and reshape or contour the area. Body contouring does not usually help you lose weight. Instead, it helps shape the body and address specific areas where weight loss isn't effective or after significant weight loss results in extra skin.

Risks of RF: RF radiation has lower energy than some other types of non-ionizing radiation, like visible light and infrared, but it has higher energy than extremely low-frequency (ELF) radiation. If RF radiation is absorbed by the body in large enough amounts, it can produce heat. This can lead to burns and body tissue damage. Although RF radiation is not thought to cause cancer by damaging the DNA in cells the way ionizing radiation does, there has been concern that in some circumstances, some forms of non-ionizing radiation might still have other effects on cells that might somehow result in cancer (25).

Color-light-therapy: This involves exposing your skin to various wavelengths of light, including red and blue, to address a wide range of concerns. LED light therapy is a skin treatment that doesn't use ultraviolet light. Instead, it uses skin-safe, low-level light in different wavelengths and colors. These include:

- Amber
- Blue
- Red
- Green

Sometimes different LED lights are combined with a photosensitive drug called 5-aminolevulinic acid. This medicine is applied to the skin and used in combination with LED light.

Light devices: Hair regrowth devices use both laser and LED light to treat androgenic alopecia, and some of these products are designed to be used at home. These devices work by re-energizing the cells in hair follicles, and essentially starting the regrowth of hair. These products are Class II medical devices, as defined by the FDA. As an aside, the hair regrowth market is estimated at $3.5 billion in the United

States, as hair loss affects so many men and women. Several LED light facial devices are available for at-home use. These include:

- Light facial masks
- Light wands for targeted spot treatment
- Ultrasonic devices
- Mesotherapy electroporation devices
- Professional LED light machines

Laser and LED light devices have been designed for other beauty issues, ranging from acne to wrinkles. This is based on the knowledge that visible blue light in the range of 407–420 nm is effective in killing bacteria. Similar to hair growth devices, Tria Blue Light is considered a Class II medical device by the FDA. Red is used for anti-aging, stimulating collagen synthesis, while blue is used for acne treatment which kills *Propionibacterium acnes*, the acne-causing bacteria. Both red and near-infrared light treat the outer layer of skin and stimulate collagen proteins. The idea is that more collagen means smoother, fuller skin, i.e., fewer fine lines and wrinkles. Experts say that red light reduces inflammation while improving circulation, which gives you a healthy glow over time. Blue light makes oil glands less active, which may help reduce acne breakouts. It can also kill acne-causing bacteria under the skin, which can help treat severe pimples like cysts and nodules. Light blue (cyan) light can improve the energy of the cells gradually and has a good effect in facilitating balance. This therapy can help treat a variety of skin problems, including acne, dermatitis, dull skin, eczema, psoriasis, rosacea, scarring, and signs of aging, including wrinkles and age spots.

Risks of LED Light Therapy

While several medical studies note the benefits of LED light therapy for the skin, there isn't enough research available yet to know for sure how well these treatments work. LED light facials might be a better choice compared to other options, like lasers, because they generally have fewer side effects. They can cause mild reactions though, including:

- Redness
- Swelling
- Itching
- Dryness

Indoor tanning beds remain popular, despite counter indication from the dermatological and cosmetic industries. These devices emit UV radiation to cause skin tanning. This US industry is valued at over $5 billion, and tanning beds are considered medical devices. Until recently, these devices were identified as Class I instruments but due to public outcry in Canada and the United States over their negative health effects, they were recently changed to Class II medical devices.

Cosmetic ultrasound: Ultrasound for face tightening is a fairly new treatment option for people with loose and sagging skin. The procedure helps rejuvenate the skin around the face without leaving behind surgical scars. It also minimizes downtime, as recovery is fast. The procedure, also known as high-intensity focused ultrasound (HIFU), is noninvasive and painless. It relies on ultrasound energy to promote the creation of collagen, which is essential for firmer skin. HIFU is also effective in treating tumors, for brow lifts, and for refining wrinkles. The device used in ultrasound skin tightening is much more helpful than laser devices. It penetrates 5 mm deep under the skin, reaching the second layer of muscle under the facial muscles. The ability to go this deep is crucial, as collage production takes place in these lower layers.

The skin's dermis layer contains most of the specialized structures and cells of the skin. It has less capability to synthesize collagen once you hit the age of 20. For women, the estrogen levels decrease as they age, making the skin thinner and drier. Through the ultrasound procedure, the dermis is stimulated to produce new collagen. The result is younger and tighter-looking skin as the tissue provides more support to the skin (26).

Fat reduction: Fat reduction belts are devices that use electrical impulses to draw out muscle contractions. This process mirrors a real workout of the abdomen and oblique muscles. The current standard for fat loss is bariatric surgery, which is invasive and poses risks typical of surgical procedures. This device technology paves the way for new innovative fat loss products that can be marketed for household use. These products are FDA approved as Class II medical devices.

Newer Techniques and Device Formulations

For thousands of years, people have applied various substances on their skin to obtain therapeutic effects, and in the modern era, various topical formulations have been developed to enhance the skin appearance and treat various conditions. Currently, with the increased consumer interest in healthy-looking skin, there is an increasing demand for products that supply multiple benefits with minimal effort. Modern consumers expect the latest technological advances with innovative formulations that contain various proven actives. As a result, formulations that promote skin permeability by actives are driving new product development in the cosmetic industry. Following the placement of a therapeutic formulation on the skin, the actives are required to penetrate through the stratum corneum (SC) into the viable tissue. To understand the transdermal delivery of actives within the skin structure, some understanding of skin physiology and the factors affecting transdermal delivery is required. For the effective delivery of beneficial ingredients into the skin cells, the barrier function of the skin must be selectively overcome. The most common and convenient method for overcoming this barrier function is the use of additives such as chemical enhancers. These compounds can "piggyback" the actives into the SC or make changes in the SC structure that increase its permeability to the actives. To date, most research on chemical penetration enhancers has studied their addition to formulations to influence the permeability of various active compounds (27).

Physical enhancers: Active methods are beyond the focus of this article, but they have been the subject of a number of recent reviews. Physical forces such as electrical voltage (iontophoresis, electroporation), ultrasound (sonophoresis), microneedles, thermal ablation, magnetophoresis, photomechanical waves, and electron beam irradiation have all been used to overcome the skin barrier. Device-based approaches to increase skin permeability or provide a driving force for transport appear to be broadly effective at increasing the transdermal delivery of macromolecules. Physical mechanisms generally create micron-scale pores in the SC, enabling the transport of very large molecules.

Vesicular Delivery Systems

The dermal application of cosmetic actives with properties such as high molecular weight, hydrophilicity, polarity, or susceptibility to enzymatic degradation remains highly challenging. Nano-sized vesicular delivery systems used for drug delivery are of particular interest to the cosmetic industry for this purpose. Liquid nano-sized systems are significantly more effective as vehicles for extremely hydrophilic agents than classical enhancer emulsions. Liposomes are the most widely used vehicle in the development and production of permeation delivery systems, but several other vehicles have also been investigated.

Liposomes

Liposomes are well known and often used as vesicular delivery systems for active ingredients in cosmetics. They comprise phospholipid membranes arranged in a sphere and are used to encapsulate polar and non-polar actives. First described by Bangham in 1965, liposomes have been prepared with a variety of phospholipids and have been extensively studied in the pharmaceutical and cosmetic industries. Liposomes are used in cosmetic applications or for transdermal delivery in particular with the expectation that their use will result in an increase in the concentration of active agents within the skin. For example, liposomes encapsulating CoQ10, a powerful antioxidant, have been shown to be beneficial to the skin. Larger vitamins, such as vitamin E, water-soluble vitamins, fat-soluble amino acids, and even chemically formulated active ingredients, can also be successfully encapsulated in liposomes to formulate various skincare products. However, although phospholipids offer the advantages of being biodegradable and non-toxic amphiphiles, liposomes have low physical and chemical stability and poor skin permeation limits when used for topical delivery. To increase the stability of liposomes, the concept of proliposomes has been proposed. Proliposomes and proniosomes, which are respectively converted to liposomes and niosomes upon simple hydration, have, therefore, been investigated for transdermal drug delivery. This approach was also extended to transfersomes and ethosomes, which exhibit superior stability compared to liposomes. These vesicular delivery vehicles are discussed further below (28).

Ethosomes

Ethosomes are composed mainly of phospholipids (phosphatidylcholine, phosphatidylserine, and phosphatidic acid) and high concentrations of ethanol and water. The incorporation of ethanol in the lipid vesicles is an alternative approach to fluidize the lipid membrane and thus enhance drug delivery. Because of the high ethanol concentration present, the lipid membrane of ethosomes is less tightly packed than conventional vesicles but has equivalent stability, allowing a more malleable structure and improved distribution among SC lipid. The size of ethosome vesicles can be modulated from tens of nanometers to microns.

Transfersomes

Transfersomes, first proposed by Cevc et al. in 1995, are proprietary lipid aggregations that can penetrate efficiently through pores or other biological constrictions that would be confining for other particulates of a comparable size. These malleable vesicles can stretch up to 500 nm in length to penetrate the SC barrier. This capability is due to the self-adaptability and extremely high deformability of the transfersome membrane. Transfersomes and ethosomes incorporating edge activators, such as surfactants, and penetration enhancers, such as alcohols, limonene, oleic acid, and polyols, have been shown to influence the properties of these vesicles and their permeation of the SC.

Niosomes

Niosomes are nonionic surfactant vesicles that self-assemble from hydrated surfactant monomers and have the capacity to deliver hydrophilic, lipophilic, and amphiphilic substances. Niosomes are similar to liposomes in terms of their structure and physical properties, as they comprise single or double alkyl chain nonionic surfactants with cholesterol. Niosomes have the ability to modify the structure of the SC through their surfactant properties, resulting in the layer becoming looser and more permeable. Niosomes are an effective alternative to liposomes, as they possess greater stability and alleviate other disadvantages associated with liposomes, such as the variable purity of the phospholipid constituents and high cost. Recent advances in liposome modifications appear to have generated increased therapeutic potential. Alterations in their composition and structure result in vesicles with tailored properties. For example, marinosomes are liposomes made with natural marine lipids that have a high concentration of polyunsaturated fatty acids and intrinsic anti-inflammatory properties. Ultrasomes are liposomes encapsulating a UV-endonuclease enzyme that recognizes sun damage to the skin and initiates the repair of UV-damaged DNA as well as inhibiting the expression of pro-inflammatory cytokines. Photosomes protect sun-exposed skin by releasing a light-activated enzyme (photolyase) extracted from a marine plant, *Anacystis nidulans*, which helps repair DNA damage. Photosomes encapsulate the photolyase in liposomes and are incorporated in sunscreen products (29).

Formulations: It has been recognized that the vehicle in which the permeant is applied to the skin has a distinct effect on the dermal and transdermal delivery of active ingredients. Cosmetic and pharmaceutical formulations for topical application are multifaceted and can range from aqueous solutions and suspensions to solid systems. Many studies have been performed to investigate the effect of various formulations such as gels, microemulsions, nanoemulsions, multiple emulsions, and liquid crystals on transdermal delivery. The type of formulation, the droplet size, the emollient, and the emulsifier, as well as the surfactant organization in the emulsion, may all affect the transdermal absorption of formulations. Some of the most widely used formulations for transdermal delivery systems (TDS) such as gels, emulsions, and vesicular delivery systems are discussed below.

Gels

Gels are semisolid formulations that usually consist of two components: A liquid component that acts as a solvent and a solid component (mostly termed a "gelator") that acts as a gelling agent. Gels are exceptional materials that are both rigid and elastic in nature and have a broad range of applications in cosmetics, medicines, and the food industry. Gels hydrate the skin by retaining a significant amount of water, thereby permitting greater dissolution of actives and facilitating their transepidermal migration.

Hydrogels

Hydrogels are three-dimensional hydrophilic polymeric networks, which have the ability to absorb large quantities of water or biological fluids. They consist of an aqueous dispersion medium that is gelled with a suitable hydrophilic agent. Many therapeutic agents are loaded in hydrogels for the purpose of efficient wound healing.

Organogels

Organogels are a class of gel composed of a liquid organic phase within a three-dimensional cross-linked network that contains oil or non-polar liquids as a dispersion medium. Many typical organogel components are known to be permeation enhancers, and organogels are thought to act by creating partitions in the lipid bilayers of the SC.

Bigels

Bigels are biphasic systems produced by mixing an organogel and a hydrogel together at high shear rates. The key feature of bigels that makes them useful for controlled drug delivery is their ability to deliver both hydrophilic and lipophilic active agents across the SC. Bigels are also easy to prepare and have a good stability. Their enhancement of skin hydration results in cooling and moisturizing effects.

Emulgels

The presence of a gelling agent in the water phase converts a classical emulsion into an emulgel. Although traditional gels have many advantages, the delivery of hydrophobic drugs has consistently been a point of concern. To overcome this limitation, emulgels were introduced. Furthermore, emulgels have the benefits of spreadability, adhesion, viscosity, and the highest drug release. Recently, nanosuspension-based gels (also called "nanogels") have received considerable attention in the development of topical applications because of their ability to enhance delivery into the skin. Proniosomal gels are primarily formulated based on either hydrogels or organogels. Organogel-based niosomal gels have mainly been investigated as vehicles of actives.

Emulsions

Emulsions are liquid or semisolid mixtures of lipophilic and hydrophilic constituents that have been stabilized into a homogeneous dispersion by a surface-active agent. Emulsions are widely used in cosmetic and pharmaceutical formulations because of their excellent solubilizing capacities for lipophilic and hydrophilic active ingredients and their application acceptability.

Microemulsions

A microemulsion is a mixture of water, oil, and an amphiphile that forms an optically isotropic and thermodynamically stable liquid solution. Microemulsions are thermodynamically stable and transparent (or translucent). The oil and water dispersion is stabilized by the amphiphile, which forms an interfacial film of surfactant molecules with a diameter of < 100 nm (usually 10–50 nm). Microemulsions are classified into three types: Oil-in-water, bicontinuous, and water-in-oil. Several recent reports have detailed microemulsion formulations designed for topical or transdermal application. Microemulsions form spontaneously or with a very low energy input but require a greater amount of surfactant compared with emulsions, which may lead to increased irritancy. Naturally occurring surfactants and oils remain an attractive option, and the phase behavior and microstructure of microemulsions based on soybean phosphatidylcholine and triglycerides have recently been reported, although propanol was used as the cosurfactant. The preparation of non-toxic microemulsions has also been described for mixtures of isopropyl myristate or orange oil with lecithin. An interesting alternative approach for the stabilization of microemulsions of octyl monoglucoside has been to employ geraniol, a perfume alcohol ($C10H17OH$), as a cosurfactant/cosolvent.

Nanoemulsions

Nanoemulsions consist of very fine oil-in-water dispersions, with a droplet diameter in the range of 20–200 nm and narrow size distributions. Nanoemulsions are kinetically but not thermodynamically stable, and their preparation requires expensive, high-energy input methods as they are formed with relatively small amounts of surfactants. The efficacy of nanoemulsions is enhanced by the nature and type of surfactant and cosurfactant used. Because nanoemulsions are transparent and typically very fluid, the slightest sign of destabilization is readily apparent. The very small size of the droplets (~ 50 nm in diameter) gives them characteristic properties that are highly valued in cosmetics. As they are transparent, consumers associate nanoemulsions with freshness, purity, and simplicity, and they are easily absorbed by the skin.

Liquid Crystals

Liquid crystals are an intermediate state between solid and liquid. This is often called a mesomorphic state, where the degree of molecular order is intermediate between that of isotropic liquids, gases, and amorphous solids. Liquid crystals form multilayers around emulsion droplets, decreasing the van der Waals force and increasing the viscosity, which increases emulsion stability. Various bioactive molecules such as chemical drugs, peptides, and proteins can be solubilized in either the aqueous or oil phase of liquid crystals for protection from hydrolysis and oxidation. Several studies have demonstrated how advantageous it is for formulations to form liquid crystals because they improve the formulation in several aspects: They increase skin hydration, which increases formulation viscosity as a result of molecular reorganization, and they increase the permeability and prolong the release of actives. A study by Otto et al. described how emulsifiers arranged in liquid crystalline structures in the water phase enhanced the skin penetration of active ingredients.

Multiple Emulsions

Multiple emulsions consist either of oil globules dispersed within water globules in an oily continuous phase (o/w/o) or of water globules dispersed within oil globules in a continuous water phase (w/o/w). Multiple emulsions, especially w/o/w systems, have shown a potential applicability in controlled release systems for the delivery of active ingredients. Several studies using different active ingredients have been performed to compare different types of emulsions (o/w, w/o, and w/o/w) with identical composition. This allowed the investigation of the effect of the type of emulsion alone without the influence of different formulation ingredients. It was found that the level of skin uptake of glucose and lactic acid, which are both water-soluble compounds, as well as the flux of glucose across the skin, decreased in the following order: o/w > w/o/w > w/o.

Skin Analysis Devices

There are several types of skin analysis devices, each with its own uses and benefits.

Magnifying lamps: Virtually every dermatologist and aesthetician commences with a magnifying light, also known as a "mag light," "mag lamp," or "loupe." This gives a good start for seeing things that are hard to view with the naked eye. Sometimes, it helps to reposition the lamp to get a good view of an area. Magnifying lamps help prevent guesswork, and they eliminate shadows and color distortion. They also make life infinitely easier for the professional by preventing squinting, neck strain, and back problems. Newer magnifying lamps offer many features, such as reduced weight, improved stability, adjustable arms and lamp heads, one-touch or hands-free positioning, dimmable LED lights that last 50,000 hours, and multiple magnification levels. When selecting a magnifying lamp, one should look for one with a durable but ergonomic arm design, with a head that can be easily repositioned and self-tightening knobs. While there are lamps with fluorescent or halogen lighting, LED lighting has become the new standard, as it provides far superior color rendering. If portability is important, there are models that can be mounted on a rolling stand for ease of use.

The diopters of the lamp determine the instrument's magnification. Diopters are fixed, so if different levels of magnification are needed, select a lamp that allows a choice between several replaceable lenses, much like changing the eyepiece on a telescope or the lens on a camera. The diopter of a lens is the reciprocal of its focal length. The higher the number of a magnifying lamp's diopters, the thicker the lens and the more it is curved. Also, the higher the number of diopters, the greater the magnification.

It is simple to convert given diopters to the lamp's magnification: Divide the diopter by four and add one. For example, a three-diopter magnifying lamp (the most common strength) gives 175% magnification:

- $3/4 = 0.75$
- $75 + 1 = 1.75$

The distance from the lens center to the point where the rays of light meet is the focal length of the lamp, and it is where the subject comes into perfect focus. The focal length of the lamp is the working distance between the lamp and the client's face. The greater the magnification, the shorter the working distance, which must be considered to allow room for hands, tools, and the like.

Wood's lamp: A Wood's lamp is another common tool used by both dermatologists and aestheticians. It is a handheld device that uses completely safe, long wave, ultraviolet light to help detect bacteria and fungi on the surface of the skin, as well as certain skin conditions. Bacteria like *Pseudomonas* species, *P. acnes*, and *Corynebacterium minutissimum*, as well as fungi, will light up as a different color (luminesce) under a Wood's lamp, usually appearing greenish, alerting the professional to their presence. A Wood's lamp can also be used to diagnose:

- Pityriasis versicolor
- Vitiligo
- Melasma
- Erythrasma
- Scabies

The normal wavelength of a Wood's lamp is 320 to 450 nm; however, newer models with a specific wavelength of 395 nm are being used to detect tumors, like basal cell carcinoma and actinic keratosis.

Dermascopes

A professional may wish to invest in a dermascope, a small skin microscope resembling an otoscope. These instruments are used primarily for further evaluation of suspicious skin lesions. With the magnification of a dermascope, a professional can quickly determine if a lesion is melanocytic (pigmented by melanin) and if it necessitates a referral outside their facility or an in-house biopsy. A dermascope may also be handy in identifying small psoriatic patches on the skin. Dermascopes have come down in price since first introduced to the market, and they are no longer the sole purview of dermatologists. In fact, they have increased the ability of professionals of all types to identify problematic lesions, so the right next steps and treatment can be commenced. It takes some practice to use a dermascope properly but, in the right hands, this tool is invaluable. There is a range of dermoscopes available on the market today, so it is essential to shop around based on use. Those who refer clients outside their facility for lesion follow-up will likely prefer a small scope that provides basic magnification. There are even smartphone dermascope attachments.

For dermatology practices, more sophisticated systems may be appropriate, including those with associated camera and video systems, perfect for telemedicine. This type of dermascope offers superior optics with adjustable magnification and field of view and usually includes a built-in scale for measuring lesions and tracking their growth. A removable reticle plate makes cleaning easier.

Full-Face Analysis

A new frontier of skin analysis tools involves full-face analysis. These instruments allow the client to place their face in a module for viewing the entire face at once. Some systems rotate around the client's face, much like a panoramic dental X-ray. Images from the analysis are transmitted to a camera or video system and can be helpful for both the professional and client. Full-face skin analysis, like traditional skin analysis with a magnifying lamp and Wood's lamp, can identify and color map issues like:

- Fine lines and wrinkles
- Spots and areas of discoloration
- Redness
- Ultraviolet damage
- Subsurface melanin
- Vascular conditions

Some offer a magnifying loupe element and aging simulation. Before and after imaging can be helpful in assessing the success of various treatments. Some practices use this type of imaging in helping clients decide on invasive procedures. These systems are still in the clinical trials phase, awaiting FDA approval, and they are not considered standard skin analysis devices yet. But they present an exciting opportunity for skin analysis in the future.

Breast Implants

A breast implant is a prosthesis used to change the size, shape, and contour of a person's breast. In reconstructive plastic surgery, breast implants can be placed to restore a natural-looking breast following a mastectomy, to correct congenital defects and deformities of the chest wall, or, cosmetically, to enlarge the appearance of the breast through breast augmentation surgery.

Saline Breast Implants

Saline breast implants are filled with sterile salt water. Should the implant shell leak, a saline implant will collapse and the saline will be absorbed and naturally expelled by the body. Saline breast implants provide a uniform shape, firmness, and feel, and are FDA-approved for augmentation in women aged 18 or older.

Structured Saline Breast Implants

Structured implants are filled with sterile salt water, and contain an inner structure which aims to make the implant feel more natural.

Silicone Breast Implants

Silicone breast implants are filled with silicone gel. The gel feels a bit more like natural breast tissue. If the implant leaks, the gel may remain within the implant shell, or may escape into the breast implant pocket. A leaking implant filled with silicone gel will not collapse. If you choose silicone implants, you may need to visit your plastic surgeon regularly to make sure the implants are functioning properly. An ultrasound or MRI screening can assess the condition of breast implants. Silicone breast implants are FDA-approved for augmentation in women aged 22 or older.

Gummy Bear Breast Implants

Form-stable implants are sometimes referred to as gummy bear breast implants because they maintain their shape even when the implant shell is broken. The consistency of the silicone gel inside the implant is thicker than traditional silicone gel implants. These implants are also firmer than traditional implants. Shaped gummy bear breast implants have more projection at the bottom and are tapered towards the top. If a shaped implant rotates, it may lead to an unusual appearance of the breast that requires a separate procedure to correct.

Round Breast Implants

Round breast implants have a tendency to make breasts appear fuller than form-stable implants. Higher profile options can achieve even more projection. Because round implants are the same shape all over, there is less concern about them rotating out of place.

Smooth Breast Implants

Smooth breast implants are the softest feeling. They can move with the breast implant pocket, which may give more natural movement. Smooth implants may have some palpable or visible rippling under the skin. Textured breast implants develop scar tissue to stick to the implant, making them less likely to move around inside of the breast and become repositioned. Texturing offers some advantage in diminishing the risk of a tight scar capsule.

Testicular Implants

Testicular implants may be performed after the testes have been surgically removed or are absent because of birth defect, illness, or trauma. Testicular implants may also be performed in certain cosmetic cases. An implant is sized to match the normal testicle, or when both testes are absent, sized to fill the scrotum to restore symmetry.

Testicular implants are filled with saline and placed inside the scrotum. They are soft to the touch to provide a realistic look and feel. Testicular implants are performed as an outpatient and can be done with minimal anesthesia. Currently, Torosa is the only FDA-approved testicular implant. It is manufactured by Coloplast, a world leader in prosthetic technology.

Vaginal Wall Implants

Vaginal prolapse may recur after it has been treated by conventional surgery. This is especially true when the prolapse involves the front wall of the vagina ("bladder prolapse"/"cystocele") and in the presence of risk factors such as obesity, chronic cough, constipation, or occupations that involve excessive abdominal straining or heavy lifting. This is known as a recurrent prolapse.

Currently available evidence suggests that surgery with mesh may be more effective than traditional surgery, in certain circumstances, in reducing the chance of recurrent prolapse. Mesh can be particularly useful in the treatment of bladder prolapse (cystocele) and vaginal vault prolapse. However, there is not much good evidence about how well this procedure works in the long term (over two years), and there is some concern regarding potential complications that are unique to permanent synthetic mesh placed through the vagina (see further details in complications section).

The aim of a mesh implant is to reinforce natural tissue which has failed to support the pelvic organs, restoring support to the bladder, uterus, or bowel and so preventing further bulging of these organs towards the vagina. The term "mesh" may refer to different types of materials including biologic grafts (derived from humans or animals), synthetic, absorbable (dissolves slowly over time), or permanent (stays in the body forever). Mesh can be used to repair prolapse of the front vaginal wall ("cystocele") or the back vaginal wall ("rectocele") in isolation or both in the same surgery. It can also be used to support the uterus (womb) in women suffering from uterine prolapse or to treat vaginal vault prolapse.

Mesh Types, Manufacturers, and Brands

The FDA categorizes mesh into four categories for gynecological use based on how the mesh reacts inside of the body.

The four categories include:
- **Non-absorbable synthetic**: Non-absorbable synthetic meshes are made from synthetic materials, such as plastic or polyester. Most mesh devices are made of polypropylene.
- **Absorbable synthetic**: The body absorbs absorbable synthetic mesh, and tissue grows at the implant site. This helps strengthen the ligaments in the pelvis.
- **Biologic**: Biologic meshes are natural products derived from animal tissue that has been disinfected. These products degrade over time and are usually made from cow (bovine) or pig (porcine) tissue.
- **Composite**: Composite mesh is made from a combination of non-absorbable synthetic, absorbable synthetic, or biologic mesh.

Cosmetic Devices Regulation

Personalized or customized cosmetics are increasing in popularity. While compliance with the EU Cosmetics Regulation 1223/2009 is mandatory, there are no clear guidelines to ensure their compliance. While cosmetic products are subject to numerous regulations, permitting their sale within the European single market, this article focuses on the requirements of the Cosmetics Regulation 1223/2009. Certain provisions of the Regulation are considered, and possible solutions proposed to enable the safe use of personalized cosmetics placed on the market.

The legal framework for cosmetics in the European Union (EU) is Regulation 1223/2009 (the Regulation). While the Regulation does not explicitly mention or address personalized products, if the definition of cosmetic is met (a product intended to be placed in contact with the external parts of the human body with the intention of cleaning them, perfuming them, changing their appearance, protecting them, keeping them in good condition, or correcting body odors), then the product must comply with the Regulation. This poses several challenges to retailers and/or manufacturers. These include ensuring good manufacturing practice (including the identification of manufacturing site or sites) and assessing the safety of a product that has a variable composition. Domestic blending devices are also available on the market. These devices mix the contents of several cartridges containing a base cream and cosmetic active ingredients in the proportion determined to be optimal for the customer according to their skin characteristics. The final formula and mixing concentrations are designed before the device and cartridges are sent to the customer, so the customer receives a cosmetic kit.

Article 8 of the Cosmetics Regulation

Good manufacturing practice: Cosmetic manufacturing facilities must work according to good manufacturing practice (GMP). This ought not to present a challenge to products formulated or manufactured in regular manufacturing facilities (i.e., personalized products that are purchased online). However, the challenge is significant when preparing the cosmetic product in situ (i.e., at the retailer's store). If a device is used, the device becomes the "manufacturing facility" and should thus comply with good manufacturing practices. This means the device should be regularly calibrated and standardized in order to ensure that volumes dispensed are accurate and consistent. Devices should also be kept in a good hygienic condition, and people using the device should be adequately trained to ensure proper use and maintenance. If no device is being used, but a person is preparing the product at the store, efforts should be directed towards ensuring that person is properly trained, dispensing materials are calibrated, and the environment is clean. If the device is used at home, a high level of automation is expected, but GMP compliance is still expected (again, the device becomes the manufacturing facility). The device should be designed to ensure accuracy and hygiene when manipulated by the consumer at home. Additionally, clear and accurate directions for use should be provided to the consumer to ensure the manufacturing process results in a safe cosmetic product.

Article 10 of the Cosmetics Regulation

A safety assessment must be performed prior to placing a cosmetic product on the market, that is, before the customer takes the product home or the product is received at home. If the customized cosmetic product is ordered online and shipped home, the timeframe is manageable, as the product's composition is well known before the final product reaches the consumer and the safety assessment can be prepared in advance. A bigger challenge exists if the exact product composition is not known in advance, i.e., if the product is designed and blended at the retail store. In this case, Responsible Persons should be able to foresee all possible combinations of ingredients their cosmetic products can have and prepare a safety assessment for each combination, so that any possible product they place on the market is covered. Using concentration ranges for the safety assessment is a possibility, but this approach becomes unfeasible if variable concentrations are possible for more than one ingredient, as ingredient interactions become challenging to predict. Alternatively, a good IT tool to perform the safety assessment in situ might be the solution, but some limitations exist, e.g., the time needed to complete the assessment and the need for a safety assessor to sign the document. Nevertheless, a safety issue may arise with this type of product (blended at the retailer's store): Microbiological quality of the product will most probably not be checked, due to practical reasons, and it is therefore questionable if a safety assessor will consider a product is safe if these data are lacking. When a device is used at home, the final product composition after mixing the contents of the several cartridges will be known. As already mentioned above, this can be considered a cosmetic kit, and therefore a safety assessment can be performed before the product reaches the consumer.

Finally, when actives or boosters are used, important safety issues may arise. Actives or boosters should have their own safety assessment (as they represent individual products) before they are placed on the market, but an additional assessment is needed for the product resulting from the combination of the active or booster with the regular cosmetic product (which we can call the "base"). If the base and booster are manufactured by the same brand, then the properties of the resulting combination can be anticipated, and the safety assessment can be performed in advance. However, if the base is manufactured by another brand, such an approach is limited. Therefore, a safety assessment is unlikely to be performed for such a combination, and the resulting product is non-compliant (and more importantly, may have associated safety issues). Thus, if actives or boosters are to be marketed, they should be prescribed for their use only with bases manufactured by the same brand, unless those brands co-operate.

References

1. https://www.aslms.org/for-the-public/general-information/devices---radiofrequency
2. https://www.fda.gov/medical-devices/aesthetic-cosmetic-devices/microneedling-devices
3. https://www.ananyaaesthetics.com/what-is-the-difference-between-microneedling-devices.html
4. https://www.health.harvard.edu/blog/dermal-fillers-the-good-the-bad-and-the-dangerous-201907152561
5. https://www.plasticsurgery.org/cosmetic-procedures/dermal-fillers/safety
6. https://www.normanrappaportmd.com/5-benefits-of-plastic-surgery/
7. https://www.healthline.com/health/microdermabrasion
8. https://www.medicinenet.com/microdermabrasion/article.htm
9. https://www.sciencedirect.com/science/article/pii/S1578219010706600
10. https://www.ncbi.nlm.nih.gov/pmc/articles/PMC7647541/
11. https://www.ncbi.nlm.nih.gov/pmc/articles/PMC4075221/
12. https://www.healthline.com/health/facial-exercises-are-they-bogus#What-does-work?
13. https://pubmed.ncbi.nlm.nih.gov/27363770/
14. https://www.webmd.com/beauty/what-is-led-light-therapy-for-skin
15. https://sci-hub.hkvisa.net/10.1007/s00266-008-9195-x
16. https://www.ncbi.nlm.nih.gov/pmc/articles/PMC3583892/
17. https://sci-hub.hkvisa.net/10.4155/tde.15.64
18. https://www.ajronline.org/doi/full/10.2214/AJR.11.6719
19. https://www.plasticsurgery.org/cosmetic-procedures/breast-augmentation/implants
20. https://www.drugwatch.com/transvaginal-mesh/
21. https://www.fda.gov/medical-devices/aesthetic-cosmetic-devices/microneedling
22. Sasaki G. Micro-needling depth penetration,presence of pigment particles and fluorescein-stained platelets: Clinical usage for asthetic concerns. *Aesthet Surg J* 2017;37(1):71–83.
23. https://www.healthline.com/health/beauty-skin-care/do-derma-rollers-work
24. Lewis W. Is microneedling really the next big thing? Wendy Lewis explores the buzz surrounding skin needling. *Plast Surg Pract* 2014;7:24–8. 21.
25. Sahni K, Kassir M. Dermafrac™: An innovative new treatment for periorbital melanosis in a darkskinned male patient. *J Cutan Aesthet Surg* 2013;6:158.
26. Chandrashekar BS, Sriram R, Mysore R, Bhaskar S, Shetty A. Evaluation of microneedling fractional radiofrequency device for treatment of acne scars. *J Cutan Aesthet Surg* 2014;7:93–7.
27. Seonguk MI, Park SY, Yoon JY, Kwon HH, Dae Hun SU. Fractional microneedling radiofrequency treatment for acnerelated postinflammatory erythema. *Acta Derm Venereol* 2016;96:87–91.
28. Oh JH, Park HH, Do KY, Han M, Hyun DH, Kim CG, et al. Influence of the delivery systems using a microneedle array on the permeation of a hydrophilic molecule, calcein. *EurJ Pharm Biopharm* 2008;69:1040–5.
29. Badran MM, Kuntsche J, Fahr A. Skin penetration enhancement by a microneedle device (Dermaroller®) in vitro: Dependency on needle size and applied formulation. *Eur J Pharm Sci* 2009;36:511–23.

General Hospital Devices and Supplies

3

Pugazhenthan Thangaraju and Hemasri Velmurugan

INTRODUCTION

The expanded use of hospital devices has provided clinicians with ready access for diagnosing as well as treating patients. The convenience of carrying these devices into patient rooms for point-of-care, real-time application cannot be ignored or underestimated.[1] The association between hospital characteristics and the utilization of high-tech medical equipment has received a large amount of attention for its complicated consequences for health care costs and quality.[2] Here, we will discuss some medical devices approved by the FDA.[3]

PERSONAL PROTECTIVE EQUIPMENT

Personal protective equipment (PPE) includes protective gloves, face shields, facemasks, clothing, helmets, and/or respirators or other equipment which is designed to protect from injury or control the spread of infection or illness.[4] It lowers the risk of self-contamination or infection for health care workers and blocks the transmission of infection through body fluids, blood, or respiratory secretions. The correct usage and proper handling of PPE in terms of donning and doffing help in the protection of health care workers from infection.[3] Coronavirus disease is mostly transmitted through droplets or contact, and PPE is a highly important component for reducing the risk of disease transmission.

Components of PPE

Medical Gloves

Medical gloves are used during examination or medical or surgical procedures.

- Before starting the procedure, gloves must fit properly and must be changed whenever they are ripped or torn.

DOI: 10.1201/9781003220671-3

- Some gloves are made of rubber latex, and some may be allergic to it. They can use gloves made of other synthetic materials (such as polyvinyl chloride (PVC), nitrile, or polyurethane).
- Wash hands before and after using them.
- Never reuse or share medical gloves with others[3] (Figure 3.1).

Masks

For preventing airborne transmission a combination of interventions is needed, not just PPE alone (Table 3.1) (Figure 3.2).

Medical Gowns

Like medical gloves they are used during examination or medical or surgical procedures and prevent the transmission of micro-organisms from patients to health care workers (HCWs) (Table 3.2).

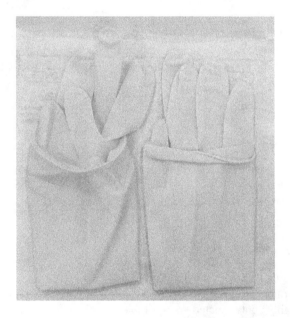

FIGURE 3.1   Medical gloves.

TABLE 3.1   Difference between N95 Respirators and Surgical Masks

NO.	N95 RESPIRATOR	SURGICAL MASK
1	• It protects HCWs by filtering the airborne particles in the environment like bacteria, viruses, dust, allergens, irritants, and others. • It acts like a protective mask around the nose and mouth.	• It is an interference device that acts the same as an N95 mask and is also known as a face mask. • Available in different thicknesses.
2	• Not for children or people with facial hair. • Breathing is difficult for patients with chronic respiratory, cardiac, or other medical conditions. • Mask with exhalation valves should not be used in sterile areas.[3]	• Less protective compared to N95 masks due to its loose fit.[3]

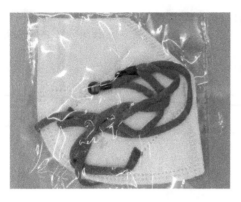 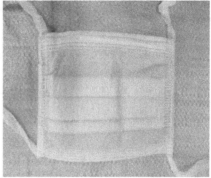

FIGURE 3.2   N95 respirator and surgical mask.

TABLE 3.2   Levels of Protection Issued by FDA in 2004

LEVELS	RISK	EXAMPLES
1	Minimal	Regular care, wards, for patient care takers, or standard isolation
2	Low	While taking blood samples, laboratory, or intensive care unit (ICU)
3	Moderate	While taking arterial blood, inserting central line or IV line, trauma and emergency department
4	High	During surgery or other long procedures (non-airborne)[3]

Surgical Gowns

- A surgical gown is a garment worn by health care workers to protect them from contamination during surgical procedures.
- They are regulated by the FDA under Class II devices for high risk (Levels 1–4).
- They are also used in normal medical units with an increased risk of contamination.

Non-Surgical Gowns

- They are regulated under Class I devices d.
- It is a garment worn by HCWs to protect themselves from contamination in minimal risk areas but not used in highly contaminated areas[3] (Table 3.3).
- Contact precaution PPE – for health care workers in the same room as patients and where aerosol generating procedures are not undertaken.

TABLE 3.3   Transmission Mode and Matched PPE

NO.	TRANSMISSION MODE	PPE
1	Airborne precaution (prevents droplet and contact transmission)	• FFP3 mask • Gloves • Goggles • Fluid-repellent long-sleeved gown
2	Droplet precaution (prevents contact transmission)	• Gloves • Apron • Fluid-resistant surgical mask • ± Goggles (risk assess)
3	Contact precaution	• Gloves • Apron

- Droplet precaution PPE – it offers protection for 2 meters' distance. Goggles are added additionally for assessing risk. The patient should also wear a fluid-resistant surgical facemask.
- Airborne precaution PPE – used in aerosol generating procedures till air exchanges have reduced the virus sufficiently[5] (Figure 3.3).

Precautions

- Proper donning, doffing, and disposal of PPE.
- Proper waste management.
- Proper cleaning of the contaminated zone (Figure 3.4).

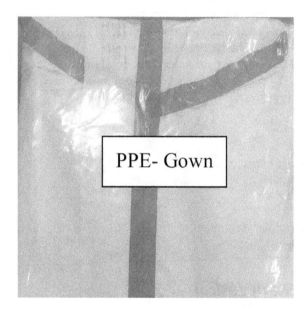

FIGURE 3.3   Fluid-repellent long-sleeved gown.

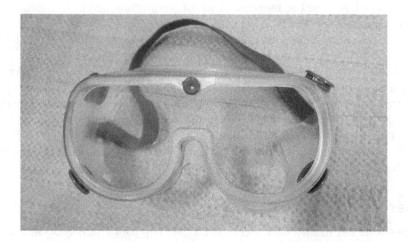

FIGURE 3.4   PPE – goggles.

Limitations

We should keep in mind that this PPE is only one part of a system to prevent disease transmission.

- Flat foldable particulate (FFP3) is only included in airborne PPE.
- Overuse of PPE creates global demand as in COVID-19, and this is a form of misuse.
- Using PPE in unnecessary situations is also a form of misuse.[5]

STERILIZATION OF MEDICAL DEVICES

Medical devices will be helpful in both diagnosing and treating patients. For proper usage of medical devices we need to sterilize them regularly. Sterilization plays a major role in the protection of medical devices from micro-organisms. This includes multiple radiation options, ethylene oxide, liquid chemical sterilization, etc.

Efficacy of Sterilization

This depends on

- Medical device and machine contact time.
- Composition of material.
- Presence of organic matter.
- Temperature.
- Type and number of micro-organisms.
- Physio-chemical environment.[6]

Ethylene Oxide Sterilization

- This is an important sterilization method that manufacturers widely use and that does not damage the device during the process.
- It has bactericidal, virucidal, and fungicidal activity.
- It is introduced and used in hospital setups for sterilization due to emerging new medical devices.
- Devices made up of polymers, glass, or metals, or devices with multiple layers or hard-to-reach places (for example, catheters) are likely to be sterilized with ethylene oxide.[7]
- If processed at a range of 40°C to 60°C for more than 3–24 h, some thermal degradation may occur.
- Components with low boiling points (e.g., 10.7°C) might evaporate due to vacuum pulses.
- After sterilization there are acceptable levels of residual ethylene oxide and ethylene chlorohydrin on the device which will help to ensure the levels are within the safe limits so that long-term and occupational exposure-related problems like cancer will be prevented.[6]
- The FDA announced a Master File Pilot Program for using fixed chamber ethylene oxide on November 25, 2019.[3]

Advantages

- Ethylene oxide sterilization is an ideal gaseous sterilant with effectiveness and compatibility as well as flexibility.
- It depends on concentration, temperature, humidity, time, and their combinations.

- It can be used for heat-, moisture-, or radiation-sensitive medical devices.
- The system consists of closed, automated, and controlled machines.
- Recently, aeration in addition to sterilization has been introduced in the same chamber or in a continuous chamber which reduces the potential occupational exposure to the gases.[6]

Disadvantages

- The problem with ethylene oxide sterilization is its complexity and hazardous and toxic potential.
- A properly designed area is needed due to its inflammable property.
- Trained staff and safe work practices are required.
- Detectors or monitors are required to protect staff since the gas is colorless and odorless until a level of 430 ppm.
- The penetration of gases in liquids or powders due to limitations of penetration depths makes it practically impossible to use them.
- Lastly, the careful aeration of medical devices absorbed gas can leave toxic residues on them.[6]

Liquid Chemical Sterilization/High Level Disinfectants

Liquid chemical sterilization is commonly used to disinfect medical devices used for invasive procedures. It does not give assurance as sterilization using thermal or low temperature sterilization methods.[7]

It consists of hydrogen peroxide, glutaraldehyde, peracetic acid and chlorine compounds.

Liquid chemical sterilization involves a two-part process:

1. Medical devices are treated with a liquid chemical germicide (LCG).
2. For the removal of chemical residues, the processed devices are rinsed with water.

Advantages

Used for endoscopes, cystoscopes, and surgical instruments with plastic components.

Limitations

The rinse water used is not sterile, and devices rinsed cannot be assured to be sterile. This shows that there is no way to maintain sterility.

Recommendation

The FDA recommends that the use of liquid chemical sterilants be limited to reprocessing only critical devices that are heat-sensitive and incompatible with other sterilization methods. The FDA has not cleared any biological indicators, but chemical indicators are appropriate and are required for monitoring the minimum required concentration of most liquid chemical sterilants.[3]

NON-CONTACT INFRARED THERMOMETERS

These are used for measuring a patient's surface temperature with the help of minimal (tympanic) or no (non-contact infrared thermometer [NCIT] and thermal scanner). As the temperature is measured from a distance from the patient it helps in disease transmission. Normal temperature is 98.6°F but some reports show between 97°F and 99°F.[3]

Types

- Non-contact infrared thermometers.
- Tympanic thermometers.
- Thermal scanners.

Procedure

- Non-contact infrared thermometers are kept at a distance from the patient's forehead and measure by thermal radiation emitted from the patient's body. This increases the accuracy as well as compliance.
- Tympanic thermometers measure the heat coming from the tympanic membrane. Later the heat is converted into a temperature. These are very easy to use.
- Handheld thermal scanners are kept at a greater distance than other non-contact thermometers and are used for mass screening.

Temperature cut off differs for each device.[8]

Advantages

- Ease of use.
- No discomfort like a normal thermometer.
- Lack of contact.
- Quick results.
- Helps to screen large numbers of people.
- Reusable.
- No risk of contamination.[3]

Limitations

- Sometimes changes in the value may be due to head coverings, head position, environment, etc.
- Risk of contamination in case of taking measurements closely.[3]
- Not everyone will have a fever due to a disease, and using antipyretics makes it difficult to measure the temperature.

Procedure

- Make the patient stand in an erect posture and take temperature by placing the thermometer perpendicular to the head.
- Avoid touching the sensing area of the thermometer.
- Before use make sure it is clean and dry.[3]

Difference between Thermal Imaging Systems and Non-Contact Infrared Thermometers (NCIT)

Both will help to measure surface skin temperatures without contact. NCIT measures in a single location, whereas a thermal imaging system measures across multiple locations which helps to create a temperature map of a region of the body.[3]

THERMAL IMAGING SYSTEMS (INFRARED THERMOGRAPHIC SYSTEMS)

- Thermal imaging systems are used for accurate measurement of temperature without any contact with the patients.
- It is one of the most advanced inventions for temperature measurement by infrared radiation.
- The principle is the conversion of invisible infrared radiation into visible two-dimensional temperature emitted by the objects.
- It prevents closer proximity or contact with the patients.[3]

Advantages

- Measures temperature faster than the typical forehead or oral (mouth) thermometer.
- The health care worker who handles the thermal imaging system is not required to be in physical contact with the patient.
- Scientific studies show evidence for the accuracy of thermal imaging systems.[3]

Limitations

- Not effective when used to take the temperature of multiple people at the same time (for example, airports, businesses, and sporting events), Thus, it is not suitable for mass temperature screening.
- Measured temperature is usually lower than a temperature measured orally.
- Needs proper adjustment for the correction in the measurements.

Precautions

- Right environment or location.
- Properly trained person.
- Proper setup and operated correctly according to the instructions.[3]

SURGICAL STAPLERS AND VASCULAR SEALING DEVICES

Surgical Stapling Instruments

Recent advances like stapling instrumentation and vascular sealing devices have improved the efficiency of surgery with hemorrhagic control. They are used for connecting two hollow visceral or tubular structures internally during surgeries and also used to close wounds externally. The range of staplers includes circular, linear, linear cutting, ligating, and skin staplers. They can decrease tissue trauma, contamination, and the anesthetic period in multiple body systems, including gastrointestinal, urogenital, cardiovascular, pulmonary, and skin.[9]

They are used in visceral and other surgeries. Examples:

- Resection – removal of part of gut surgically.
- Transection – in organs, it cuts between the two rows.
- Anastomoses – joins two hollow structures.[3]

Types

- Thoraco-abdominal staplers.
- Gastrointestinal anastomosis and intestinal linear anastomosis staplers.
- End-to-end anastomotic (EEA) staplers.
- Endoscopic stapling devices.
- Surgical skin staples.

Precautions

1. Not for use in inflamed, edematous, or lack a vascular supply.
2. Should penetrate all tissue layers.
3. Accurate size – not too thick to be penetrated or too thin to support the staple.
4. Proper checkup before use and no capturing of inadvertent tissues.
5. Careful removal is needed to avoid disrupting the staples and check for hemorrhage, leakage, or loose staples.[9]

Advantages

- Low cost.
- Strength.
- Maintain homeostasis and reduce tissue reaction.
- Ease of use.
- Reduce the risk of contamination.

Disadvantages

- Incomplete ligation of vascular tissue.
- Decrease in lumen size.
- Leakage of air or fluid.
- Technical errors.

Complications

- Intestinal leakage.
- Infection and inflammatory reactions.
- Abscess formation.

Vessel Sealing Devices

These are designed for providing effective hemostasis of vascular tissues by coagulating vessels and hemorrhagic tissues in open and minimally invasive procedures. They are an alternative to ligatures and stapling instruments. They use electrothermal bipolar electrosurgery energy and pressure to induce denaturing and fusion of collagen and elastin within the vessel wall and surrounding tissues for vascular occlusion.[9]

Ligasure System

Ligasure System is made of two jaws designed to deliver bipolar energy into the grasped tissues. Benefits that have been noted include efficient and complete hemostasis of vessels, adequate arterial bursting pressure, absence of foreign material, and no need for additional ligation support.[9]

DEVICES USED FOR IV THERAPY

Components

- **Tubing set and solution bag** – may be glass or plastic. Ranges from 50 mL to 1000 mL and needle size range from 0.5 to 1.5 inches in length with 16 to 26 G[10] (Figure 3.5).
- **IV pole and/or pump** – a smart electronic infusion pump is automated and equipped with safety features and alerts health care workers while setting the pump.[7] They can be large or small volume pumps. An IV pole is about 18–24 inches in height.[10]
- **Small-bore connectors** – they connect medical devices such as tubing, syringes and other accessories that deliver fluids and gases for patient care. Small-bore refers to the small size, with the opening of the connector less than 8.5 mm.[3]

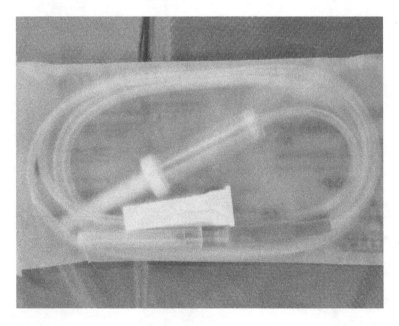

FIGURE 3.5   IV set.

Site Selection

The most frequently used sites are in the forearm veins as the bones in the forearm act as a natural support and splint.

- Adults – hand (cephalic vein), forearm (basilic vein), antecubital fossa.
- Infants – veins in the scalp and feet (saphenous vein).

Procedure

- Open and hang the IV fluid bag.
- Connect the infusion set and IV fluid bag.
- Squeeze the dripping chamber to fill two-thirds of it.
- Micro drip chamber delivers about 60 drops/mL.
- Macro drip chamber delivers 15 (10–20) drops/mL.
- Screening of the drip chamber for any faults or functional.
- The IV cannula on the patient is connected to the infusion set.
- Re-set after use (Figure 3.6).

Factors Affecting the Procedure

1) Position of the needle in the vein.
2) Gravity affects the flow rate.
3) Height of the infusion pole.
4) Position of the limbs.
5) Position of the intravenous tube.

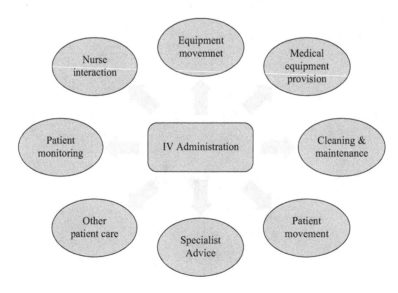

FIGURE 3.6   Steps to follow during IV therapy.

Advantages

- Large capacity and wide range of flow rates.
- Single injections at a time.
- Better patient compliance.
- More precise and safe administration is achieved.
- Emergency situations.
- Low dosage will be needed.[10, 11]

BLOOD PRESSURE MEASUREMENT

The sphygmomanometer is used for measuring blood pressure.
It consists of

1) Cuff containing a distensible bladder.
2) Rubber bulb with an adjustable valve for inflation.
3) Connecting tube.
4) Manometer to display the pressure level.

Indications

- Hypertension.
- Causes of hypertension – heart failure, coronary heart disease, stroke, cerebral hemorrhage, chronic kidney disease, hypertensive encephalopathy, retinopathy, peripheral vascular disease, aortic aneurysm, left ventricular hypertrophy, myocardial infarction (Figure 3.7).

Contraindications

- Arterial-venous shunt.
- Recent axillary node dissection.
- Deformity or surgical history of that arm.
- Misinterpretation in conditions like arrhythmias and dysrhythmias, persistent systole.

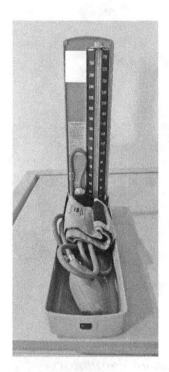

FIGURE 3.7 BP apparatus.

Procedure

- Place the cuff 2 cm above the elbow crease which will be directly over the brachial artery.
- Bell of the stethoscope should be placed over the brachial artery.
- Start auscultating blood pressure by inflating the cuff to a level 20–30 mmHg above the pulse obliteration pressure.
- Deflate at a rate of 2 mmHg per second and finally measure the average blood pressure (BP).

Precautions

- Avoid undersized cuffs – assessment of arm circumference at the midpoint of the upper arm is required to assure that a properly fitted cuff is used.
- It can be selected based on arm measurement and inspection of the match between the index and range lines once the cuff is placed on the patient.[12]

BREATHING OR RESPIRATORY SYSTEMS

Anesthetic machines and ventilators used to improve a patient's breathing. Work on the international standard for breathing and respiratory systems is still underway, and the FDA anticipates recognizing this standard once it is finalized.[8]

Pulse Oximeter

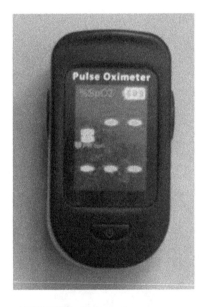

FIGURE 3.8   Pulse oximeter.

Oxygen saturation measures how much hemoglobin is bound to oxygen and how much remains unbound. Due to the critical nature of tissue oxygen consumption in the body, it is essential to be able to monitor current oxygen saturation. A pulse oximeter is used to measure the oxygen saturation[13] (Figure 3.8).

- A low oxygen level is a warning sign for the management of COVID-19.
- If the patient has signs of COVID-19 or has been close to someone who has it, a pulse oximeter may help in detecting oxygen levels. But this is not the only way to know how sick someone is.
- Pulse oximetry results may not be as accurate for people with skin pigmentation.
- Their levels according to the oximeter can be higher than they really are.[13, 14]
- Oxygen levels measured by a pulse oximeter can be normal even if the patient complains of shortness of breath or is breathing faster than usual or feels too sick to do their usual daily activities.[13–15]

Ventilators

Invasive Ventilators

These are patient ventilators for intensive care units and patient ventilators for transport/mass-casualty care.

Non-Invasive Ventilators

- Continuous positive airway pressure (CPAP).
- Bi-level positive airway pressure (BPAP).
- High-flow nasal cannula (HFNC).
- High-flow nasal oxygen (HFNO).

Spirometry

Spirometry is used to measure basic lung function. It is a non-invasive technique and helpful in diagnosing obstructive and restrictive lung diseases (Figure 3.9).

Procedure

- Before performing the forced expiration, the patient should be comfortable, sit calmly in a normal position and then take a deep breath followed by quick, full inspiration.
- Alternatively, a deep breath can be taken in, then the mouth placed tightly around the mouthpiece before a full expiration is performed.
- The patient can be asked to completely empty their lungs, then take in a quick full inspiration, followed by a full expiration.

Indications

Obstructive and restrictive lung diseases.

Contraindications

- Hemoptysis of unknown origin.
- Pneumothorax.
- Unstable cardiovascular status, recent myocardial infarction, or pulmonary embolism.
- Thoracic, abdominal, or cerebral aneurysms.
- Acute disorders affecting test performance, such as nausea or vomiting.
- Recent thoracic or abdominal surgical procedures.[16]

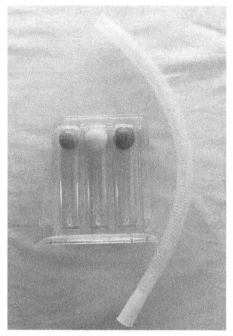

FIGURE 3.9   Spirometry.

EMERGENCY DEPARTMENT

Defibrillator

An automated external defibrillator (AED) is a portable type of defibrillator that automatically diagnoses the ventricular fibrillation in a patient and generates an electrical shock to the affected heart (fibrillated heart or other shockable rhythm). This helps in increasing the force of contraction of the heart to produce a more normal cardiac rhythm. There are semi-automated and fully automated defibrillators. AED improves both the survival rate and quality of life of the patient after discharge. It reduces the burden of Out of Hospital Cardiac Arrest (OHCA).[16]

Principle

Energy is generated at a slow rate from an AC line and stored in the capacitor.

Stored energy in the capacitor is then delivered at a rapid rate to the chest of the patient through the patient's own resistance.

Efficacy of AED

The working of AED depends on trans-thoracic resistance like:

- Chest width and configuration.
- Phases of ventilation.
- Skin and electrode interaction.
- Position and size of the electrodes.
- Force of electrode application.
- Rate of energy supply.
- Time interval between the shocks.

Indications

- Atrial flutter and atrial fibrillation.
- Re-entry supra ventricular tachycardia (SVT).
- Monomorphic and polymorphic ventricular tachycardia (VT).

Contraindications

- Digitalis-induced dysrhythmias.
- Junctional tachycardia or ectopics or multilocal atrial tachycardia.

Advantages

- Used in emergencies, such as a patient with sudden cardiac arrest.
- Speed of operation – the first shock can be delivered within 1 minute of patient arrival.
- Safe and easy to use.
- Recommended by current resuscitation guidelines.

Disadvantages

- Untrained people cannot use this.
- Difficult to synchronize with CPR.
- Longer times until shock delivery.
- No possibility to override the device.
- Risk of electrocution for the rescuer if inappropriately used.[16,17]

ENTERAL DEVICES

These are used to deliver medicine or liquid nutrients to the stomach or intestines in patients who are unable to eat or drink by mouth or need supplemental nutrition. Feeding tubes are inserted into the

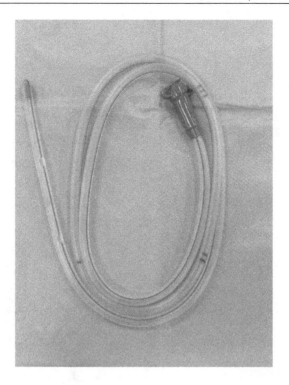

FIGURE 3.10 Ryle's tube.

patient's abdomen. Some use pre-packaged food purchased from nutrition manufacturers or blend their own diets at home. New standards have been framed for the misconnection issue and to reduce the risk of misconnections between enteral and non-enteral devices[3] (Figure 3.10).

INTRAVASCULAR OR HYPODERMIC DEVICES

Intravascular or hypodermic devices, such as arterial or intravenous (IV) lines, are generally used to deliver medications or fluids through a patient's neck, chest, or veins in the arm[3] (Figure 3.11).

NEURAXIAL DEVICES

Neuraxial devices, such as epidural catheters, are used to deliver medicines or anesthesia to neuraxial sites, such as the epidural space, or are used to monitor or remove cerebral-spinal fluid for therapeutic or diagnostic purposes.[3]

LIMB TOURNIQUET CUFFS

Limb tourniquet cuffs are compression devices used to apply pressure, such as to the radial artery, to help stop bleeding after a procedure.[3]

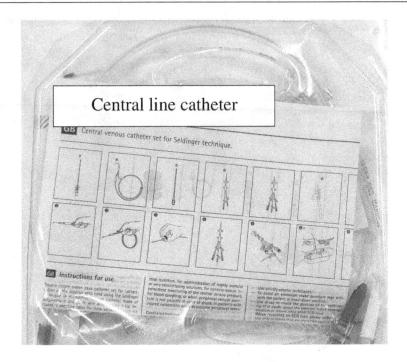

FIGURE 3.11   Central line catheter.

MEDICAL DEVICE DATA SYSTEMS

Medical device data systems (MDDS) are hardware or software products intended to transfer, store, convert formats, and display medical device data and do not modify the data or modify the display of the data. They may or may not be intended for active patient monitoring.[3]

HOSPITAL SETUP

Hospital Beds

- A hospital bed system includes the head end and food end with bed side rails and mattress cover.
- Hospital beds are classified as Class I and Class II devices and are used for patients in acute care, long-term care, or home care settings[3] (Figure 3.12).

Hospital Bed Mattress Cover

- The Centers for Disease Control and Prevention (CDC) have developed an inspection plan to inspect and remove and replace damaged, worn, or stained mattresses.
- If the damaged mattress is not replaced it allows the passage of infectious fluids into the bed.
- A patient who comes in contact with those contaminated covers will have an increased chance of getting an infection.
- Undamaged hospital bed mattress covers should be clean and disinfected according to the manufacturer's guidelines.[3]

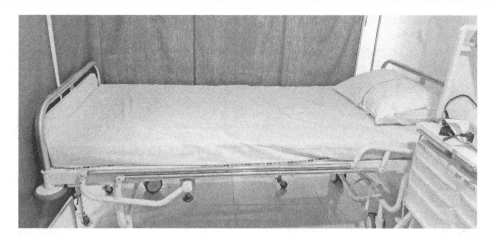

FIGURE 3.12   Hospital bed.

Patient Lifts

- Patient lifts are designed to lift and transfer patients (Figure 3.13) from one place to another (e.g., from bed to bath, chair to stretcher), not to be confused with stairway chair lifts or elevators.
- They may be operated using a power source or manually.
- When properly used they can reduce the risk of injury to patients and caregivers.

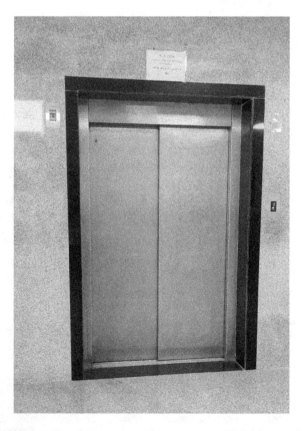

FIGURE 3.13   Patient's lift.

- However, improper use of patient lifts can pose significant public health risks including head traumas, fractures, and deaths.
- In several states, safe patient handling laws have been passed to make use of the patient lifts.
- It is expected that the use of patient lifts will increase because of these laws and the clinical community's goal of reducing patient and caregiver injury during patient transfer.[3]

HOSPITAL DEVICES AND COVID-19

- During the COVID-19 pandemic, the FDA issued the Enforcement Policy for Telethermographic Systems in the Public Health Emergency guidance to help expand the availability of thermal imaging systems and mitigate thermometer shortages.[3]
- COVID-19 can be spread by presymptomatic and asymptomatic individuals, and universal face masking has been recommended worldwide.[18]
- Temperature-based screening does not effectively determine if someone definitively has COVID-19 because a person with COVID-19 may not have a fever. It is not accurate when used for multiple people at the same time, and the accuracy depends on careful setup and operation, as well as proper preparation of the person being evaluated.[3]
- PPE can reduce the risk by covering exposed parts, but health care workers should train in donning and doffing the kit.[4]
- Globally, there is a shortage of devices like ventilators, and many companies have volunteered to develop emergency devices.[10]

CONCLUSION

These medical devices are used widely in the health care setting, and these devices represent a potential vector for various micro-organisms.[1] Some studies show that hospital devices can also act as a vector for bacterial colonization and potential risk factors for disease transmission.[1] Thus, infection control should not only focus on hand hygiene but also give equal attention to handheld devices that come into close proximity to patients. We should conduct more awareness and training programs for the usage of some medical devices by normal people in the community. Additional studies are necessary to determine the safety risks to patients and identify best practices and infection control policies as this technology expands in the health care system.[1]

References

1. Khan A, Rao A, Reyes-Sacin C, Hayakawa K, Szpunar S, Riederer K, Kaye K, Fishbain JT, Levine D. Use of portable electronic devices in a hospital setting and their potential for bacterial colonization. *Am J Infect Control*. 2015 Mar 1;43(3):286–8. doi: 10.1016/j.ajic.2014.11.013. Epub 2015 Jan 1. PMID: 25557772.
2. Health C for D and R. General hospital devices and supplies [Internet]. *FDA*. FDA; 2021 [cited 2021 Jun 30]. Available from: https://www.fda.gov/medical-devices/products-and-medical-procedures/general-hospital-devices-and-supplies
3. Wei Y, Yu H, Geng J, Wu B, Guo Z, He L, et al. Hospital efficiency and utilization of high-technology medical equipment: A panel data analysis. *Health Policy Technol*. 2018 Mar 1;7(1):65–72.
4. Verbeek JH, Ijaz S, Mischke C, Ruotsalainen JH, Mäkelä E, Neuvonen K, Edmond MB, Sauni R, Kilinc Balci FS, Mihalache RC. Personal protective equipment for preventing highly infectious diseases due to exposure to contaminated body fluids in healthcare staff. *Cochrane Database Syst Rev*. 2016 Apr 19;4:CD011621.

5. Cook TM. Personal protective equipment during the coronavirus disease (COVID) 2019 pandemic: A narrative review. *Anaesthesia*. 2020 Jul;75(7):920–7.
6. Shintani H. Ethylene oxide gas sterilization of medical devices. *Biocontrol Sci*. 2017;22(1):1–16.
7. Rutala WA, Weber DJ. Disinfection and sterilization: An overview. *Am J Infect Control*. 2013 May 1;41(5) Supplement:S2–5.
8. *Non-Contact Thermometers for Detecting Fever: A Review of Clinical Effectiveness* [Internet]. Ottawa (ON): Canadian Agency for Drugs and Technologies in Health; 2014 Nov 20.
9. Peycke LE. Facilitation of soft tissue surgery: Surgical staplers and vessel sealing devices. *Vet Clin North Am Small Anim Pract*. 2015 May;45(3):451–61.
10. Hoffman L, Bacon O. *Infusion Pumps Making Healthcare Safer III: A Critical Analysis of Existing and Emerging Patient Safety Practices* [Internet]. Rockville, MD: Agency for Healthcare Researcher and Quality. 2020 March.
11. Rajkomar A, Blandford A. Understanding infusion administration in the ICU through Distributed Cognition. *J Biomed Inf*. 2020 June;45(3):580–90.
12. Williams JS, Brown SM, Conlin PR. Videos in clinical medicine. Blood-pressure measurement. *N Engl J Med*. 2009 Jan 29;360(5):6.
13. Hafen B, Sharma S. *Oxygen Saturation*. StatPearls [Internet]. 2021 May 7 [cited 2021 Jun 25]; Available from: https://www.statpearls.com/ArticleLibrary/viewarticle/26491
14. Health C for D and R. *Pulse Oximeter Accuracy and Limitations: FDA Safety Communication*. FDA [Internet]. 2021 Feb 19 [cited 2021 Jun 26]; Available from: https://www.fda.gov/medical-devices/safety-communications/pulse-oximeter-accuracy-and-limitations-fda-safety-communication
15. Pons-Odena M, Valls A, Grifols J, Farre R, Cambra Lasosa FJ, Rubin BK. COVID-19 and respiratory support devices. *Paediatr Respir Rev*. 2020 Sep;35:61–3.
16. M.V.C. Spirometry: Step by step. *ERS J*. 2012;8:232–40.
17. Delhommea C, Njeime M, Varlet E, Pechmajoua L, Benameur N, Cassani P, Derkennej C, Jostj D, Lamhaut L, Marijona E, Jouvena Xavier, Karama Nicole. Automated external defibrillator use in out-of-hospital cardiac arrest: Current limitations and solutions. *Arch Cardiovasc Dis*. 2019;112:217–22.
18. Ju JTJ, Boisvert LN, Zuo YY. Face masks against COVID-19: Standards, efficacy, testing and decontamination methods. *Adv Colloid Interface Sci*. 2021 Jun;292:102435.

Home Health and Consumer Devices

4

Sree Sudha T Y, Hemasri Velmurugan,
K. S. B. S. Krishna Sasanka, T. Y. Sri Hari,
Yakaiah Vangoori, and Pugazhenthan Thangaraju

HOME DEVICES

Blood Glucose Meters

Glucometers (glucose meters) are medical devices employed universally for approximately estimating the blood glucose concentration; they are utilized in the management of hyperglycemic (diabetes) and hypoglycemic disorders. Testing blood sugar accurately helps in planning lifestyle changes if needed to lower the risk of blindness, neuropathies and kidney diseases associated with diabetes.

Principle of Blood Glucose Detection

The two key elements of a glucometer are an enzyme essential for reaction and a detector. The enzymatic part is packaged in a desiccated form on a disposable strip or reaction cuvette. The patient's sample contains glucose which can react with the enzymes, and the resultant product is identified by the detector. Hydrogen peroxide or an intermediate product may be produced in some devices that the coloring dye binds to causing a color change depending on the glucose concentration in the sample, whereas in other glucose meters, the biosensor-linked enzymes cause electron release that is detected by the meter. The three enzyme-linked principles of blood glucose meters are glucose oxidase, glucose dehydrogenase, and hexokinase; each of these methods has advantages and disadvantages (Figure 4.1).

Steps to Follow in Monitoring Blood Glucose

Though these devices are simple to operate, flaws may creep in if proper caution is not maintained. To get the most accurate results, follow the below tips while using a blood glucose meter.

DOI: 10.1201/9781003220671-4

- Carefully read the instructions on the packaging to confirm if the strips will work with that particular device.
- If the blood dropped on the test strip is insufficient, the glucose meter may not give an accurate reading. So, use adequate blood drop size. Repeat the test if in doubt.
- Do not squeeze the finger selected for collecting blood.
- Always use a complete test strip every time.

These devices are generally reliable and help to manage diabetes, but they are not error free, unlike the accurate technology that is used in an established lab in a hospital or clinic. A glucometer may give an erroneous reading due to dehydration, shock, elevated hematocrit value, etc. Incorrect readings are also seen in cases of precariously low blood glucose. Even if the meter reads normal blood sugar values, if the patient feels uneasy and suspects high or low sugars, it is always better to get clinical care and treatment under a qualified doctor.

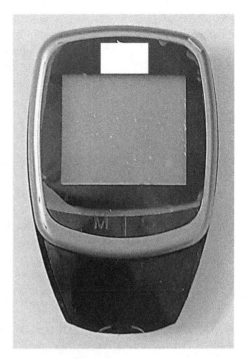

FIGURE 4.1 Glucometer.

Hemopiezometer

Blood pressure (BP) is the most essential cardiopulmonary metric, which measures the pressure imposed by blood against the artery wall. When the heart contracts (systole) and relaxes (diastole), BP gives indirect information about blood flow and can also represent cellular oxygen delivery.

The most common cause of cardiovascular disease that may be avoided is hypertension. Home blood pressure monitoring (HBPM) is a self-monitoring technology that is suggested by major guidelines and can be added into the management of hypertensive patients. Research supports the advantages of patient HBPM over office-based monitoring, including improved blood pressure control, white-coat hypertension diagnosis, and cardiovascular risk assessment. Furthermore, HBPM is less expensive and less time consuming than 24-hour ambulatory blood pressure monitoring (ABPM). However, all HBPM devices must be validated, as a large percentage of monitors provide false alarms. A longer inflatable region within the cuff wraps all the way around the arm with new technology, widening the "acceptable range" of placement and thereby lowering the impact of cuff placement on reading accuracy, surpassing the limits of current systems.

Types of BP Monitoring Devices

Electronic Monitors for Self-Monitoring of Blood Pressure
The majority of home monitoring studies at the time used aneroid sphygmomanometers [1]. Automatic electronic devices, on the other hand, have become increasingly popular in recent years. An oscillometric device that measures pressure from the brachial artery is now the typical type of monitor for home use. These are easier to operate than devices that employ a Korotkoff sound microphone since cuff placement is not as crucial, and the oscillometric method has been found to be as reliable as the Korotkoff sound method in practice. Early versions were frequently inaccurate [2], but contemporary versions are frequently adequate [3–4].

Wrist Monitors [5]

Because the wrist diameter is unaffected by obesity, these monitors are smaller than arm devices and can be utilized by people with larger arm diameters. The systematic error produced by the hydrostatic impact of changes in the location of the wrist relative to the heart [6] is a possible concern with wrist monitors. This can be prevented if the wrist is always at heart level when the measurements are recorded; however there is no way to determine whether this was done subsequently when reviewing a series of readings. Wrist monitors offer potential, but further research is needed [7–8].

Finger Monitors

Despite their convenience, these monitors have been proven to be inaccurate and should not be used [9].

Ambulatory Monitors

Ambulatory blood pressure monitoring, which was first introduced about 40 years ago, is just now gaining acceptance as a clinically valuable tool. Patients wear ambulatory blood pressure monitoring (ABPM) devices for 24 hours with repeated measures, and they are regarded as the gold standard for blood pressure measurement [10]. Recent technological advancements have resulted in the advent of compact, modest monitors that can capture up to 100 blood pressure measurements over the course of 24 hours while patients go about their daily activities [11].

Advantages and Limitations of Home Blood Pressure Monitoring [12]

Advantages

1. Suitable for taking multiple readings over a longer period.
2. Prevents the white-coat reaction in blood pressure measurements.
3. Replicable and precise.
4. Predicts cardiovascular (CV) morbidity and mortality more accurately than office blood pressure.
5. Is able to distinguish between white-coat and disguised hypertension.
6. Enables individuals to gain a better understanding of how to manage their hypertension.
7. Telemonitoring allows healthcare practitioners to watch patients remotely.
8. Recognizes an increase in BP variability.

Limitations

1. Cuff location can influence accuracy.
2. Can cause anxiety and over-monitoring.
3. A few devices have been shown to be inappropriate.
4. Inadequate nocturnal tracking.
5. The risk of people changing their treatment plans based on haphazard home measures without consulting their doctors.

Hearing Aids

Hearing aids are sound-amplifying devices that help people with hearing loss.

Almost all hearing aids have

1. A microphone – that catches audio.
2. An amplifier – that makes the sound louder.
3. A speaker (receiver) – that transmits the enhanced sound into the ear canal.
4. Batteries – that run the electronic circuits (Figure 4.2).

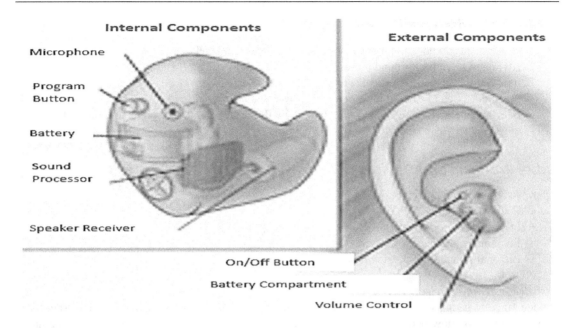

FIGURE 4.2 Hearing aid.

Different Models or Styles of Hearing Aids [13]

Behind-the-Ear (BTE) Type

This form is popular with young children since it supports a variety of earmold types; it has to be replaced as the child develops. The hearing aid parts are kept in a tiny plastic shell that sits behind the ear, with the support of a transparent tube connecting it to an ear canal. The BTE hearing aids are durable and simple to clean and operate.

Mini BTE/on-the-Ear Type

This is a newer small aid which can be placed on the ear and also behind the ear as well. The mini aid is connected to the ear canal via an extremely thin, nearly undetectable tube. Mini BTEs improve comfort, reduce occlusion or "blocked up" sensations in the ear canal and solve cosmetic concerns.

In-the-Ear (ITE) Type

ITE type aids fit over the ear's outer portion. The ITE aids are bigger than in-the-canal and completely-in-the-canal devices and may be easy to handle.

In-the-Canal (ITC) and Completely-in-the-Canal (CIC) Type

These are the tiniest hearing aids, with both cosmetic and hearing benefits. Because of their small size people face difficulty using and handling them.

Advantages of Hearing Aids

1. Able to hear sounds that were previously too quiet to hear.
2. Able to hear voice clearly over the phone.
3. Able to communicate even in noisy environments.

Limitations with Hearing Aids

1. Hearing aids do not completely restore hearing to normal levels.
2. All noises, even background noise, are amplified with hearing aids.
3. It takes time, sometimes months, to adjust hearing clarity.
4. Small noises can be heard in resound while wearing hearing aids.
5. Hearing aids with more advanced technology will require you to learn how to modify the settings, and they can be costly.

Other Products and Devices to Improve Hearing

- Assistive listening devices
- Cochlear implants
- Implantable middle ear hearing devices
- Bone-anchored hearing aids
- Personal sound amplification products

Assistive Listening Devices

A wide range of gadgets known as assistive listening devices (ALDs) or assistive listening systems has been developed to allow people to hear noises in everyday situations. Public places like meeting halls, auditoriums, movie theatres and houses of worship have ALDs. They help in promoting sound clarity for normal hearing people as well as those with hearing loss. With the ALDs, one can clearly hear sound at a distance.

Cochlear Implants

A cochlear implant is a surgically implanted electrical device that stimulates nerves in the inner ear to provide usable auditory perceptions. Cochlear implants include two components:

a. External component: an externally worn microphone, sound processor and transmitter system.
b. Internal component: a receiver and an electrode system, which contains the electronic circuits that receive signals from the external system and transmit electrical impulses to the inner ear (Figure 4.3).

Implantable Middle Ear Hearing Devices (IMEHD)

These devices are helpful in sensorineural hearing loss patients. IMEHDs transmit sounds to the inner ear. These are tiny devices which will be attached to the middle ear's small bones. When sound waves

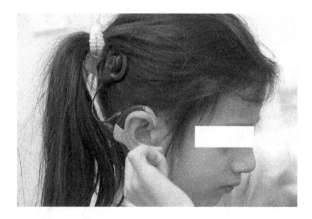

FIGURE 4.3   Cochlear implant.

start, IMEHD begins to vibrate and move along the middle ear cavity. This forms vibrations in the inner ear allowing the sound to be identified.

Bone-Anchored Hearing Aids (BAHA)

BAHAs are similar to cochlear implants, consist of both external and internal components and also work by the same mechanism. These devices are suggested for people with middle ear disease or with hearing impairment unilaterally.

Personal Sound Amplification Products (PSAPs)

PSAPs enhance distant sound in high clarity. These are primarily used to listen to sounds clearly for non-hearing-impaired consumers but are not used as hearing aids.

Contact Lenses

For people who require vision correction, contact lenses are the preferred option. Contact lenses provide ease and convenience for many people. There are a wide range of lenses designed to match a wide range of needs and interests. Myopia (near-sightedness), hyperopia (farsightedness), astigmatism and presbyopia are all vision abnormalities that can be corrected with contact lenses (Figure 4.4).

Types of Contact Lenses [14]

    1) Soft contact lenses
    2) Rigid gas permeable (RGP) contact lenses
    3) Extended wear contact lenses
    4) Disposable (replacement schedule) contact lenses
    5) Specialized uses of contact lenses
        a)   Orthokeratology (Ortho-K)
        b)   Decorative (plano) contact lenses

Soft Contact Lenses

Soft contact lenses are comprised of flexible, soft polymers that let oxygen pass through to the cornea. Soft contact lenses are more comfortable and simpler to adjust to than hard gas permeable lenses. Silicone-hydrogels are used in newer soft lens materials to deliver more oxygen to your eyes while you wear your lenses.

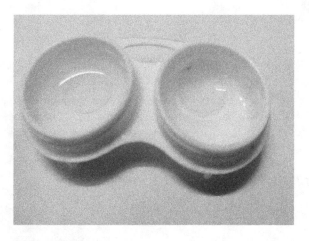

FIGURE 4.4   Contact lenses.

Rigid Gas Permeable (RGP) Contact Lenses

Rigid gas permeable contact lenses (RGPs) are more durable and less likely to accumulate deposits, and they provide finer vision. Because they last longer than soft contact lenses, they tend to be less expensive over time. They are less likely to tear and are easy to handle. However, they are not as pleasant as soft contacts at first, and it may take a few weeks to become used to wearing RGPs instead of a few days.

Extended Wear Contact Lenses

Prolonged use contact lenses can be worn overnight or continuously for 1 to 6 nights or up to 30 days. Soft contact lenses are typically used for extended wear. They're made of flexible polymers that let oxygen reach the cornea. Only a few RGP lenses are designed and authorized for night-time use.

Disposable (Replacement Schedule) Contact Lenses

The term "disposable" refers to something that is only utilized once and then discarded. A whole new pair of lenses is utilized every day with a true daily wear disposable schedule.

Specialized Uses of Contact Lenses

Traditional contact lenses work in the same manner as glasses do, but they are in direct contact with the eye. Orthokeratology lenses and decorative lenses are two types of lenses that serve various purposes.

Orthokeratology (Ortho-K)   Ortho-K is a lens fitting process that involves changing the curvature of the cornea with specially designed RGP contact lenses to momentarily enhance the eye's ability to focus on things. This treatment is most commonly used to address myopia (near-sightedness). The most frequent form of Ortho-K lenses is overnight Ortho-K. Some Ortho-K lenses are only recommended for use during the day. Ortho-K lenses are usually suggested to be used for at least eight hours every night during sleeping. They are taken off when you wake up and are therefore not used during the day. The effects of vision correction are only temporary. The corneas will return to their original shape once Ortho-K is stopped, which will cause the eye's nearsightedness to disappear. To preserve the therapy effect, Ortho-K lenses must be worn every night or on some other approved maintenance plan.

Decorative Contact Lenses   These are used for Halloween or to imitate a favorite film star or artist.
Other names for decorative contact lenses:

- Halloween contact lenses
- Fashion contact lenses
- Colored contact lenses
- Cosmetic contact lenses
- Theatre contact lenses

The appearance of your eyes can be altered using decorative contact lenses. They might not be able to correct your vision. For Halloween, they can temporarily convert your brown eyes to blue or make them look like cat or monster eyes.

Complications of Decorative Contact Lenses

- Corneal abrasion
- Itching
- Redness

- Pain in the eye
- Watering of eyes
- Reduced vision
- Foreign body infection
- Loss of vision

Precautions to Be Taken While Wearing Contact Lenses

- Before handling contact lenses, always wash your hands to avoid the risk of infection.
- If your eyes become red, inflamed or your vision changes, remove the lenses right away.
- For proper contact lens and lens care product use, always follow your eye care professional's instructions as well as all labeling instructions.
- Do not use expired or discarded contact lens solutions.
- Rinse only with sterile saline solutions.
- Follow all labeling instructions provided with your lens care products while cleaning and disinfecting lenses.
- After each use, throw away any remaining contact lens solution. Lens solution should never be reused.
- Avoid putting your contact lenses in any type of water, including tap, bottled, distilled, lake or ocean water. Use only sterilized water. Acanthamoeba keratitis, a corneal infection that is resistant to treatment and cure, has been linked to contact lens exposure to water.
- Change your contact lens storage case every three months or as directed by the manufacturer.

Hydrogen Peroxide Solution

By splitting up and eliminating accumulated debris, protein and fatty deposits, hydrogen peroxide and multipurpose solutions clean and disinfect contact lenses (lipids). Hydrogen peroxide solutions, unlike multipurpose solutions, are preservative-free, making them a good choice for people who are allergic to or sensitive to the preservatives included in multipurpose solutions. They are not without risk.

Breast Pumps

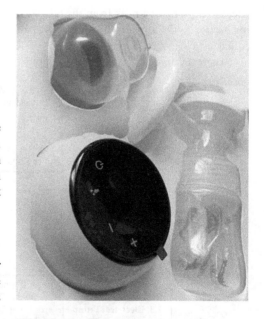

1) Indications and uses of breast pumps
2) Types of breast pump
3) Parts of breast pumps
4) Pumping types

A breast pump is a mechanical device that mothers use to extract milk from their breasts while breastfeeding. When a mother is unable to nurse her infant directly from the breast for any reason, this device is employed. Even if a mother intends to solely breastfeed her child, a breast pump is a highly useful tool (Figure 4.5).

Indications and Uses of Breast Pumps

1.1. To assist working women in solely feeding their babies breast milk. The woman can use a device to pump and store her milk. While the mother is at work, a caretaker can feed the baby that milk.

FIGURE 4.5 Breast pump.

1.2.   To avoid formula feeding at all costs. A breast pump allows a mother to exclusively feed her infant breast milk. If the mother and the infant are unable to be together at all times during the feeding, pumping can help to eliminate the need for formula.

1.3.   To maintain milk production by stimulating the breasts. A negative signal is given to the body to decrease or cease milk production if the infant does not suckle or milk is not withdrawn from the breast on a regular basis. Pumping ensures that milk does not build up in the breast and that the body produces enough milk.

1.4.   To nurse an ill or preterm baby. Pumped breast milk can be given to a premature or unwell baby who is unable to suck effectively.

1.5.   To prevent breast engorgement pain. The mother is relieved of discomfort as a result of this. The milk can then be fed to the baby at a later time.

1.6.   Pumping draws out flat or inverted nipples? Latching to flat or inverted nipples might be difficult for a baby.

1.7.   To make sure you have enough backup or extra supplies. The mother may become ill and have to take medication or the mother's health can be harmed by difficult delivery or surgery, as well as a demanding feeding schedule. Instead of feeding the infant during the mother's very dangerous situation, she can pump and keep appropriate supplement.

1.9.   To breastfeed while weaning the baby off the mother's milk. When the mother wants to wean the infant off the breast, breastfeeding can be used as a supplement or add-on feed.

1.10.   Gives mothers room to breathe. An infant is fed every two to three hours. By pumping and allowing someone else to look after the baby, the mother can relax for a short period of time.

1.11.   To provide breast milk to a large number of infants. When a mother has twins or many kids, extracting breast milk and feeding it to all of them is a better option than nursing them all the time.

1.12.   To allow the parent and kid to form a bond. Feeding the kid expressed milk allows other family members, particularly the father, to form a special bond with the child.

1.13.   It's possible that some women produce significantly more milk than their newborns require. Such moms may choose to give their excess milk to milk banks, which will be used to nourish babies whose mothers are unable to provide them with their own milk.

Types of Breast Pumps [15]

Breast pumps extract milk from the breasts by creating a seal around the nipple and applying and releasing suction to the nipple, which expresses milk from the breast. Each suction and release combination is called a cycle.

There are three types of breast pumps.

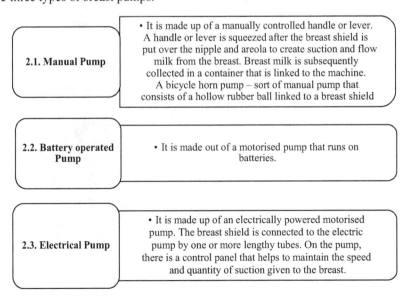

2.1. Manual Pump
• It is made up of a manually controlled handle or lever. A handle or lever is squeezed after the breast shield is put over the nipple and areola to create suction and flow milk from the breast. Breast milk is subsequently collected in a container that is linked to the machine. A bicycle horn pump – sort of manual pump that consists of a hollow rubber ball linked to a breast shield

2.2. Battery operated Pump
• It is made out of a motorised pump that runs on batteries.

2.3. Electrical Pump
• It is made up of an electrically powered motorised pump. The breast shield is connected to the electric pump by one or more lengthy tubes. On the pump, there is a control panel that helps to maintain the speed and quantity of suction given to the breast.

Two types of electrical pumps are known.

Electric Breast Pump of Hospital Quality
This is commonly utilized in hospitals and can be used by several ladies at the same time. It's the most effective, simple and quick type of pump available. It's a dual pump, which means it can empty both breasts at once. It can, however, be used to drain a single breast at a time. Using this pump, emptying both breasts takes approximately 10–15 minutes.

Electric Pump for Individual Use
This is only for one person's use. It's a bit slimmer. Working women or travelers will find it more practical and convenient to use. When compared to a hospital-grade pump, however, it is less efficient.

All Breast Pumps Consist of a Few Basic Parts

A seal is formed around the nipple by the breast shield. Using the pump to apply and release suction on the nipple expresses milk from the breast. A cycle is the term coined for each suction and release combination. The expressed milk is collected and kept in a separable jar.

1. **Breast shield**: a circular region enclosing the nipple and a cone-shaped cup that fits over it (the areola).
2. **Pump**: provides a mild vacuum that allows milk to be expressed. The breast shield may be attached to the pump, or the pump may be connected to the breast shield with plastic tubing.
3. **Milk container**: a removable container that sits beneath the breast shield and accumulates milk when it is pumped. The container is usually a reusable bottle or a disposable bag that can be used to store milk or to feed a baby when attached to a nipple.

Pumping Types

There are two different pumping types: single and double.

1. **Single-breast pumping**: milk is extracted from one breast at a time. Single-breast pumps make up the majority of manual breast pumps. Single-pump battery-powered pumps are the most common.
2. **Double-pumping type**: can extract milk from both breasts at once. To stimulate both nipples at the same time, a separate breast shield can be mounted to each breast. Some electric pumps have two motors.

Thermometers

The measurement of human body temperature is of remarkable significance in medicine, especially in the treatment of fever. Normally, the temperature of the human body is found to be about 37 degrees Celsius (°C) or 98.6 degrees Fahrenheit (°F) but with diurnal variations such as a lower temperature in the morning, eventually increasing with the passing of the day, with the highest during late afternoon or evening time. In human adults, a temperature of 100.4°F (38°C) or above is considered a "fever".

Integral tools for measuring body temperature are thermometers, probes or non-contact devices. Some forms contain mercury and generally, the newer ones are mercury free. A typical thermometer consists of two primary components: the temperature sensor and the numerical reading to make the temperature measurement visible in numerical value.

Types of Thermometer

- **Contact thermometers**
- **Digital thermometer**

Using a digital thermometer, body temperature can be noted in a simple, quick and accurate way. Contact thermometers can be placed in various body parts:

- **Oral**: the thermometer is kept under the tongue and is advised only for adults and children above four years who can cooperate to hold the device in the mouth for a while.
- **Axillary**: here, the thermometer is rested in the armpit for adults and young children in whom oral placement of the thermometer isn't feasible. This is not as accurate as oral or rectal measurement, yet it helps as a rapid first check (Figure 4.6).
- **Rectal**: in this method, the thermometer is inserted into the rectum gently, and it is often preferred in infants and small children, probably up to three years of age. This is the most accurate way to measure body temperature [16].
- A non-contact thermometer is a way to record a person's temperature without touching them.
- **Tympanic (ear) thermometer**: this measures the temperature inside of the ear by reading the internal infrared heat. It has a low cost but is not recommended in babies younger than three months. It should not be used if the person has an ear ache or excessive earwax.
- **Temporal (Forehead) thermometer**: "infrared (IR) guns" are non-invasive thermometers for fever screening, placed on the temporal artery of the forehead; they measure the invisible infra-red heat emitted from the head above absolute zero, and the energy is converted to an electrical signal which after processing will be displayed in the appropriate units.

    IR thermometers are usually more expensive and their recordings may not be as reliable as digital thermometers. New studies during the COVID pandemic show that the non-touch thermometers miss 80% of fever cases; hence they may not be the most accurate device for fever mass screening during a pandemic.
- **Pacifier thermometer**: if a baby uses a pacifier, this type of temperature measurement may be an easy way to record an approximate temperature. The ease of use is the biggest benefit of the pacifier thermometer; the drawback is that it must be kept in the mouth, without moving, for about six minutes to provide an approximate temperature, probably close to an exact reading.
- **Mercury (liquid in glass) thermometer**: once upon a time, mercury thermometers were the only option available for taking temperature. They are no longer widely available due to safety issues and may even be illegal in some parts of the world. The advantages of mercury thermometers are that they provide accurate temperature readings; they do not require batteries and can be used orally, rectally or under the arm. Their main drawback is the glass body which can break easily, allowing toxic mercury to escape, and they can cause cuts or glass splinters if broken. Proper disposal must be ensured, meaning they cannot be thrown into the trash, as they contain a hazardous substance. Mercury thermometers must be kept steady for at least three minutes, and they can be hard to read for some people (Figure 4.7).
- **Phase-Change or Dot Matrix Thermometers (Liquid Crystal, Chemical)**
    Disposable single-phase thermometers are plastic strips, in which the recesses are stamped at the same intervals. In each of them there is a mixture of substances that change color depending on the temperature.
- **Telethermographic system or thermal scanner** cameras can measure temperature from a reasonable distance. They are not used as a primary diagnostic tool, yet for screening multiple

individuals in an uncontrolled environment, such as an airport, they are quite handy [17,18]. Results may not be as accurate as non-contact infrared thermometers (NCITs), and they may be more difficult to use effectively.

Syringes

Syringes are devices used to inject medication into the body or aspirate body fluids. The word "syringe" comes from the Greek syrinx, which means tube. There are three common types of syringe tips: Slip-Tip, Luer-Lok and eccentric. Slip-Tips allow the needle to be held on the syringe by friction. The needle is reasonably secure, but it may come off if not properly attached or if considerable pressure is used. Luer-Lok tips incorporate a collar with grooves that lock the needle in place and allow the removal and reattachment of the needle. Eccentric tips, which are off-center, are used when the needle must be parallel to the plane of injection such as in an intradermal injection.

Syringes come in different sizes ranging from 1 to 60 mL. As a rule, select a syringe whose capacity is the next size larger than the volume to be measured (Figure 4.8).

Plastic syringes are cheap, disposable and sterile. The major drawback is that the syringe plungers and barrels are malleable under pressure leading to inaccurate injection volumes. Glass syringes are reusable, compatible with most applications, more accurate, but costly, and they can be used for syringe pumps [19]. Stainless steel syringes are the most durable syringe, used for high-pressure dosing applications that

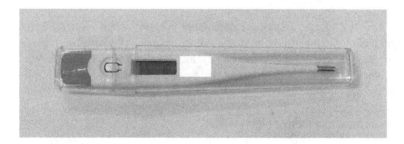

FIGURE 4.6 Digital thermometer.

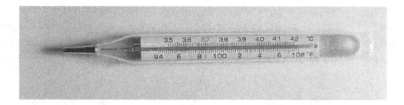

FIGURE 4.7 Mercury thermometer.

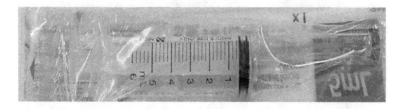

FIGURE 4.8 Syringe with needle.

would cause a glass or plastic syringe to burst. Their dosing accuracy is the same as glass syringes, and they are expensive. Typically they do not come in sizes much smaller than 5 mL, thus minimizing their application for smaller scale use. Relatively, these are not as user friendly as other syringes because they are not transparent, making loading and removing air bubbles more challenging.

The new loss-of-resistance (LOR) syringe is spring-loaded with Luer slip and Luer-Lok configurations which works with a pressure guided or LOR technique. Automatic LOR syringes are routinely used for the quick, reliable identification of epidural space. They have an internal compression spring that applies constant pressure on the plunger, allowing the operator to use both hands while continuously advancing the epidural needle. The syringe plunger has a locking system (safely locking trippets) to ensure the injection of the exact amount of fluids at four different levels and automatically depresses when the needle enters epidural space, providing an objective, visual confirmation of LOR.

Automatic Retractable Needle Safety Syringes

Automatic retractable needle safety syringes are easy to use, require no additional steps, and allow for single-handed activation. After activation, they require less disposal space than most other safety needles/syringes and prevent disposal-related needle stick injuries. The needle is automatically retracted directly from the patient into the barrel of the syringe when the plunger handle is fully depressed. The pre-removal, automated retraction virtually eliminates exposure to the contaminated needle, effectively reducing the risk of needle stick injury.

AutoInjectors
Autoinjector devices (AIDs) are single-use, disposable syringes filled with fluid medication that are designed for rapid and painless self-administration of drugs and antidotes [20]. It can also be used even by medically untrained personnel for any emergency and mass casualty management without any hesitation. An AID has a drug cartridge with an embedded needle for subcutaneous or intramuscular injection. Examples of AID use are atropine and pralidoxime for nerve agent poisoning, epinephrine for anaphylactic shock and allergy, insulin pens, diazepam for seizures, sumatriptan for migraine, buprenorphine for pain relief and monoclonal antibodies (Figure 4.9).

Infusion Sets
An intravenous (IV) infusion set is a tubing system with a needle that is used for delivering or infusing drugs and nutrients from the infusion bag/bottle into the vein of the patient. Since the medication is directly infused into the circulatory system, it is the fastest mode of drug delivery. The IV set operates on the action of gravity. When the infusion bag is fixed at a higher position compared to the patient level, the gravitational force pulls down the fluid and the fluid flows into the veins of the patients. The rate of flow of fluids is controlled with the help of the roller clamp and must be checked from time to time. The mode

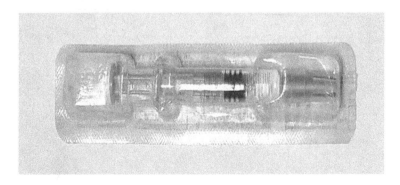

FIGURE 4.9   Pre-filled syringe.

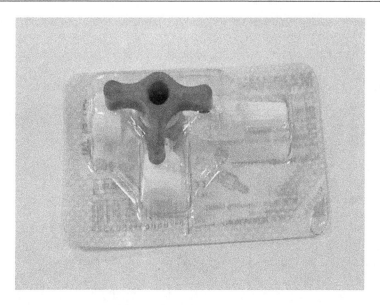

FIGURE 4.10   Connection set.

of infusion can be bolus, drip or extended infusion. Multiple drugs can be administered through the injection site of the IV set. The disadvantages are pain at the site and chances of extravasation or infiltration.

- **Connection needles/sets**: Needles that connect to a tube used to transfer fluids in and out of the body. This is generally used for patients on home hemodialysis (Figure 4.10).

Precautions While Handling and Disposing of Sharps

- Follow hand hygiene.
- Prefer a syringe with a safety shield.
- Recap the needles.
- After use, all sharps should be immediately placed in a sharps disposal container.
- Used needles and other sharps must be disposed of safely because they can injure people and spread common infections like hepatitis B or C (HCV) and human immunodeficiency virus (HIV).
- In case of an accidental needle or sharp stick injury, right away wash the exposed area thoroughly with water and soap or use an antiseptic such as rubbing alcohol or hand sanitizer.

Nebulizer

A nebulizer is a type of medical electronic instrument that converts liquid medication into a fine spray or mist (aerosol) so that it can be inhaled, and the drug reaches the lungs easily when a nebulizer is used for 5–15 minutes. They can also prevent or slow the accumulation of phlegm and mucus. These breathing machines nebulize medications, both for the prevention and treatment of asthma [21]. Drugs administered via nebulizer are as follows:

- **Inhalational steroids** like fluticasone, budesonide, flunisolide, triamcinolone, etc., to combat inflammatory sequelae in respiratory disorders.

- **Bronchodilators** such as salbutamol, terbutaline, salmeterol and ipratropium to keep airways open.
- Others: acetyl cysteine, hypertonic saline solution to loosen up mucus, certain antibiotics.

Based on the size, compactness and portable nature, nebulizers can be either stationary (tabletop) or portable (mobile).

Types of Nebulizers

The three main types of nebulizers are as follows:

- **Jet nebulizers**: with the help of compressed gas in a compressor, fine particles of medication called aerosols are produced. These are less expensive.
- **Ultrasonic nebulizers**: these use high-frequency ultrasonic waves and vibrations to aerosolize the liquid medicament, and the particles formed are relatively larger than with a jet nebulizer. Being portable, compact and battery operated, these are the best for domestic purposes (for children as well as adults).
- **Mesh nebulizer**: liquid passes through a very fine vibrating mesh (membrane) to form the smallest monodisperse aerosol particles. This is the most expensive type and requires proper care, careful handling and thorough cleaning as the membrane is prone to getting blocked. The mesh can be replaced after some time (Figure 4.11).

Nebulizer vs. Inhaler

Inhalers and nebulizers deliver drugs directly into the lungs [22].

- A nebulizer is often preferred in young children due to its ease of use. It takes longer to deliver medicine: at least five or ten minutes. Nebulizers can be bulky, hard to carry around and expensive.
- Inhaler use necessitates training, but most people quickly learn to use it. It delivers an exact dose of medication. These are cheaper, produce lesser side effects than nebulizers and can be carried in a pocket or bag.

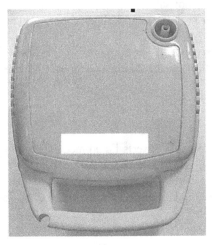
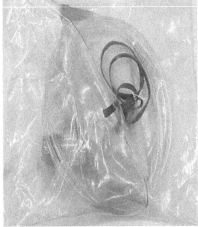

FIGURE 4.11   Nebulizer and mask.

Clinical Uses of Nebulizers

Nebulizers are useful in the management of exacerbations and long-term treatment of chronic obstructive pulmonary disease (COPD), bronchiectasis, cystic fibrosis and bronchial asthma and for symptomatic relief in palliative care [23]. Bronchial asthma and COPD can be treated with an inhaler to the same effectiveness as with a nebulizer. Conditions such as cystic fibrosis and bronchiectasis can be better treated with nebulizers.

Disadvantages of Nebulizers

Nebulized aerosol particles can carry bacteria and viruses deep into the lungs. The transmission of infection by droplet nuclei and aerosols can increase during nebulizer treatment due to the high concentration of aerosols.

CONSUMER DEVICES

Infusion Pumps

Definition

An infusion pump is a device that delivers a measured and controlled amount of fluids like nutrients or drugs into the circulatory system at a predetermined rate. They are suitable for intravenous, subcutaneous, enteral and epidural infusion [24]. They are designed to be portable or wearable.

Types of Infusion

See Table 4.1.

Types of Pumps

- Large volume pumps
- Small volume pumps

Application

- Dehydration.
- To replace blood or blood products.

TABLE 4.1 Types of Infusion

S. NO.	TYPES	DESCRIPTION
1.	Continuous infusion	It is designed for the continuous flow of fluid between 20 nanoliters and 100 microliters with programmed speed of infusion.
2.	Intermittent infusion	It is designed for the intermittent flow of fluid to keep the cannula open with programmed timing.
3.	Patient-controlled infusion	It is designed to stop the flow of fluid once it reaches the desired level to avoid toxicity.
4.	Total parental infusion	It provides nutrition required for daily meals.

- Chemotherapy for cancer patients.
- Pain management:
  - Acute conditions – epidural analgesia.
  - Chronic conditions – patient-controlled analgesia (PCA).
- Total parental nutrition.
- Anesthetic or sedation during surgery.
- To deliver insulin to patients with diabetes, anti-arithmetic drugs for cardiac patients and oxytocic agents for inducing labor.

Indications

- For the intravenous administration of a specific amount of a pharmacological agent into the bloodstream.
- Prevention of fluid overload.

Contraindications

- If a peripheral venous assessment is not possible, infected, injured, or burned extremities should be avoided.
- Extremities with renal shunts or fistulas.
- No absolute contraindications for pediatric cannulation.

Advantages

- Large capacity and wide range of flow rates.
- No need for repeated injections.
- Patient can remain ambulant.
- More precise and safe administration is achieved.
- For management of unexpected events [25].

Disadvantages

- Relatively expensive.
- Staff training and daily monitoring required.
- Allergic reaction at the infused area which will act as a source of transmission of secondary bacterial infection.
- Infusion site availability will be difficult in emaciated patients.
- Cannot give all the drugs in the medical field.
- Human error.
- Machine-made errors like false pump alarms or old pumps, etc.
- Need for prolonged disconnection.

Conclusion

Infusion pumps are very helpful in healthcare settings for both doctors and patients. But they also have some disadvantages in drug administration and can result in adverse drug reactions. With the recent development of smart infusion pumps there is a reduction in side effects caused by normal infusion pumps; however the machine-related errors and equipment failures have not been eliminated.

Infusion Therapy [26–28]

Definition

This is the administration of fluid or medication directly into the bloodstream through an intravenous catheter or needle, which cannot be taken orally by the patient.

Types of Solutions

See Table 4.2 (Figure 4.12).

Infusion Devices

Cannula IV: if the gauge number is small then the cannula's diameter will be large.
    See Table 4.3.

For calculating dripping rate:
    FORMULA = (*mL*)/*minute* × dripping factor (Figure 4.13).

TABLE 4.2   Types of Solutions

S. NO.	OSMOLALITY	EXAMPLES
1	**Isotonic solution** Similar to the osmolality in body fluids and increases extracellular volume. Due to same osmolality, they cannot enter the cells as there is no osmotic force between the fluids.	1) **0.9% normal saline** • Increases plasma volume • Replaces fluid loss without changing its concentration • Replaces Na^+ 2) **5% dextrose in water (D_5W) – "physiologically hypotonic"** • Increases total fluid volume • Useful in rehydrating 3) **Lactated ringers** • Replaces fluid • Buffers pH
2	**Hypotonic solution** Diluted or has less osmolality than body fluids. Due to less osmolality, it enters the cells by osmosis and can prevent edema.	1) **0.45% saline (1/2 NS)** • Increases total fluid volume • Helps in maintaining body fluids • Stabilizes renal function • Fluid replacement in diabetic patients 2) **0.225% saline (1/4 NS)** 3) **0.33% saline (1/3 NS)**
3	**Hypertonic solution** Concentrated or has more osmolality than body fluids. Due to high osmolality water will move out of the cells and enter into the extracellular fluid. Should check for fluid overload.	1) **3% saline** 2) **5% saline** 3) **10% dextrose in water (D10W)** 4) **5% dextrose in 0.9% saline** • Replaces fluid Na^+, Cl^- and calories 5) **5% dextrose in 0.45% saline** • Helps in maintaining body • Useful rehydrating postoperative patients 6) **5% dextrose in lactated ringers** • Same as lactated ringer

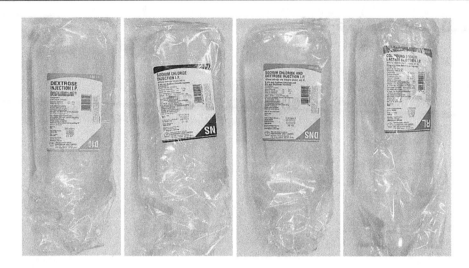

FIGURE 4.12   IV fluids – dextrose (D10), normal saline, dextrose normal saline (DNS) and ringer lactate.

TABLE 4.3   Infusion Devices Particulars

SIZE	COLOR CODING	FLOW RATE	USES
14G	Orange	240 mL/min	In need of large volume replacement
16G	Gray	180 mL/min	In emergency situations like in trauma patients or during or after surgery or intra-partum/post-partum, gastrointestinal bleeding, multiple blood transfusions, etc.
17G	White	125 mL/min	New
18G	Green	90 mL/min	For delivery of blood and blood-related products, irritant drugs, etc.
20G	Pink	60 mL/min	Generally used (universal)
22G	Blue	36 mL/min	Small and fragile veins
24G	Yellow	20 mL/min	Used in children
26G	Violet	13 mL/min	New

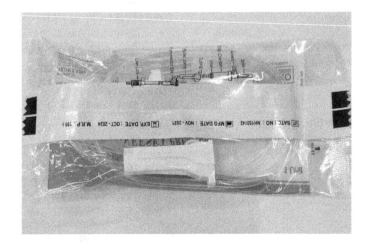

FIGURE 4.13   Infusion set.

Uses

- For unresponsive patients
- Restricted oral intake
- For infusing drugs and chemotherapeutic agents
- To take blood samples or for transfusing blood
- Total parenteral nutrition
- When rapid absorption is necessary

Complications

- Fluid overload
- Phlebitis and thrombophlebitis
- Infection and infiltration
- Air embolism
- Localized or systemic tissue damage
- Hematoma

Indication

See Figure 4.14.

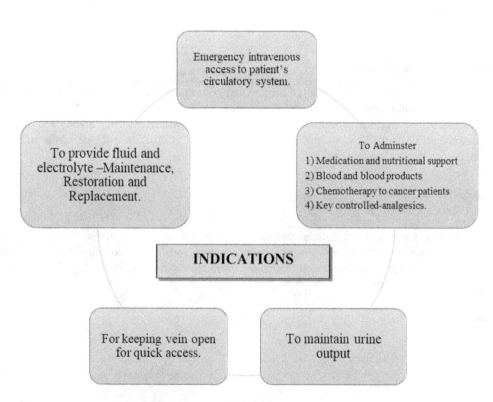

FIGURE 4.14 Indications of infusion route.

Contraindication

- Liver disease, severe hypoxia, shock, CHF, lactic acidosis, Addison's disease
- Vomiting or non-gastrointestinal tract induced alkalosis
- Certain drugs like amphotericin, thiopentone, doxycycline, etc.
- Surgically compromised or injured extremities

Conclusion

Intravenous drug administration is a mode of treatment in patient care and is in high demand in emergency and ICU settings. Infusion therapy will be useful in healthcare settings.

Electrical Muscle Stimulators

Definition

Electro muscle stimulation (EMS) is also known neuromuscular electrical stimulation (NMES) or electromyostimulation. It is a device which uses electrical pulses to stimulate the muscles particularly by targeting a motor nerve. This results in the contraction of that particular muscle and helps in the tightening and toning of that muscle [29].

Types of Electrodes

- A hand-held electrode
- Disc electrodes

How Does an EMS Unit Work?

- The circuit generates an interrupted direct current with low frequency between 10 and 120 Hz. The current is transmitted by the electrodes, and they are placed on the skin. A circuit generates the current to stimulate either sensory or motor nerves. The current flow will be regulated and controlled, so that the required amount of current with the same intensity will reach the nerve.

Mechanism

- The normal mechanism of muscle contraction is due to an impulse generated from the brain by a sensory nerve; the impulse reaches the motor nerve resulting in contraction. But in EMS, the motor nerve is activated directly to cause contraction without any impulse from the brain or sensory nerve [30].

See Figure 4.15.

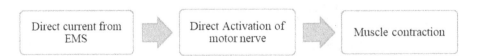

FIGURE 4.15   Flowchart showing how EMS works.

Uses

- Muscle tightening.
- Can reduce the occurrence of aging on the face.
- Can be used in a healthcare setting to give stimulus to critically ill and postoperative patients.
- Patients with a history of severe congestive heart failure (CHF) or COPD can benefit from EMS.

Indication

See Figure 4.16.

Contraindication

- Over the carotid sinus
- During pregnancy
- Individuals with pacemakers
- Sensitivity to electricity
- When active range of movement is contraindicated
- Problems in treating patients with conditions like

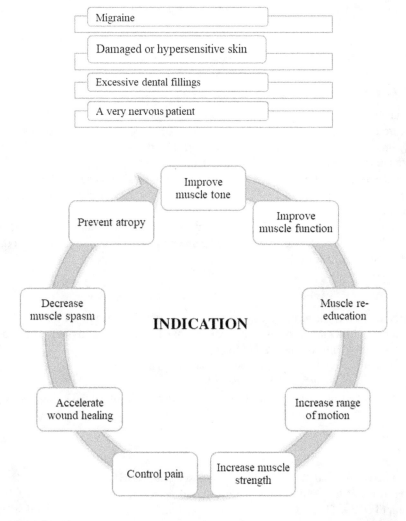

FIGURE 4.16   Uses of EMS.

Complications

- Muscle fatigue or muscle spasm due to over-treatment in a particular area.
- Some may feel a claustrophobic effect while using face masks.
- In case of any discomfort, stop the treatment immediately and massage the muscle.

Conclusion

EMS exercise helps in increasing muscle strength in both normal and ICU patients. This kind of innovation in the medical field helps clinicians in the improvement of patient care. But still, we need more new development for the betterment of mankind.

Endeavor Game-Based Digital Therapeutic Devices in ADHD

Introduction

The endeavor game-based device is used for children with attention deficit hyperactivity disorder (ADHD). This software was designed by Adam Gazzaley, a neuroscientist, who named the device Neuroracer. This will be helpful for physicians in treating children with symptoms of ADHD. It has yet to receive clearance from the FDA as it is designed for use for a limited time. In some developed countries game-based therapy has been using for ADHD in pediatric patients [31]. This will be helpful for children between 8 and 12 years of age diagnosed with primarily inattentive or combined type ADHD.

How Does It Work?

The endeavor game-based device is a software program connected to the mobile phone of the user which is called software-as-medical device (SaMD). The technology uses adaptive algorithms also known as the Selective Stimulus Management Engine (SSMETM). It is designed so that the difficulty level can be adjusted for the personalized treatment experience that is needed for each individual child. This game is like a video game with colorful pictures, art and cartoons with music. These will help the children to pay more attention to the game and increase their concentration. By using it frequently, children will adapt to the game and move to the next level of difficulty. The software consists of a screen with audio and high-resolution display. Clinicians usually prescribe using it for approximately 25 minutes per day for 5 days per week including lock-out after the allocated game play, as well as reminders for both children and parents to maximize compliance [32,33].

Uses

- The difficulty level will be changed according to the performance of the child.
- Whenever the child plays the game, it makes them engaged and stimulates some specific centers in the brain to improve concentration and attention.
- Any child that is eligible as per clinical indication can access it.
- Younger children may enjoy playing games.
- It can be included in a therapeutic program for children with ADHD along with physician-based therapy or medication.

Indications

- Children between 8 and 12 years of age diagnosed with ADHD.
- Children using it have improvement in a digital assessment known as Test of Variables of Attention (TOVA). This test is to check sustained and selective attention but does not display benefits in behavioral symptoms like hyperactivity.

Limitations

- Color blindness
- Eye problems
- Eye or ear deformity
- Photo-sensitive epilepsy
- Physical limitations that restrict use of devices

Conclusion

It will be a challenge for healthcare workers to diagnose and treat this kind of disorder. Only developed countries are prescribing devices like this, for example the United States. Still, we need programs or campaigns for developing countries to make use of the devices. But this can never be considered as a main or standard therapy. This endeavor game-based device is only an additional therapy for children with ADHD to improve their concentration and attention power.

Automated External Defibrillator

Definition

An automated external defibrillator (AED) is an automatic external defibrillator mostly used to diagnose ventricular fibrillation; it generates an electrical shock to the damaged heart (fibrillated heart or other shockable rhythm). This makes the heart increase the force of contraction and helps to produce normal cardiac rhythm. It is available with self-adhesive electrodes in the market (Figure 4.17) [34,35].

Types

- Semi-automated defibrillators
- Fully automated defibrillators
- Public access AEDs
- Professional use AEDs (Figure 4.18)

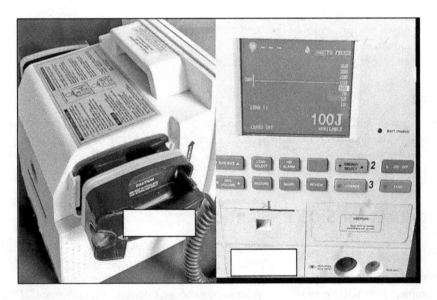

FIGURE 4.17 Automated external defibrillator.

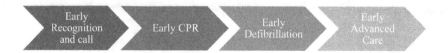

FIGURE 4.18   Steps and early approach of CPR.

Indications [36]

- Atrial flutter/atrial fibrillation
- Re-entry supra ventricular tachycardia
- Monomorphic and polymorphic VT
- Re-entrant tachycardia with narrow or wide QRS complex

Contraindications [36]

- Junctional tachycardia or ectopics or multilocal atrial tachycardia
- Dysrhythmias due to digitalis toxicity

Advantages [36]

- In emergency situations – speed of operation: the first shock can be delivered within one minute of patient arrival.
- Remote defibrillation through adhesive pads.
- Can also be used manually for the delivery of shocks by professionals.
- Safe and easy to use.
- Good compliance with instructive protocols.
- Recommended by current resuscitation guidelines.

Disadvantages [36]

- Difficulty in usage by untrained people.
- Difficulty in matching with CPR maneuvers for normal people.
- Takes time for shock delivery.
- An automated device cannot be operated manually by professionals.
- Not recommended by current guidelines except for special situations.
- If not used properly then there is risk of electrocution.

Conclusion

Since the invention of AEDs there has been a decrease in mortality rates in healthcare settings and also an improvement in the quality of life of the patient after discharge. Many deaths happening in the world outside the hospital are termed out of hospital cardiac arrests (OHCA). Thus, we need to increase the usage of AEDs along with their deployment is healthcare settings.

Baby Products for SIDS Prevention

Definition

The sudden or ill-defined death of an infant less than one year of age whose cause cannot be identified even after complete investigation or autopsy is known as sudden infant death syndrome (SIDS). The main causes may be asphyxia, accidental suffocation or strangulation in the bed [37]. This can be due to the baby sleeping prone on uneven surfaces, being premature or being exposed to smoke. To prevent SIDS there are lots of products available on the market.

Types of Baby Products [38,39]

- Baby monitors
- Mattresses
- Crib tents or beds
- Sleep positioners

Crib

- A crib or bassinet is used in developed countries which meets the recommended safety standards of the Consumer Product Safety Commission (CPSC).
- CPSC demands that proper cribs or bassinets should have spacing with no drop sides.
- Cribs should be small, easy to care for and more portable.
- They should have a facility for attachment to the parental bed so that it will be easy for the parents to monitor the baby.
- Cribs should have a firm surface covered with a mattress so that the baby can sleep in a supine position and avoid the risk of SIDS and suffocation.

Mattresses

- Mattresses should be firm and clean.
- Place in the crib without any gap between the crib and mattress.
- Baby should be kept on the firm surface of the crib covered by a clean mattress.
- Each crib has a specific mattress.
- Don't substitute the mattress with pillows or cushions.
- Don't use any objects, even pillows or quilts, etc., in the crib.

Sitting Devices

- Due to convenience, these are used by most parents and caregivers even when they are not traveling.
- Some studies show that usage of these devices can lead to suffocation in babies younger than four months old.
- Position – the infant's head is up and above the fabric, the face is visible, and the nose and mouth are clear of obstructions while using infant slings.
- If an infant falls asleep in a sitting device, he or she should be shifted and moved to a crib or other appropriate flat surface as soon as is safe and practical.

Beneficial for

- Brain abnormalities
- Low birth weight babies
- Respiratory infections
- Babies sleeping on stomachs or sides

Drawbacks

- Mattress cannot be used for babies younger than one year of age.
- There are fewer reports of reduction in SIDS.
- Product itself can cause suffocation.

- For some families with financial burden or reduced space in living area, the use of a crib may not be possible.
- But the CPSC does not recommend safety standards for bedside sleepers.
- Bedside rails can increase the risk of strangulation.

Conclusion

To date the FDA has not approved or cleared any baby products for the prevention and reduction of SIDS. Currently, there are new crib mattresses available in the market with the special feature of rebreathing carbon dioxide when the baby sleeps in a prone position. Every healthcare worker should have knowledge about these baby products so they can educate the parents, which can reduce the risk related to these products. At the community level, many programs and campaigns should be conducted to create awareness about the devices and increase their usage.

Nasal Rinsing Devices

Definition

Nasal irrigation is a technique that uses saline to flush the nasal cavity and help in thinning of nasal mucosa. Nasal irrigation also helps to remove more effectively micro-organisms and other irritants from the nasal cavity. It is also known as Jala Neti, Neti Pot therapy, nasal lavage or hypertonic saline lavage [40]. Devices used for nasal irrigation are known as nasal rinsing devices.

Types

- Bulb syringe
- Neti pot – looks like a small teapot
- Squeeze/spray bottle
- SinuCleanse Rhinomer
- Naso cup

Mechanism of Action

- The nasal rinsing devices will remove the infectious particles in the nasal cavity and reduce swelling.
- The fluid poured in one nostril can enter the other nostril.
- It helps in the cleaning and removal of infectious particles and also improvement in the mucociliary function of nasal mucosa (Figure 4.19).

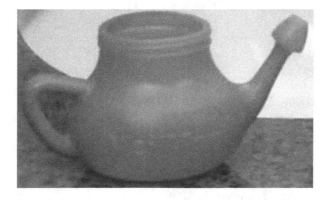

FIGURE 4.19   Nasal rinsing device.

Indications

- Chronic rhinosinusitis (more than 12 weeks) [41].
- Failure of conservative management or endoscopic surgeries.
- Allergic rhinitis and rhinitis of pregnancy (mild and moderate cases).
- Children older than two years can use it for allergies.
- Sarcoidosis and Wegener granulomatosis.

Contraindications

- Incompletely healed facial injury, as it increases the risk of infection.
- Neurologic or musculoskeletal problems like intentional tremor – increases the risk of aspiration.
- Patients prone to nasal bleeding.

Advantages

- Clears nasal passages and improves breathing.
- Relieves cold and allergic symptoms.
- Prevents or reduces sinus infection.
- Helps to stop snoring.

Disadvantages

- Discomfort or nervousness during its use.
- Danger of forcing infected matter into eustachian tubes or sinuses or both.
- Can be counterproductive if used frequently for a long time.
- Tap water should not be used for nasal irrigation.
- Improper usage of devices can lead to secondary infection.

Conclusion

Nasal irrigation is an effective way to get rid of infectious particles from the nasal cavity and improve mucociliary function. So, it is helpful in patients with sinusitis and with traditional sinus treatments such as antibiotics and nasal steroids. It should be used with caution, because of the potential hazards of forcing infected material into the adjacent cavities. But it is simple to use and inexpensive which increases patient compliance.

Pulse Oximeter and Oxygen Concentration

Introduction

A pulse oximeter is an automatic device used for measuring oxygen saturation in the blood which has become an important parameter in the diagnosis and management of patients. It is a non-invasive device used for measuring oxygen in the blood [42]. It works by clipping onto a finger, or another part of the body, and wavelengths are measured to get the ratio of the current levels of oxygenated hemoglobin to deoxygenated hemoglobin in the blood. The readings on a pulse oximeter are the oxygen percentage in the patient's blood (Figure 4.20).

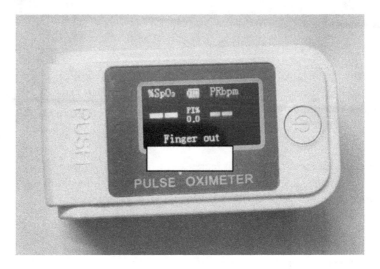

FIGURE 4.20   Pulse oximeter.

Normal Readings

- No sharp cut value or range for hypoxemia to occur.
- A normal value is usually 95% or higher; COPD or sleep apneic patients have normal levels around 90%.
- 80% to 85% oxyhemoglobin saturation can damage the brain.

How Does It Work?

- A pulse oximeter follows the Beer-Lambert law of light absorption which states that light from LEDs is absorbed when it is transmitted through clear fluid example plasma with solute at a specific wavelength like hemoglobin.
- Arterial blood appears to be red and venous blood appears to be blue because their spectrums of absorption are different.
- The value is changed into an algorithm in a microprocessor where the oxyhemoglobin saturation is calculated and eventually displayed to the user.

Indications

- All hospital settings
- Patients with lung or heart conditions
- Any clinical condition where hypoxemia occurs

Contraindications

- Abnormal hemoglobin eg. carbon monoxide toxicity
- Blisters or damage to nail bed
- Burns patients

Complications [43]

The accuracy of pulse oximeter signals can be decreased by

- Pigmentation of the skin or nail polish or intravascular dyes
- Saturations below 83%

- High-intensity ambient lighting
- Abnormal hemoglobin like carboxyhemoglobin

False Positive Readings

- Abnormal hemoglobin like oxyhemoglobin results in false positive readings.
- Always correlate with clinical features for diagnosis, e.g. carbon monoxide poisoning.
- Diabetic patients with HbA1 higher than 7 have high arterial oxygen saturation.

False Negative Readings May Occur

- Abnormal hemoglobin like sulfhemoglobin or methemoglobin
- Abnormal inherited hemoglobin
- Venous congestion
- Severe anemia or sickle cell anemia

Clinical Significance

- Sensitivity – 92% and specificity – 90% at oxygen saturation – 92%.
- Convenient, easy to use and non-invasive technique.
- Patients can use it even at home.
- Helpful for continuous monitoring.

Conclusion

Pulse oximetry is an effective and rapid tool for assessing oxygen saturation mostly during emergency situations. But the problem is that blue discoloration of the tongue and mucus membrane known as cyanosis may not be visibly noticed till oxygen saturation reaches 67% [44]. That is we should have a basic knowledge about its limitations. We have to conduct lots of programs and campaigns to create awareness among people so they can make use of it, like in developed countries (Table 4.4).

TABLE 4.4 Weight Classification

WEIGHT STATUS	BMI (KG/M²)
Normal	18.5–24.9
Overweight	≥25.0
Preobese	25.0–29.9
Obese	≥30.0
Class – I	30.0–34.9
Class – II	35.0–39.9
Class – III	≥40.0

Weight Management Devices

Obesity is an abnormal collection or accumulation of fat in the body which is not good for health. It is measured in body mass index and expressed as kilogram per meter square. Body mass index helps in the classification of overweight and obesity [45]. So, obesity has become a major problem in both developing and developed countries. Lots of weight loss foods, devices and therapies are available on the market.

Types of Devices [46]

See Table 4.5.

Gastric Band
The gastric band is adjustable and made up of silicone placed on the upper part of the stomach.

TABLE 4.5 Types of Devices

NO.	DEVICES	EXAMPLES
1	Gastric banding system	Lap-Band Adjustable Gastric Banding System
2	Electrical stimulation systems	Maestro Rechargeable System
3	Gastric balloon systems	• Orbera Intragastric Balloon System • Obalon Balloon System • Transpyloric Shuttle Delivery Device
4	Gastric emptying systems	Aspire Assist
5	Oral removable palatal space-occupying device	Sensor Monitored Alimentary Restriction Therapy (SMART) Device
6	Ingested, transient, space-occupying device	Plenty

Indication
- Severely obese for more than five years with a BMI 40 or BMI of 35 with other co-morbid conditions

Contraindication
- People who are not willing or who cannot afford it.
- Patients with certain stomach or intestinal disorders or infections.
- Medication with aspirin.
- Addiction to alcohol or drugs.

Electrical Stimulator – Maestro Rechargeable System
Indication
- Severe obesity with a BMI of 40 to 45 or BMI of 35 to 39.9 with other co-morbid conditions

Contraindication
- Liver cirrhosis
- Portal hypertension
- Esophageal bleeding
- Hiatal hernia
- Patients with any other permanently placed implants

Gastric Balloon
These are kept in the stomach and inflated to reduce the available space to reduce gastric emptying (Table 4.6).

TABLE 4.6 Types of Gastric Balloon

S. NO.	DEVICE	INDICATION	WORKING	REMOVAL
1	Orbera Balloon System	BMI 30–40 kg/m^2	Gastric balloon is inflated with saline in the stomach through endoscopic procedure. So, the space will be reduced which helps in weight loss.	After 6 months.
2	Obalon Balloon System	BMI of 30–40 kg/m^2	Same as Orbera balloon except that the balloon is ingested as a swallowable capsule. But later the balloons will be removed under endoscopy.	After 6 months.
3	Transpyloric Shuttle Delivery Device	BMI of 35–40 kg/m^2 or BMI of 30.0 to 34.9 kg/m^2 *with other co-morbid conditions*	Large balloon is kept in the stomach and small balloon can either be placed in stomach or small intestine to reduce the gastric emptying.	After 12 months.

Contraindication
- Patients who have undergone any previous surgeries in the gastrointestinal tract
- Anatomical abnormality in the esophagus or pharynx
- Abnormality of stomach like ulcer or mass or varices or hiatus hernia (> 4cm)
- *Helicobacter pylori* infection
- Stomach or intestinal ulcers or inflammatory disorders
- Overuse of NSAIDs like aspirin
- Bleeding disorder
- Portal hypertension
- Patients with a psychiatric disorder like bulimia nervosa
- Pregnant women or women planning pregnancy
- Patients with history of allergic reaction

Gastric Emptying System – Aspire Assist

Indication   Obese individuals equal to or more than 22 years of age with BMI 35–55 kg/m^2.

Contraindication   Same as for gastric balloon.

Sensor Monitored Alimentary Restriction Therapy (SMART) Device
This is useful in people with a BMI of 27–35 kg/m^2, but should be used along with behavioral modification.

Plenity
There are also space-occupying devices that are placed in the stomach (natural gastrointestinal tract) instead of the mouth. These will be useful in people with a BMI of 25–40 kg/m^2.

Conclusion

Weight management devices should be prescribed by a physician and should follow the instruction given by them regularly. They are used widely in developing countries. Health care professionals should have a basic understanding of these devices and should advise patients to follow a healthy diet and regular exercise regimen before considering surgery.

References

1. http://www.fda.gov/diabetes.
2. http://www.fda.gov/cdrh/oivd.
3. Kleinert HD, Harshfield GA, Pickering TG, et al. What is the value of home blood pressure measurement in patients with mild hypertension? *Hypertension.* 1984;6:574. [PubMed: 6235190]
4. van Egmond J, Lenders JW, Weernink E, et al. Accuracy and reproducibility of 30 devices for self-measurement of arterial blood pressure. *Am J Hypertens.* 1993;6:873. [PubMed: 8267944]
5. Foster C, McKinlay S, Cruickshank JM, et al. Accuracy of the Omron HEM 706 portable monitor for home measurement of blood pressure. *J Hum Hypertens.* 1994;8:661. [PubMed: 7807495]
6. O'Brien E, Waeber B, Parati G, et al. Blood pressure measuring devices: Recommendations of the European Society of Hypertension. *BMJ.* 2001;322:531. [PubMed: 11230071]
7. Mitchell PL, Parlin RW, Blackburn H. Effect of Vertical Displacement of the Arm on Indirect Blood-Pressure Measurement. *N Engl J Med.* 1964;271:72. [PubMed: 14149257]
8. Eckert S, Gleichmann S, Gleichmann U. Blood pressure self-measurement in upper arm and in wrist for treatment control of arterial hypertension compared to ABPM. *Z Kardiol.* 1996;85 (Suppl 3):109. [PubMed: 8896310]
9. Wonka F, Thummler M, Schoppe A. Clinical test of a blood pressure measurement device with a wrist cuff. *Blood Press Monit.* 1996;1:361. [PubMed: 10226260]

10. Pickering TG, Miller NH, Ogedegbe G, et al. Call to action on use and reimbursement for home blood pressure monitoring: Executive summary: A joint scientific statement from the American Heart Association, American Society Of Hypertension, and Preventive Cardiovascular Nurses Association. *Hypertension*. 2008;52:1. [PubMed: 18497371]

11. Little P, Barnett J, Barnsley L, et al. Comparison of agreement between different measures of blood pressure in primary care and daytime ambulatory blood pressure. *BMJ* 2002;325:254

12. Parati G, Stergiou GS, Asmar R, et al. European Society of Hypertension practice guidelines for home blood pressure monitoring. *J Hum Hypertens*. 2010;24:779–85.

13. http://www.fda.gov/hearing aids.

14. http://www.fda.gov/contact lenses.

15. http://www.fda.gov/breast pumps.

16. American Academy of Pediatrics. *How to Take a Child's Temperature*. https://www.healthychildren.org/English/health-issues/conditions/fever/Pages/How-to-Take-a-Childs-Temperature.aspx (Accessed 3/23/2020).

17. Braun. *Braun Thermometers*. https://www.braunhealthcare.com/uk_en/ (Accessed 3/23/2020).

18. https://medyczny-rzeszow.pl/_blog/10-Rodzaje_termometrow_medycznych_i_ich_zastosowanie.html.

19. Joseph EJ, Pachaimuthu E, Arokyamuthu V, Muthukrishnan M, Kannan DK, Dhanalakshmi B. Comparative study of Episure™ AutoDetect™ syringe versus glass syringe for identification of epidural space in lower thoracic epidural. *Indian J Anaesth*. 2015;59:406–10.

20. Vijayaraghavan R. Autoinjector device for rapid administration of drugs and antidotes in emergency situations and in mass casualty management. *J Int Med Res*. 2020;48(5):300060520926019. doi: 10.1177/0300060520926019

21. British Guideline on the management of asthma; Scottish Intercollegiate Guidelines Network - SIGN (2016) https://www.brit-thoracic.org.uk/document-library/guidelines/asthma/btssign-asthma-guideline-2016/

22. Cates CJ, Welsh EJ, Rowe BH. Holding chambers (spacers) versus nebulisers for beta-agonist treatment of acute asthma. *Cochrane Database Syst Rev*. 2013 Sep;139:CD000052. doi: 10.1002/14651858.CD000052.pub3.

23. Boyter AC, Carter R. How do patients use their nebuliser in the community? *Respir Med*. 2005 Nov;99(11):1413–7. Epub 2005 Apr 21.

24. Hall KK, Shoemaker-Hunt S, Hoffman L, Richard S, Gall E, Schoyer E, Costar D, Gale B, Schiff G, Miller K, Earl T, Katapodis N, Sheedy C, Wyant B, Bacon O, Hassol A, Schneiderman S, Woo M, LeRoy L, Fitall E, Long A, Holmes A, Riggs J, Lim A. *Making Healthcare Safer III: A Critical Analysis of Existing and Emerging Patient Safety Practices [Internet]*. Rockville, MD: Agency for Healthcare Research and Quality (US). 2020 Mar. Report No.: 20-0029-EF. PMID: 32255576.

25. Rothschild JM. A controlled trial of smart infusion pumps to improve medication safety in critically ill patients. *Crit Care Med*. 2005 Mar;33(3):533–40.

26. Rajkomar A, Blandford A. Understanding infusion administration in the ICU through Distributed Cognition. *J Biomed Inf. June*2020;45(3):580–590.

27. Nickel B. Peripheral intravenous access: Applying infusion therapy standards of practice to improve patient safety. *Crit Care Nurse*. 2019 Feb;39(1):61–71.

28. *Intravenous Fluid Therapy in Adults in Hospital*. London: National Institute for Health and Care Excellence; 2017 May.

29. Karatzanos E, Gerovasili V, Zervakis D, Tripodaki ES, Apostolou K, Vasileiadis L, Papadopoulos E, Mitsiou G, Tsimpouki D, Routsi C, Nanas S. Clinical study electrical muscle stimulation: An effective form of exercise and early mobilization to preserve muscle strength in critically Ill patients. *Crit Care Res Pract*. 2012 Jan;2012:1–8. doi: 10.1155/2012/432752. Epub 2012 Apr 1. PMID: 22545212; PMCID: PMC3321528.

30. Available (https://www.accessdata.fda.gov/cdrh_docs/reviews/DEN200026.pdf)

31. Anguera JA et al. Video game training enhances cognitive control in older adults. *Nature*. 2013 Sept 5;501(7465):97–101. doi: 10.1038/nature12486.

32. Constance L. FDA OKs ADHD video game therapy for emergency release during the pandemic [Internet]. *ADDitude*; 2020 [cited 2021 Jul 1]. Available from: https://www.additudemag.com/akili-adhd-video-game-treatment-release-pandemic/

33. Austerman J. ADHD and behavioral disorders: Assessment, management, and an update from DSM-5. *Cleve Clin J Med*. 2015 Nov 1;82(11 suppl 1):S2–7.

34. https://www.nhlbi.nih.gov/health- topics/defibrillators.

35. https://www.webmd.com/heart-disease/heart-failure/qa/what-is-the-definition-of- defibrillator.

36. Delhommea C, Njeime M, Varlet E, Pechmajoua L, Benameur N, Cassani P, Derkennej C, Jostj D, Lamhaut L, Marijona E, Jouvena Xavier, Karama Nicole. Automated external defibrillator use in out-of-hospital cardiac arrest: Current limitations and solutions. *Arch Cardiovasc Dis*. 2019;112:217–222.

37. Pretorius K, Choi E, Kang S, Mackert M. Sudden infant death syndrome on facebook: Qualitative descriptive content analysis to guide prevention efforts. *J Med Internet Res*. 2020 Jul 30;22(7):e18474.

38. Moon RY, Task Force on Sudden Infant Death Syndrome. SIDS and other sleep-related infant deaths: Evidence base for 2016 updated recommendations for a safe infant sleeping environment. *Pediatrics*. 2016 Nov;138(5):e20162940.

39. *Baby Products with SIDS Prevention Claims*. FDA. https://www.fda.gov/medical-devices/products-and-medical-procedures/baby-products-sids-prevention-claims.

40. Principi N, Esposito S. Nasal irrigation: An imprecisely defined medical procedure. *Int J Environ Res Public Health*. 2012 May;14(5): 516.

41. Harvey R, Hannan SA, Badia L, Scadding G. Nasal saline irrigations of chronic rhinosinusitis. *Cochrane Database Syst Rev*. 2007;(3):CD006394.

42. Hafen B, Sharma S. Oxygen saturation. *StatPearls* [Internet]; 2021 May 7 [cited 2021 Jun 25]; Available from: https://www.statpearls.com/ArticleLibrary/viewarticle/26491

43. Health C for D and R. *Pulse Oximeter Accuracy and Limitations: FDA Safety Communication*. FDA [Internet]; 2021 Feb 19 [cited 2021 Jun 26]; Available from: https://www.fda.gov/medical-devices/safety-communications/pulse-oximeter-accuracy-and-limitations-fda-safety-communication

44. Enoch AJ, English M, Shepperd S. Does pulse oximeter use impact health outcomes? A systematic review. *Arch Dis Child*. 2016 Aug;101(8):694–700.

45. Marrone AK. Food and drug administration's perspective on medical devices intended for weight loss: A guide for the interventional radiologist. *Tech Vasc Interv Radiol*. 2020 Mar;23(1):100661.

46. Health C for D and R. Weight-loss and weight-management devices [Internet]. *FDA*. FDA; 2021 [cited 2021 Jun 23]. Available from: https://www.fda.gov/medical-devices/products-and-medical-procedures/weight-loss-and-weight-management-devices

Further Reading

1. Healthlink BC. *How to Take a Temperature: Children and Adults.* . https://www.healthlinkbc.ca/healthlinkbc-files/how-take-temperature-children-and-adults (Accessed 3/23/2020).

2. Massachusetts Department of Health. *Flu: What you can do: Caring for People at Home*. https://blog.mass.gov/publichealth/flu-facts/flu-what-you-can-do-caring-for-people-at-home/ (Accessed 3/23/2020).

3. https://infekcje.mp.pl/publikacje/122369,rodzaje-termometrow-lekarskich-i-ich-cechy

4. NHS Choices. *How to Take Someone's Temperature*. https://www.nhs.uk/common-health-questions/accidents-first-aid-and-treatments/how-do-i-take-someones-temperature/ (Accessed 3/23/2020).

Implants and Prosthetics

5

Sree Sudha T Y, Anjaly Mary Varghese, Z. Naveen Kumar, K. S. B. S. Krishna Sasanka, T. Y. Sri Hari, and Pugazhenthan Thangaraju

BREAST IMPLANTS

Breast implants are highly popular medical devices employed by a plastic surgeon to revamp the breast's size and contour for cosmetic and reconstructive reasons or as part of gender reassignment surgery. Some women opt for breast implants for cosmetic breast augmentation while some others get it done for reconstructive purposes, as in the case of post-mastectomy in breast cancer patients or trauma or severe congenital deformities. These are also employed in the recorrection or revision of an original flawed surgery. To use or not to use implants in reconstructive and breast augmentation procedures is solely the choice of the patient and comes with age specifications from the FDA: minimum 22 years or above in case of breast augmentation for women and breast reconstruction for women of any age [1].

Saline Implants

The prototype of modern breast implants was comprised of a sterile saline-filled silicone rubber (elastomer) shell, an empty, balloon-like device, smooth or textured, permitting suitable alterations in size for asymmetrical breasts. Saline-filled breast implants may be single or double, barrier coated or covered with polyurethane foam; they may be either pre-filled or filled during the surgical implantation and distended with sterile isotonic saline to the optimal desired size. Saline-based implants may rupture, start leaking (consequently the saline may be absorbed by the body), deflate and pose unwarranted inconvenience.

Silicone Gel Implants [2]

Silicone gel implants contain a silicone gel-like material enclosed in a silicone shell. These implants are available in smooth or textured shells and in various sizes. They are filled with a fixed amount of silicone gel with varying viscosity among the different implants and manufacturers. Popularly, doctors and

DOI: 10.1201/9781003220671-5

patients tend to choose silicone gel over saline implants as they offer quality results, smoother texture and feel more like real breasts, making them the implants of choice.

Three generations of these devices with numerous modifications in each type have been marketed.

First Generation

Among the earliest designs to hit the market was the silicone elastomer with a smooth polished finish in two parts like thick envelopes glued together, holding a viscous silicone gel material (dimethylsiloxane) (Figure 5.1) [3].

Second Generation

Thinner shells and less viscous gel were tried to control capsular contracture, but failed. Many such implants crumbled and were rendered useless within ten years of device fixation.

Third Generation

Novel and modern devices have a stronger shell, the gel content more viscous and cohesive, and they are accompanied by diphenyl silicone as a barrier coat preventing the silicone gel from leaking through the implant shell.

Presently implants include the silicone gel filler called Memory Gel with approval from the FDA, with a thicker gel constituency with a doughy feel; it is more cohesive to minimize the gel spread if the device ruptures and to reduce the chances of contour deformity due to scar shrinkage.

Local complications may include pain in the bust region, visible deflation, altered sensation in the nipple and breast, rupture, bleeding, scarring, formation of a hardened mass or area around the site of implant, disfigurement, serious post-surgical infection of the incision site, asymmetrical abnormal breasts and the need for medical interventions and repeat surgeries. In silicone gel implants, a distinctive capsular contracture due to the hardening from scar shrinkage is observed. A silent rupture of the silicone implant may discharge the contents into the shell itself or may leak outside of the implant, without any obvious symptoms. Hence the FDA recommends adopting screening by MRI and ultrasound, for between five and six years post-surgery with repeat screening two to three years afterwards.

There is an increased risk for breast cancer undoubtedly in implant users. Textured implants may be linked with breast implant-associated anaplastic large cell lymphoma (BIA ALCL), a non-Hodgkin's lymphoma, with symptoms of persistent swelling, lump or pain in the implanted area occurring several years after the implantation. "Breast implant illness" is described as having systemic symptoms like chronic fatigue, rash, pain in the joints, memory loss, "brain fog" and autoimmune diseases. Practically, getting a mammogram done is difficult with implants; hence alternatively special X-ray views may be called for to detect silent ruptures or filler leakage. Breastfeeding may not be feasible for women with breast implants. Such implants do not last a lifetime and may need replacement if any complications arise or any changes in size or shape are observed over time.

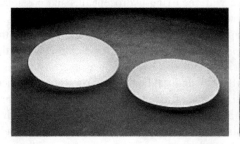 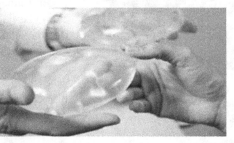

FIGURE 5.1 Saline-filled breast implant and silicone gel-filled prosthesis model.

CEREBROSPINAL FLUID SHUNT

A cerebrospinal fluid (CSF) shunt is a life-saving medical device utilized in hydrocephalus, a condition where excessive CSF is stored up in the brain and must be drained. CSF protects the brain and spinal cord as these organs are immersed in this normally colorless clear fluid. Sometimes, CSF accumulates overabundantly due to a blockage in the system that regulates CSF, hence causing an undue increase in intracranial pressure which may fatally affect the brain with intracranial hematoma, cerebral edema and herniation. A CSF shunt is a surgically inserted tube that drains overloading fluid into the abdomen or heart and thus prevents the impending brain damage. The excess CSF is sucked up into the circulation. The three important parts of CSF shunts are namely an in-flow catheter tube, a fluid flow-regulating valve and an out-flow tube which transfers the fluid into the abdomen or heart where eventually it is harmlessly mopped up.

CSF shunt valves can be of two types:

- **Fixed shunt valves** work by permitting the draining of CSF fluid when a certain "fixed" threshold for fluid pressure is exceeded.
- **Adjustable shunt valves** accept fluctuations in volume of the fluid flowing through the valve.

Again, adjustable CSF shunt valves may be of two categories.

Magnetic Externally Adjustable Shunt Valves

The mechanical components can be operated externally. A magnetic tool may be placed on the skin near the valve to rotate to adjust these valves manually. Patients implanted with magnetic externally programmable CSF shunt valves may have a risk of experiencing an unintended change in their valve setting when exposed to strong magnetic fields from external magnetic sources and implanted medical devices that use magnets.

Non-Magnetic Externally Adjustable Valves

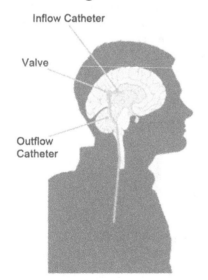

Inflow Catheter

Valve

Outflow Catheter

These may either possess self-adjusting flow-regulating valves or possibly minimally invasive surgical procedure-based adjustments. Such shunts are not dependent on an external magnetic field for valve adjustments (Figure 5.2) (Table 5.1) [4].

Typically, these systems require repeated monitoring and regular medical follow-up as infection, shunt malfunction and improper drainage are common risks. **Shunt malfunction** may occur due to any obstruction within the device resulting in CSF under-drainage with recurring hydrocephalus and possible surgical replacement of the blocked component or components. **Over-drainage happens** when CSF drains from the ventricles through the shunt disproportionately to CSF formation causing the collapse of ventricles, blood vessel damage manifesting as headaches, hemorrhages (subdural hematomas) or a sharp reduction in the ventricle size (slit ventricle syndrome). The drainage pressure of the shunt valve can be modified to resolve the over-drainage and under-drainage of CSF. Adverse effects of the shunt and blood clots can also occur in some patients.

FIGURE 5.2 CSF shunt system and its parts.

TABLE 5.1   Variants of CSF Shunts and Their Functionality

Lumboperitoneal (LP) shunt	CSF drained from subarachnoid space in the lumbar spine (lower back) into the abdomen.
Ventriculoatrial (VA) shunt	CSF drained from ventricles of the brain into the right atrium of the heart.
Ventriculoperitoneal (VP) shunt	CSF drained from ventricles of the brain into abdominal peritoneal cavity.
Ventriculo-pleural (VPL) shunt	CSF drained into the pleural cavity.
Ventriculo-cisternal (VC) shunt	CSF drained into the cistern magna.

IMPLANTABLE HEARING DEVICES

The hearing devices typically implanted in the ear are of different types, namely:

1. Cochlear implants
2. Auditory brainstem implants
3. Bone conduction devices
4. Middle ear implants

These are indicated in patients with sensorineural, conductive or mixed hearing loss or in patients with a damaged auditory nerve or those unable to wear hearing aids. None of the implants cure deafness; they only give a useful portrayal of sounds in the environment and considerable aid in understanding speech.

Cochlear Implants (CIs) [5]

The cochlea or the inner ear is called the organ of hearing. As sound is transmitted through the external and middle ear, the minute hair cells in the cochlea vibrate, converting acoustic waves into electrical signals that finally reach the brain through the auditory nerve and we perceive the sound. A CI is an electronic hearing prosthesis which bypasses the damaged hair cells in the inner ear and transmits electrical signals directly to the brain via the auditory nerve. A CI is designed to restore or provide hearing in adults or children with sensorineural hearing loss (SNHL) or impairment in both the ears in whom hearing aids provide limited benefit.

The two main components of cochlear implants are: [6]

1. **External components** including the **headpiece/microphone** to pick up the sound, a **speech or sound processor** that filters sound to recognizable audible speech and passes on the electrical acoustic signals to the transmitter and a **transmitter coil**, by electromagnetic induction, forwards the processed audio impulse to the internal hardware components. The transmitter antenna is kept positioned externally behind the ear by a magnet. Implants **will definitely need** new or recharged **batteries** for functional hearing.
2. **Implanted internal components** comprise a surgically implantable **receiver, stimulator** and system of electrodes with the electronic circuits which pick up external auditory communications and convert them to electrical impulses through an internal cable to the electrodes in the inner ear.

A receiver/stimulator component is like a magnetic disk that is bone fastened behind one ear, just below the skin; the external system is retained in place next to the implanted internal system by a magnet. **With**

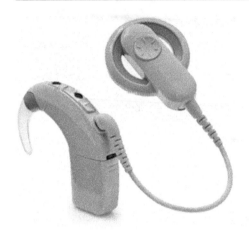

FIGURE 5.3   Cochlear implant.

advanced technology, the patient can upgrade the implant by changing only the external parts of the CI (Figure 5.3).

Mechanism of Cochlear Implants

Cochlear implants resemble the normal physiological process of hearing. Sound signals from the external environment are picked up by the microphone and forwarded to the processor, where they are converted into short electric currents that are broadcasted transcutaneously through the transmitter coil; the Implanted Internal Components take these in and send them to the cochlear electrodes. The ganglion cells in the scala tympani are stimulated; in turn the impulses are siphoned through the auditory nerve to the brain. These small currents activate the nerve and pass these signals to the central cortex where they are recognized appropriately culminating in the experience of "hearing". In a "hybrid strategy", the residual hearing may be amplified using a hearing aid on the same implanted ear.

Risks Associated with the Use of CIs [7]

Sound perceptions differ from normal hearing in implant users. There may be residual hearing loss in the implanted ear. These implants directly stimulate the auditory nerves to evoke electrical currents, and this stimulation in the long term may affect the nerve function detrimentally. The interpretation of complex auditory signals, such as those in music, may not be fully possible. Device failure may be due to short circuits in the internal component or fluid leakage, requiring reimplantation.

Localized inflammation or **reparative granuloma** may be seen if the body rejects the CI and may be unpredictable; unforeseen complications could occur with prolonged use of such implants. Though rare, if skin flap necrosis with infection occurs after the surgery, the implant may have to be temporarily or permanently removed. Engaging in active sports, unfortunate accidents and falling down may impact and damage the CI, demanding surgery or replacement. Replacing damaged or lost parts may be costly. Damage to the external part from water may require repair, so it is advised to remove the external parts of the device before taking showers, swimming or participating in water sports.

MRI imaging as a routine diagnostic method for the early detection of illness may prove dangerous because it may demagnetize the implant's internal magnet or cause dislodgement of the implant. Such an implant will interact with certain other electronic equipment like screening metal detectors or other security systems and may be adversely affected by mobile phone radiation or other electromagnetic devices and radio transmitters. It may have to be switched off during take offs and landings in aircraft as it can interact with computer networking and magnetic fields in an unpredictable fashion.

The outcomes of CI will depend on proper patient evaluation, motivating parents of children with hearing impairment and intensive auditory verbal therapy. As these implant users will have to use them for the rest of their lives, replacement parts or other future customer service must be carefully looked into. Candidates contraindicated for cochlear implantation include those with absent cochlea and cochlear nerve.

Auditory Brainstem Implants (ABIs)

ABIs, similarly to CIs, convert sounds into signals that are sent directly to the brain and cause direct stimulation of the auditory pathway by acting further downstream thus bypassing the non-functioning or non-existent auditory nerve. ABIs are best indicated in patients with absent cochlear nerve or in patients with a cochlea practically unsuitable for CIs, and in patients with neurofibromatosis type II (NF2) – a tumor on the auditory nerve or trauma following surgery.

Middle Ear Implants [8]

A middle ear implant (MEI) is a hearing device which keeps the ear canal entirely open and is used in sensorineural hearing loss (SNHL), conductive hearing loss, mixed hearing loss and obstruction of the outer or middle ear. The increasing number of cases of hearing loss may be due to exposure to loud noise, trauma, viral infections, increasing geriatric population and rising incidence of malformation of the inner ear.

Types of MEIs

Piezoelectric Middle Ear Implants
In this type of MEI, piezoelectric materials are used, which on application of voltage will result in deformation of the material that generates mechanical energy to stimulate the middle ear ossicles.

Piezoelectric devices move ossicles using a piezoelectric crystal that bends or lengthens in time with changes in a signal voltage applied across it. Piezoelectric ossicular actuators generally yield greater power and less distortion than electromagnetic devices.

Electromagnetic Middle Ear Implants
The integral components of an electromagnetic are a magnet attached to the ossicular chain or the round window membrane and an energizing coil placed in the ear canal. When the energized coil generates signals corresponding to the acoustic input as received by the amplifier, the magnetic field causes the magnet to vibrate. This creates a fluctuating magnetic field which in turn causes movement of either the ossicular chain or the cochlear fluids directly. The chief advantage of this device is convenient implantation in a minor procedure via a trans tympanic approach (through the tympanic membrane)

Electromechanical Middle Ear Implant
This design was often classified as a subtype of electromagnetic device, and was developed as a solution to the problem of inconsistent, differing distances between the magnet and coil. The main drawback of this technique is structural complexity with a higher risk for device failure due to component wear or defect.

Totally Implanted (integrated) Cochlear Amplifier (TICA) [9]

A digitally programmable processor is implanted subcutaneously on the mastoid bone and can be charged transcutaneously within 90 minutes. The signal produced is transferred to a piezoelectric coupler which is in direct contact with the body of the incus. The device battery may last for approximately five years and mandates battery replacement every five years.

Bone Anchored Hearing Aid (BAHA)

This implantable device is embedded in the bone with a processor for external attachment. A BAHA device is helpful for problems with hearing in the middle or outer ear. BAHA devices are safe and effective in those with conductive or single-sided deafness or (unilateral) mixed sensorineural hearing loss.

CONTRACEPTIVE OR BIRTH CONTROL IMPLANTS (DEVICES)

A common, effective and reversible approach to birth control is intrauterine devices (IUD) and contraceptive implants, also known as long-acting reversible contraceptives (LARC). A hormonal contraceptive implant is a type of small, flexible, non-biodegradable plastic tube about the size of a match stick, implanted to prevent pregnancy and commonly inserted subcutaneously on the inner aspect of a woman's arm. The most advantageous feature of LARC is the prompt reversal of fertility soon after the implant removal from the body. Implantable contraceptives require very little maintenance.

Intrauterine Contraception [10]

Intrauterine contraceptive devices like copper T and levonorgestrel IUDs are 99% effective in avoiding unwanted pregnancies. Their main advantages are high efficacy, cost effectiveness, longer duration of action, rapidly reversibility of fertility and convenience for use.

Non-Hormonal or Copper T Intrauterine Device (IUD)

IUDs are non-hormonal "T"-shaped minute devices that the doctor inserts inside the uterus to provide contraception for ten years or more. An IUD has a polyethylene frame with copper wire wrapped around the vertical stem and two copper sleeves of copper, placed on each of the horizontal arms. Patient may experience heavier menstrual blood loss, more cramps and random spotting.

Hormonal IUD – Levonorgestrel Intrauterine System (LNG IUD)

Similar to copper T, the levonorgestrel IUD is another tiny T-shaped contraceptive instrument placed into the uterine cavity by a doctor with the help of an inserter. It may be left in the uterus for up to six years.

Hormonal Implants

These preloaded implants are soft, flexible, single or multiple, thin, non-biodegradable rod(s) that are inserted subcutaneously on the women's non-dominant upper arm only by a trained health care professional under strict aseptic conditions. Progestin is released in minute amounts into the body from the progestin-only birth control implant over the next three to five years. Progestin-based implants are excellent for breastfeeding women and immediate postpartum administration. The chief drawback is their cost (Table 5.2).

Some experience irritation, infection or scarring at the implant site. Hormonal implants may disrupt uterine bleeding patterns, and an irregular period is a common reason for discontinuing the implant. Other side effects of contraceptive implants are acne, breast tenderness, uterine cramps, spotting, abnormal vaginal discharges, migraine headaches, weight gain, depression, mood swings and increased risk of blood clots; thrombi and emboli formation can be deleterious to the lungs, heart and brain. Throbbing headaches or any signs of a blood clot, such as chest pain, lower leg pain, breathing difficulties, tingling, malaise, inability to speak coherently or improper vision might call for immediate medical attention. Birth control implants are **not** recommended in those with a history of thromboembolic disorders, bleeding disorders, liver and kidney disease, undiagnosed vaginal bleeding, breast cancers and other hormone-dependent cancers, etc. It is imperative to screen for hypertension, diabetes, hyperlipidemia and gall bladder problems and check medical history for seizures, migraine and any relevant medical problems before the hormonal

TABLE 5.2   Types of Hormonal Norplants

NORPLANT 1	JADELLE (NORPLANT 2)	NEXPLANON AND IMPLANON
Comprised of six silastic rods of levonorgestrel 36 mg each	Two rods of levonorgestrel 75 mg each	Single rod – etonogestrel 68 mg
Replaced every 5 years	Effective contraception for 5 years	Replaced every 3 years Commonly used nowadays
Mechanism of action: acts by thickening cervical mucus, inhibiting ovulation by acting on pituitary feedback circuit	MOA: thickens cervical mucus, inhibiting ovulation by acting on pituitary feedback circuit	MOA: thickens cervical mucus, inhibiting ovulation by acting on pituitary feedback circuit

implants are prescribed. Case reports of contraceptive failure with efavirenz, carbamazepine and other cyp 450 inducers raise caution while prescribing concomitant drugs in implanted women [11].

HERNIA SURGICAL MESH IMPLANTS

Surgical mesh implants are flat sheets of prosthetic material obtained from synthetic materials or animal tissue and are an indispensable surgical tool providing additional support to promote the healing of fragile, damaged tissue in conditions like hernia. A hernia mesh serves as a flexible scaffold in surgery for hernia repair, reinforcing the weakened muscular walls, averting the fall of organs through the hernial sac and thereby reducing recurrence. A surgical mesh ideally facilitates the repair of peritoneal defects like plugging the hole, allowing regrowth of the tissue and peritoneal regeneration, and augmenting the healing process [12]. The gold standard material of hernia meshes is polypropylene (PP). Permanent synthetic PP meshes offer several advantages as they are inert, biocompatible, non-immunogenic and non-cancerogenic. Surgical mesh improves patient outcomes by minimizing operative time and shortening recovery time (Figure 5.4) [13].

Types of Mesh

Synthetic Surgical Mesh

These "classical" or "traditional" meshes were the first to be used and are the least expensive. Synthetic meshes may be absorbable, non-absorbable or a combination of absorbable and non-absorbable materials

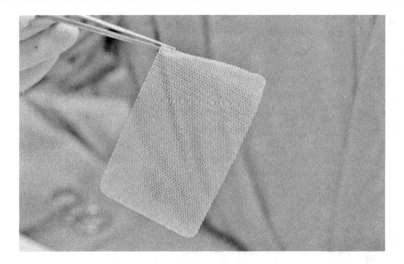

FIGURE 5.4   Herinia meshes.

and available as knitted and non-knitted or woven forms. Absorbable mesh material wears off over time; durability may be lost, and hence they are not suitable for long-term hernia repair reinforcement. As mesh degradation speeds up, new tissue will grow and strengthen the repaired tissue or scar the tissue. Non-resorbable mesh may remain standing indefinitely in the body and provides permanent reinforcement to the repaired hernia and is considered a permanent implant. Synthetic degradable materials were utilized in open abdominal wounds with decreased adhesion risks. Fully resorbable meshes minimize inflammation, but durability may be lost early due to progressive degradation of the mesh, resulting in the recurrence of hernia. Newer synthetic degradable meshes useful in hernia repair degrade over several months and have reduced recurrence, infection and pain (Figure 5.5) [13].

SYNTHETIC DEGRADABLE MESH	COMPONENT	DEGRADATION TIME
Vicryl.	Polyglactin.	1–3 months
Dexon	Polyglycolic acid	1–3 months
Gore Bio-A mesh	Polyglycolic acid Trimethylene carbonate	6 months
Phasix	Poly-4-hydroxybutyrate	12–18 months
Tigr Matrix	Polyglycolide/polylactide/trimethylene carbonate	Partially degrades in 4 months, completely degrades after 3 years

(a–e) scanning electron microscope images showing respective mesh textile structures. (e–h) scanning electron microscope images showing respective mesh textile structures.

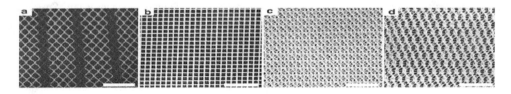

FIGURE 5.5   Synthetic meshes. (A) Polypropylene surgical mesh. (B) Propylene second generation mesh: 2D macroporous mesh. (C) second generation: 3D macroporous polyester flat sheet mesh. (D) Third generation: polyester composite mesh with a resorbable collagen barrier.

TABLE 5.3 Comparison of Advantages and Disadvantages of Classes of Mesh

CLASS OF MESH	ADVANTAGES	DISADVANTAGES
Synthetic • Non-degradable	Inexpensive Low recurrence rates Easy to shape intraoperative Long-term stability	Not recommended for contaminated or infected fields. Risk of infection, discomfort and adhesions higher
• Degradable	Fewer long-term complications than non-degradable Less expensive than biological	Recurrence high Insufficient evidence for newer meshes
Biological • Degradable	Useful in complex/infected sites	High recurrence rates. Expensive

Biological Mesh

Biological meshes obtained from allografts (human tissue) and xenografts (animal – porcine (from pig) or bovine (from cow)) are biodegradable and are less infection prone. They are biocompatible and less immunogenic and inflammatory. Human dermal scaffoldings have higher recurrences due to their lower mechanical strength in comparison to meshes of synthetic origin. A novel mesh design is the "drug-loaded mesh" where the mesh is coated with antibiotics and antiseptics to reduce infection (Table 5.3).

Like any medical device, hernia meshes also carry benefits and certain risks. The most crucial problem linked with hernial repair is the risk of peritoneal adhesions (scar-like tissue sticks together) between the mesh and the abdominal viscera. Other common and potential mesh-associated complications after hernia repair with mesh are infection, pain, bleeding, hernia recurrence, fistula and, rarely, mesh migration (extrusion) and mesh shrinkage (contraction). Bulging in the area where implantation was performed indicates that the mesh has dislodged (mesh migration) leading to inflammation. The FDA recalled certain mesh products because of associated complications like perforation and bowel obstruction in cases of hernia repair with surgical mesh [14].

HIP IMPLANTS

Deterioration of the hip joint may lead to joint stiffness, pain and effortful walking, and hip replacement (arthroplasty) options may be recommended where the bony joint structure may be replaced by prosthesis. Hip implants are medical implants employed to reinstate hip mobility and function and thus provide pain relief in those with rheumatoid arthritis, osteoarthritis, osteonecrosis, bone tumors and other hip diseases or injuries. Prosthetic implants must be durable and inert, must not provoke any unwanted tissue reaction and must permit extraordinary low-friction movement at the articulation.

Three Basic Components of Hip Implants

1. A stem – inserted into the femur.
2. A ball (femoral head component) attached to the femur top – replaces the head of the femur.
3. A cup (acetabular component) attached to a socket in the pelvis – implanted into the pelvis (Figure 5.6).

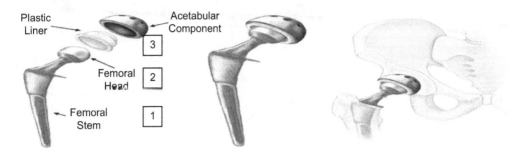

FIGURE 5.6   Parts of a hip implant.

Types of Implants

Four categories of total hip replacement devices are available:

- Metal-on-polyethylene (MoP) implants: consist of a metal ball and plastic (polyethylene) socket or with a plastic lining. MoP implants can give rise to debris (osteolysis), eventually causing implant failure.
- Ceramic-on-polyethylene (CoP): has a ceramic ball with a polyethylene socket or lined with polythene.
- Ceramic-on-ceramic (CoC): this type of device has a ceramic head and a ceramic lining on the socket. Loosening of the lining and component fractures result in device failure.
- Ceramic-on-metal (CoM): this is a new design with a ceramic ball and a socket with a metal lining (Figure 5.7).

Metal-on-Metal (MoM) Hip Implants [15]

These have a ball, a stem and a metal shell, all made of metal materials. The benefits of MoM hip implants are as follows:

- Corrosion-resistant metal alloys reduce implant degradation when the ball and socket rub against each other.
- Less dislocation of the femur (due to the larger head size of MoM total hip implants) and device fracture.
- MoM hip implants have been shown to have high implant survivorship (Figure 5.8).

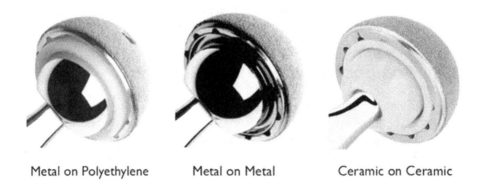

Metal on Polyethylene   Metal on Metal   Ceramic on Ceramic

FIGURE 5.7   Various types of hip implant devices.

Metal-on-Metal Hip Implant Systems

Total Hip Replacement   Hip Resurfacing

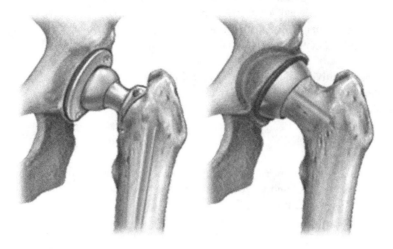

FIGURE 5.8   Total hip replacement by MoM implant.

Fixed Bearing Hip Implants [16]

It has a stem thrust into the femur, a ball replacing the femur head and a fixed shell lining the hip socket. A large number of hip implants belong to this type.

Hybrid Total Hip Implants

It has either the cup or stem part inserted without cement and the other component cemented and has high stability.

Mobile-Bearing Total Hip Implants

The insert attaches to the acetabulum tightly yet can move a little as the hip moves.

Indications for Hip Implants

- For those with excruciating pain with irreversibly damaged joints, joint instability.
- Rheumatoid arthritis, severe osteoarthritis, congenital hip defects.
- Femoral neck fracture, pathologic fractures from metastatic cancer.
- Previous reconstructive surgery failure because of non-union, avascular necrosis, etc.

Contraindications for Hip Implants

- Recent or remote infection.
- Age under 60 years, especially when alternative surgery is available.
- No manual maneuvers tried so far.

The FDA classifies MoM implants as Class III, higher risk medical devices. Complications and adverse events after surgery may be encountered such as joint infection, bone fracture, chronic pain, vein thrombosis, pulmonary embolism, osteolysis, hip dislocation, loosening or breakage of device, local nerve damage, different length of the leg, bone growth beyond normal edges of the bone, etc. Joint inflammation and local tissue damage may be associated with metal wear debris from MoM implants. Systemic effects of higher blood metal ion levels (chromium, cobalt, molybdenum, titanium) result from device wear in MoM hip implants including:

- General hypersensitivity reaction (e.g., skin rash)
- Cardiomyopathy, neurological changes including sensory changes
- Psychological status change (including depression or cognitive impairment)
- Renal function impairment
- Thyroid dysfunction (including neck discomfort, fatigue, weight gain and feeling cold)

Soft tissue imaging and metal ion testing are necessary for assessing hip implant complications. Their lifespan is commonly between 10 and 15 years; surgery may be required to remove, repair or replace the device in case of excessive wear out.

PHAKIC INTRAOCULAR LENSES (PIOL)

Phakic intraocular lenses or phakic lenses are soft, clear, flexible implantable lenses implanted permanently in the eye, bringing down the necessity for reading glasses or contact lenses. The term "phakic" points to the implantation of an artificial intraocular lens without disturbing or removing the natural crystalline lens. During the PIOL implantation surgery, a small incision is made in the front of the eye through which the phakic lens, made of clear synthetic plastic or silicone, is inserted and placed right in front of or just behind the iris; it doesn't need to be cleaned (Figure 5.9).

Types of Intraocular Implant

Angle Supported PIOLS

These are inserted in the anterior chamber, right in front of the iris. Novel PIOL design is devoid of corneal endothelial cell loss which was higher with the older versions. Patient might experience distortion of the pupil, glare and problems with night vision.

Iris Fixated PIOLs

These are also fixed in the anterior chamber and have distinctive claws to attach to the iris; thus the lens is pinned in the correct place.

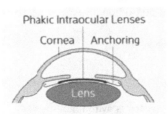
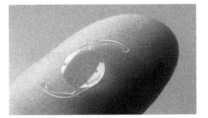

FIGURE 5.9   Phakic lens.

Posterior Chamber PIOLs

Unlike the previous PIOLs, this intraocular implant fixation is in the posterior chamber, located between the iris behind and the crystalline lens up front.

Indications

PIOLs are approved for the rectification of refractive errors like myopia (nearsightedness), presbyopia, myopic astigmatism beyond the range of laser vision correction, keratoconus, post-corneal transplant, pseudophakia for the correction of residual refraction, post-laser vision correction, etc.

Contraindications

- Eye problems like cataracts, corneal diseases or recurrent inflammation in the eye (uveitis).
- Phakic intraocular lens can elevate intraocular pressure; hence PIOL is not advised in glaucoma patients.

Complications of PIOL

Infection, endophthalmitis, uveitis and eye discomfort are common in the early months. Irreversible corneal damage by anterior chamber implants, loss of vision due to nerve damage due to a rapid rise in intraocular tension post-operation, and retinal damage and retinal detachment have been reported. Visible red blotches (subconjunctival hemorrhages) may be seen temporarily. The transient elevation of IOP can precipitate glaucoma.

UROGYNECOLOGIC SURGICAL MESH IMPLANTS

Surgical meshes are indicated in urogynecologic surgical procedures in pelvic organ prolapse (POP) and stress urinary incontinence (SUI) in males and females. Urogynecological mesh implants are permanent prostheses to repair the weak vaginal wall in POP or support the urethra or bladder neck in case of SUI and in colorectal (bowel) functional disorders. The main surgical procedures to treat pelvic floor disorders with surgical mesh are:

1. Mesh sling to treat SUI
2. Transvaginal mesh to treat POP [17]
3. Transabdominal mesh to treat POP

The surgical meshes approved for surgical procedures are commonly made up of non-absorbable synthetic polypropylene. These abide lifelong in the body and provide perpetual reinforcement of strength to the urogynecologic repair whereas absorbable meshes may disintegrate and do not fortify the repair site for a prolonged time. As the material is resorbed, new tissue grows in its place, making the repair sturdier. A larger surface area of mesh is needed for prolapse repair than for SUI.

Mesh Sling to Treat SUI [18]

SUI is the most common type of urinary incontinence in women. In this surgery, a surgical mesh in the form of a "sling" (tape) is attached permanently to hold the urethra or bladder neck up, thereby correcting the issue of SUI. Male slings are used to treat stress urinary incontinence after prostatectomy. The synthetic sling can be either adjustable or fixed. Placed under the urethra, male slings compress and support the urethra and reduce leakage by fully closing the bladder. It is designed to resist traction and allow complete tissue ingrowth (Figure 5.10) [18].

In females with SUI, vaginal sling surgery is simpler and easy to perform, having excellent overall success, durable cure rates, a shorter recovery period and minimal postoperative complications. Mid-urethral slings (MUS) are the gold standard for the surgical treatment of female SUI.

Tension-Free Vaginal Tape (TVT)

This polypropylene-meshed tape covered by a plastic sheet, propped up by two stainless-steel needles on the edges, is a recent introduction for the treatment of SUI. The TVT device is placed at the mid-urethra.

Transvaginal Mesh for Pelvic Organ Prolapse

Pelvic organ prolapse (POP) refers to the drooping of pelvic organs like the uterus (uterine prolapse), bladder (cystocele, most commonly involved organ in POP), urethra (urethrocele), cervix, vagina, (vaginal vault prolapse), rectum (rectocele) and small intestine (nterocele). A transvaginal mesh is a net-like implant used for uplifting, anchoring a feeble vaginal wall or keeping the urethra or bladder neck in its place (Figure 5.11) [17].

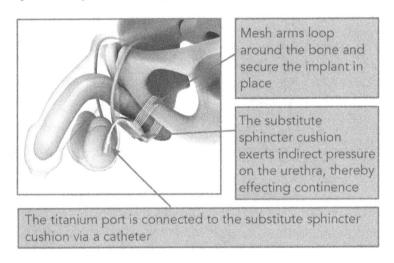

Mesh arms loop around the bone and secure the implant in place

The substitute sphincter cushion exerts indirect pressure on the urethra, thereby effecting continence

The titanium port is connected to the substitute sphincter cushion via a catheter

FIGURE 5.10   Male sling.

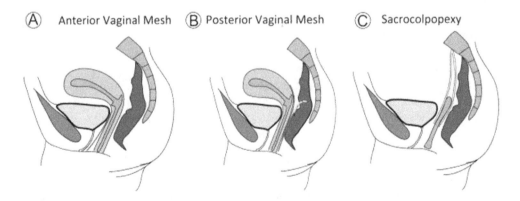

(A) Anterior Vaginal Mesh   (B) Posterior Vaginal Mesh   (C) Sacrocolpopexy

FIGURE 5.11   Various placements of vaginal mesh.

Vaginal mesh complications include:

- Intraoperative injury/safety issues like visceral and urinary tract injury and bleeding.
- Postoperative complications may include mesh erosion through vagina, scarring, infection, mesh extrusion and mesh contraction (shrinkage).
- Voiding dysfunction, bladder, bowel, blood vessel perforation.
- Sexual dysfunction/pain, vaginal/pelvic pain, pain in the buttock, leg pain.
- Failure and recurrence of prolapse or incontinence.

Women who have received transvaginal mesh for the surgical repair of prolapse must have annual or routine health follow-ups and periodic medical monitoring; any vaginal bleeding or discharge, pelvic or groin pain, or pain during sexual intercourse must be notified to the doctor. As of now, no FDA-approved surgical meshes [19] are marketed for POP or SUI in America, as the benefit-risk profile of mesh remains fairly questionable.

DRUG DELIVERING IMPLANTS

Conventional routes of drug administration have several limitations that are overcome considerably by the newer drug delivery systems (NDDS) like the implantable drug delivery systems (IDDS) which are placed inside or on the surface of the body for appropriately administering therapeutic substances at a steady rate, undoubtedly enhancing patient compliance and quality of life. With IDDS the drug release rate can be controlled precisely, releasing drugs locally to the targeted specific organ or tissue with minimal side effects. IDDS may be categorized into biodegradable and non-biodegradable implants. All biodegradable and non-biodegradable implants have a drug incorporated in them with sufficient reservoir backup to ensure steady and controlled delivery of the drug locally according to the requirements of the patient and do not affect the whole body, with minimal side effects to other healthy organs and tissues. Non-biodegradable devices can be refilled with medication (e.g., via injection), and upon removal, the drug effects may be quickly reversible.

Globally, IDDS-like hormonal implants for contraception, cardiovascular stents, insulin delivery devices for diabetes, pain management, ophthalmology and orthopedic drug delivering implants are available on the market. The special targeted action is most likely to be used in cardiology and oncology drugs.

Advantages of Implantable Drug Delivery Systems [20]

- Local drug delivery and targeted delivery to a limited specific location with higher bioavailability and reduced dose requirement. Monitoring and medical observation may be marginalized.
- Patient acceptability and tolerance improved as a result of compliance.
- Systemic side effects are minimal; fluctuations in drug concentration in the plasma are avoided.
- Drug stability is improved due to bypass of first pass metabolism.
- In case of any adverse reaction or intolerance to the drug, implant removal can cause termination of drug delivery.
- Computerized or sensor-linked pumps may deliver drugs intermittently in response to various factors such as cardiac rhythm, metabolic needs, etc.

Disadvantages of Implantable Drug Delivery Systems

- Invasive; hence scar formation is seen.
- Osmotic pump actions and non-biodegradable implants must be surgically removed when the therapy is finished.
- Implant extrusion, migration and failure: surgical removal of the device is needed.
- Biocompatibility and safety issues are still posing threats for safe drug delivery through IDDS.
- Adverse reactions: as a high concentration of drug is delivered to the implantation site with the help of the device, there is always a chance of adverse reaction due to this local high concentration.

Clinical Applications of IDDS [21]

Contraceptive Implants

Levonorgestrel sub-dermal implants are surgically inserted subcutaneously into the inner aspect of the non-dominant hand of females for contraceptive purposes and work for up to five years. Levonorgestrel Sub-dermal (Norplant) implants are comprised of six identical drug-impregnated silicone rods. Implanon, Nexplanon and the newer contraceptive implants contain etonogestrel.

Ocular Implants

An ocular insert (ocusert) is loaded with pilocarpine in a core reservoir, covered by a rate-controlling membrane, with seven days' lifespan. It is well tolerated in adult glaucoma patients where intraocular tension is reduced with minimal side effects; whereas in geriatric patients, it is poorly tolerated (Figure 5.12).

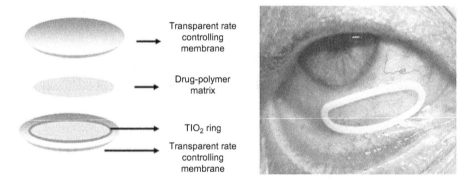

FIGURE 5.12 Photograph of patient with ocusert in lower cul-de-sac of eye.

Insulin Pumps

These are computerized mini pumps mimicking the insulin delivery function of the human pancreas. Usually, a basal insulin rate in the pump is configured by the treating physician. Some devices have in-built bolus calculators to estimate the insulin dose needed at mealtime based on the patient blood sugar levels and the consumed quantity of carbohydrates. Patch pumps are directly worn on the body and have a reservoir, pump and infusion set all incorporated in a tiny box, wirelessly controlled by a separate device permitting insulin delivery shots from the patch. Some pumps monitor blood sugar levels throughout the day (Figure 5.13).

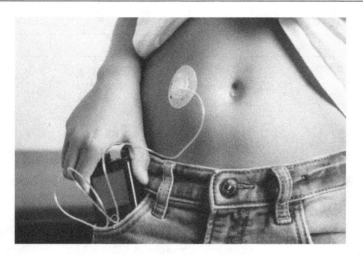

FIGURE 5.13   Insulin pumps.

Cardiac Implants – Implantable Drug-Eluting Devices [22]

Endoluminal metallic stents are used for percutaneous transluminal angioplasty (PTCA) in coronary artery disease (CAD) patients (Figure 5.14). These thwart fibrosis and clot formation and could potentially obstruct the stented artery (restenosis). To mitigate restenosis and also promote endothelial healing, attempts at the local delivery of antiproliferative drugs via stents were made. Drug-eluting stents (DES) are available delivering immunosuppressants like sirolimus, everolimus, biolimus, tacrolimus, pimecrolimus, paclitaxel, docetaxel, CD34 antibody, anti-vascular endothelial growth factor (anti VEGF), etc. (Table 5.4).

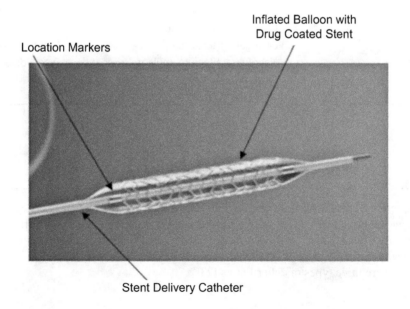

FIGURE 5.14   Cardiac implant.

TABLE 5.4 Summary of Drugs Delivered through IDDS

ROUTE	DRUG DELIVERED	INDICATION
Subcutaneous – sialistic implant	Norplant, Jadelle – levonorgestrel	Contraception
	Implanon, Nexplanon – etonogestrel	
SC – pellet implantation	Testosterone	Hormone replacement, deficiency
	Desoxy corticosterone acetate (DOCA)	Addison's disease
Vaginal ring	Medroxyprogesterone acetate	Contraception
	Nuvaring – Etonorgestrel, estradiol	
	Estring – etonogestrel	Menopause
	Levonorgestrel	Contraception
	Tenofovir	HIV prevention
	Glycerine	Vaginal dryness
Intrauterine implants	Copper T, levonorgestrel IUD	Contraception
Intraocular implants	Ocusert – pilocarpine	Open angle glaucoma
	Retisert – fluocinolone	Non-infectious uveitis
	Vitrasert – ganciclovir	CMV retinitis in AIDS
Subcutaneous	Tenofovir alafenamide	HIV prophylaxis
	Med-Launch, Risperdal consta – risperidone	Schizophrenia
	Synchromed - morphine	Cancer pain
	Hydromorphine	Chronic neuropathic pain
	Baclofen	Muscle spasticity
	Probuphine – buprenorphine HCl	Opioid abuse deterrence
Intravesical	LiRIS program – lidocaine	Interstitial cystitis
	GemRIS – gemcitabine	Non-muscle invasive Bladder cancer
Subcutaneous	Vantas – histrelin acetate	Prostate cancer
	Zoladex – goserelin	
	Prostap – leuprolide	
Intra-tumoral	Gliadel wafers – carmustine	Primary malignant glioma
	Oncogel – paclitaxel	Esophageal cancer
Subcutaneous	NanoPortal titanium implant – exenatide	Type II diabetes
	Encaptra – human embryonic stem cells (pancreatic cells)	Type I diabetes

DEFIBRILLATORS

Defibrillators, referred to as defibs, are devices that send a high-voltage electric shock (called defibrillation) to someone having a heart attack, to restore a normal heartbeat to prevent or correct arrhythmias. This device can reinstate normal cardiac functioning if the heart suddenly stops, essentially reviving life in an emergency.

Types: There are three types of defibrillators [23].

Automated External Defibrillators (AEDs)

AEDs, generally used in public spaces, are lightweight, portable battery-operated devices, which send an external shock to cardiac tissue thus restoring a normal rhythm in a sudden heart attack. These devices have sticky pads with electrodes (sensors) that can be fixed onto the chest and send information regarding the heart's rhythm to a computer digital screen which scrutinizes the cardiac rhythm and if necessary, delivers the electric shock via the external pads attached to the chest.

Implantable Cardioverter Defibrillators (ICDs)

An implantable cardiac defibrillator tracks ventricular tachyarrhythmia (rapid heartbeat) and delivers a shock from inside the body. The components of ICD are a small-sized battery-powered pulse generator and electronic circuitry. This device is fitted surgically in the chest below the collar bone, where it checks and sends a jolt of electric shock to correct the arrhythmia. ICDs are similar to pacemakers delivering low energy, but differ from them in delivering high-energy electrical shocks. ICDs are beneficial in cardiac failure as they can boost the cardiac pumping capacity. Incorporated into a cardiac resynchronization therapy defibrillator (CRT-D), these devices help resynchronize both the ventricular contractions and exhibit defibrillation properties. Patients must be advised to keep phones away from the ICD implantation site, use the opposite ear while on the phone and not keep mobile phones in a pocket over the device (Figure 5.15) [23].

Subcutaneous ICD (S-ICD) is another type of ICD placed on the side of the chest, under the armpit, with a single lead implanted under the skin. The electrodes are attached outside the heart and deliver a shock in fatal arrhythmias. ICDs are recommended for patients with high continuous risk of sudden cardiac arrest.

Wearable Cardioverter Defibrillators (WCDs)

WCDs are rechargeable external devices with a belt attached to a light-weight vest that can be worn under the clothing all day long. A portable unit is present comprising a generator and recorder. This device has skin-attached electrodes (sensors) that are connected by wires to a monitor that continuously records the heart rate, and when needed the electrodes deliver a shock repeatedly up to five times. Like ICDs, WCDs too deliver low- and high-energy shocks but WCDs are non-invasive (Figure 5.16).

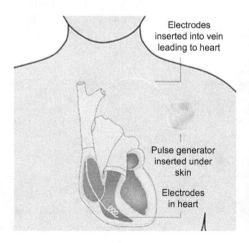
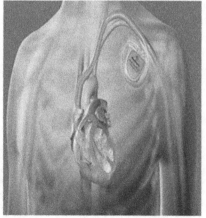

FIGURE 5.15   ICDs.

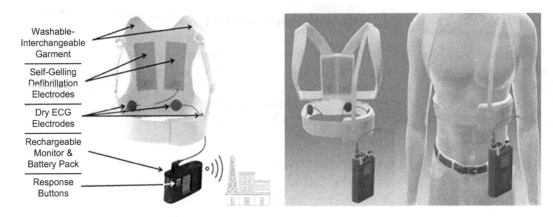

FIGURE 5.16   Wearable cardiac defibrillators (WCD).

PACEMAKERS

A pacemaker is a small life-saving electronic device used when there is an intrinsic cardiac electrical conduction disorder. It paces the heart by sending low-energy electrical pulses used to rectify any irregularity in heartbeats known as arrhythmias, helping initiate a normal heart rate and rhythm. They also help synchronize atrioventricular contractions so the heart can efficiently pump more blood if heart failure sets in. Pacemakers may be used short-term (temporary) or for a prolonged period (permanent). A temporary pacemaker is implanted through a vein in the neck and is positioned outside the body, whereas permanent pacemakers are commonly implanted in the chest (Figure 5.17) [24].

Traditional (Transvenous) Pacemakers

These transmit electrical pulses through wires (leads). The device has the ability to transmit data remotely to a doctor. This data could be used to reset a pacemaker for improved performance. A rate-responsive pacemaker has sensors that detect changes in the patient's physical activity and automatically adjust the pacing rate to cater to the body's metabolic needs. Single-chamber and dual-chamber pacemakers send pulses to the right side of the heart. A biventricular pacemaker sends pulses to both ventricles and atrium, coordinating electrical signaling between the two ventricles to help the heart pump blood. This pacemaker is also called a cardiac resynchronization therapy (CRT) device.

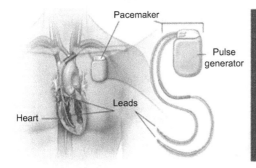
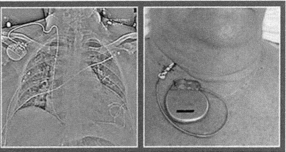

FIGURE 5.17   Pacemaker implantation.

The three main parts of a traditional pacing instrument are:

1. **Implantable pulse generator (IPG)** – generates the impulses with the help of a battery power source and circuitry controls pacemaker operations. This is inserted either in the chest or abdomen and is linked to the electronic circuit through the wires placed in the cardiac chambers.
2. **Leads (insulated wires)** are implanted inside the veins and transmit the pulses from the IPG to the heart and vice versa.
3. **Electrodes (cathode, anode)** – a conductor located at the end of the lead records the heartbeat, identifies abnormal heartbeat, and if required delivers an electrical shock to make the heart pace normal again.

Wireless Pacemakers (Leadless Cardiac Pacemakers – LCP)

Wireless pacemakers are innovative, small implantable cardiac pacing devices that can be placed in the heart without invasive surgery. They are smaller than conventional pacemakers and have all of the electrodes and the pulse generator in one unit. After it is set in the right place, the LCP transmits signals to the right ventricle and monitors overall cardiac functioning.

Indications for Pacemakers

- Heart failure.
- When a patient has a permanent or temporary reduced heart rate as in chronic atrial fibrillation with slow ventricular response.
- Fibrosis or sclerotic changes of cardiac conduction system.
- Symptomatic AV or ventricular conduction disturbance.
- Tachyarrhythmia that doesn't respond to medication.
- Third degree AV block, sick sinus syndrome.
- Hypersensitive carotid sinus syndrome.

Possible complications from a pacemaker may include:

- Hypersensitivity reaction to the device or allergy to medicines used.
- Thrombotic risks, infection around the device pocket or its extensions.
- Device failure and device-related problems. Sometimes wires get damaged, dislocated or stop working partially or completely. Misplaced cables can cause vessel or heart valve blockages and can cause perforation. Wireless pacemakers can be extruded. Always watch out for any signs of pacemaker malfunction.
- Pacemaker syndrome is when only one ventricle is stimulated and the rhythmic upper and lower chamber contraction synchrony is mismatched; consequently blood will be streamed erroneously.
- Some may develop cardiac arrest, tachyarrhythmia or cardiac-related issues post-device implantation.
- Ventricular hypertrophy and the overgrowing tissue around the device can form a hardened scar around the wires or device.
- Pleural effusion, pericarditis and pneumothorax may be seen in some patients because of fluid or air trapped around the lungs.

Precautions

Medical recommendations suggest avoiding any equipment as it may impede the pacemaker function, for example, MRI, radiotherapy, lithotripsy, electro-cautery and ultrasonic scaling equipment used by dentists, electric arc welders or going very close to high-power radar or electrical installations.

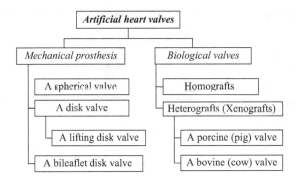

FIGURE 5.18   Artificial heart valves.

The pacemaker batteries work well for about five to ten years, depending on the pacemaker type and frequency of device activation. Most pacemakers have an elective replacement indicator (ERI) giving an alarm signal indicating when the battery is approaching depletion.

Artificial or Prosthetic Heart Valves (PHV) [24]

An artificial heart valve is a one-way valve inserted in the heart to replace a dysfunctional heart valve (valvular heart disease – aortic, mitral stenosis, regurgitation). Artificial cardiac valves can be broadly classified into mechanical heart valves, bioprosthetic tissue valves and engineered tissue valves – homografts and heterografts (bovine, porcine) (Figure 5.18).

- The typical lifespan of a mechanical prosthesis is for decades whereas the lifespan of biological prostheses is only 10–12 years.

Complications of Artificial Heart Valves

- Infection.
- Calcification can occur primarily in tissue valves where deposits of calcium phosphorus minerals cause stenosis.
- Device failure, tissue overgrowth, local reactions, tissue atrophy, sometimes requiring replacement.
- Thromboembolism, stroke and heart attack risks are high; hence lifetime anticoagulant may be advised.
- Endocarditis.

RETINAL IMPLANTS

Retinal implants are innovative implantable electronic devices which help to regain vision remarkably or improve visual perception in degenerative retinal defects like retinitis pigmentosa (RP) or age-related macular degeneration (AMD). For a retinal electronic implant to work well, the patient should have an intact optic nerve, some functional retinal cells and a visual cortex as the implant elicits neural activity in the functional retinal neurons by detecting light (bypassing degenerated photoreceptors) and converting it into electrical stimuli using artificial devices. The location of electrode implantation may be epiretinal, subretinal or suprachoroidal.

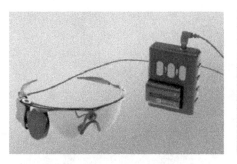
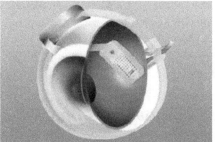

FIGURE 5.19   Retinal prosthesis system.

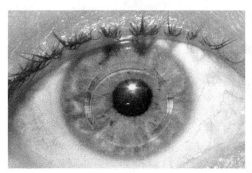
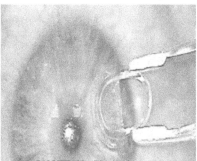

FIGURE 5.20   Intrastromal corneal ring segment and full-ring corneal implant.

Retinal prostheses may be implanted in the eye with challenged visual acuity and have both extraocular and intraocular components [25]. The extraocular part has a small camera that is mounted on a pair of eyeglasses. A visual processing unit (VPU) and a coil attached to the sidearm of the glasses transmit signals wirelessly via radio frequency telemetry to internal components. Internally, on the scleral surface is attached the receiver and transmitter (transmitting coil) and a case containing electronic components; with the help of a tack, a series of electrodes are fixed on the damaged retinal surface; they stimulate the retinal photoreceptor cells. The tiny eye glasses-mounted camera delivers wireless electrical signals to the retinal electrode array, which are further transmitted to the optic nerve and processed by the brain to induce visual perception. This device is quite expensive, yet acceptable because it lasts a lifetime (Figure 5.19) [26].

Corneal Ring Implants

Intracorneal implants (corneal inlays) are flexible synthetic implants used in corneal ectasia (abnormal corneal thinning) by delaying or deferring the need for keratoplasty or corneal transplant. Such ring implants are inserted in a minimally invasive procedure and can flatten and reshape the cornea to achieve correction in refractive errors. The FDA has approved corneal ring implants for the correction of mild nearsightedness. The main categories of corneal implants are intracorneal ring segments (ICRS) or incomplete ring and intracorneal continuous complete ring (Figure 5.20).

Indications

1. Corneal implants can be used for reconstructive purposes to reshape, preserve corneal integrity in cases of thinning of the cornea, descemetoceles or to reconstruct the eye like after a corneal perforation.

2. In corneal edema, pseudophakic bullous keratopathy, keratoconus, corneal degeneration, keratoglobus and dystrophy, as well as scarring due to keratitis and trauma, implants can improve uncorrected vision acuity.

3. Corneal scars may present with whitish or opaque cornea and may be cosmetically corrected using intracorneal implants.

Risks of Corneal Ring Implantation

The majority of patients tolerate corneal ring implantation generally well. Infection, swelling in the eye, chronic eye pain, keratitis, perforation of eye, movement or extrusion of the ring, night halos or glare may be seen sometimes.

Keratoprosthesis (Artificial Cornea) [27,28]

A keratoprosthesis (Kpro) is employed when conventional keratoplasty fails; hence a diseased, damaged or opaque cornea is replaced with an artificial cornea. The Kpro design is similar to an ocular lens with an optic and a haptic. The optical part helps in viewing; it is a polymethyl methacrylate (PMMA) cylinder placed in the cornea through a central opening like an optically clear window and retained in place. The haptic segment determines the type of the prosthesis, that is, biointegrated, non-biointegrated or biocompatible. Kpro should be the last resort in bilaterally end stage corneal blindness. Post-surgical adverse effects include infection, chronic inflammation, glaucoma and tissue necrosis. Osteo-Odonto-Keratoprosthesis (OOKP) devices have reported an increased rate of device extrusion (Figure 5.21).

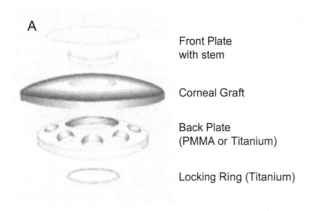

A

Front Plate with stem

Corneal Graft

Back Plate (PMMA or Titanium)

Locking Ring (Titanium)

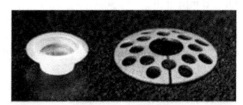
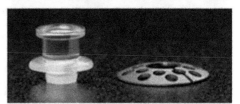

FIGURE 5.21 Keratoprosthesis.

DENTAL IMPLANTS

Dental implants (oral or endosseous implants) are the most popular treatment modality for replacing missing or diseased teeth (single, multiple or the entire jaw) and help restore their aesthetic and physiological function. Fixed or removable dental prostheses are surgically anchored in the oral cavity. These are made of biocompatible alloplastic material.

Parts of a Dental Implant

- A screw-like part fits the implant into the jawbone just like an anchor.
- An abutment bridges the artificial tooth and the dental implant.
- The crown part functioning like natural teeth is customized for each individual, matching the teeth color.

Altogether the screw, abutment and crown give a "new tooth" feel, keep the tooth aligned and enable proper eating and a confident smile.

Types of Dental Implants [29]

Transdental Implant (Endodontic Implant)
This is also called an endodontic stabilizer because it helps stabilize a mobile tooth. It may be regarded as a metallic extension of the root as it increases the root-to-crown ratio. It replaces the missing tooth and also gives better stability in the arch and preserves the remaining natural tooth.

Transosteal Implant (Mandibular Staple Implant or Transmandibular Implant)
This has a metallic layer with pins for holding onto the inferior mandible edge and two transosteal pins passing through the entire mandible. Eventually these two pins protruding through the gums can anchor an overdenture-type prosthesis (Figure 5.22).

Subperiostal Implant
This is inserted below the periosteum with the bony cortex overlying and is composed of a subperiosteal dental implant substructure, abutment and implant superstructure.

Endosteal Dental Implant
This is embedded in the basal bone to support the dental prosthesis and transect into the cortical plate (Figure 5.23) [29].

Advantages of Dental Implants

- **Aesthetic**: as the dental implant emerges directly from the soft tissue, a natural appearance of the tooth is provided, boosting the aesthetic value.
- **Bone preservation:** in addition to the aesthetic correction, these devices stimulate healthy bone development like a natural tooth and prevent facial collapse as seen in multiple teeth loss.
- **Functional improvement:** dental prosthesis design minimizes the noxious effect on the residual ridge as well as improves the chewing efficiency of the dental implant compared to other prosthetic replacements.
- Since artificial dental implants don't need to be taken out and sanitized every night, they provide comfort that feels natural and convenient.
- **Stability and retention**: because of osseintegration and bone remodeling, endosseous implants are highly stable (not moving loosely) and retentive compared to other retentive dental elements.
- They lower the risk of developing cavities and sensitivity issues in nearby teeth.

Disadvantages of Dental Implants

- More expensive than other methods of tooth replacement.
- Require more healing time and complicated fabrication procedures.

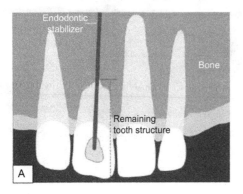
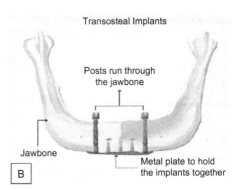

FIGURE 5.22 (A) Transdental implant. (B) Transosteal implant.

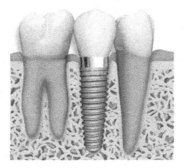
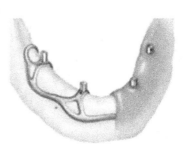

FIGURE 5.23 Endosteal implant, Subperiosteal implant.

Indications for Dental Implants

1. They are used as an alternative to complete dentures when we have completely edentulous patients who are intolerant of conventional prostheses for any reason.
2. When there is only one missing tooth and the adjacent healthy teeth need to have some of their structure reduced in order to prepare for an implant, they are used as an alternative to fixed prostheses.
3. They are used as an alternative to partial dentures when the patient refuses to use a removable type of prosthesis and is in a challenging prosthetic situation.
4. They help in retaining maxillofacial prostheses like those used in the ears, eyes and obturators.

Contraindications to Dental Implants

Oral implants must not be ventured on patients with unregulated diabetic, coagulation disorders or poor oral hygiene, heavy smokers, those on steroids or patients frequently exposed to radiation, history of mental illness and diseases of hard or soft tissue. It is perilous for patients under 18 years of age to receive this prosthesis because their bone development is not yet completed. At an extremely tender age, it is better to wait till attaining complete dental growth before inserting dental implants.

PENILE IMPLANTS

A penile prosthesis implant is a device that simulates an erection by causing penile rigidity. A surgically implanted penile prosthesis restores erectile function generally after other treatments for erectile dysfunction (ED) fail. It is recommended as the definitive treatment in severe unresponsive, refractory ED patients [30].

Mechanism of Action

The device is filled with saline and the pump is implanted under the scrotum. Saline from the reservoir is flushed into the device when the pump is pressed. The two chambers are inflated by the pump; the patient then has an erection. The implant can be deflated manually after use (Figure 5.24).

Types of Penile Prosthesis

Malleable Penile Prosthesis (MPP)/Semi-Rigid Penile Prosthesis (SRPP) [31]

These devices are always firm, non-inflatable and made of silicone, except for the distal portions which have a silver or stainless-steel central core (for stability in bending and retaining shape); hence they are technically MR conditional because of the metallic blending. There are low chances of malfunction as the implant is a very simple build.

Soft Penile Implants – Mechanical Rod

These are paired prostheses inserted into each corpus cavernosum. They are entirely made of silicone and thus "MR Safe".

Inflatable Penile Prosthesis (IPP)

Ninety percent of the currently implanted prostheses are IPP. They could be called "hydraulic" implants, because of the manual "inflation or deflation" of the pump. Most of the commonly used implants contain

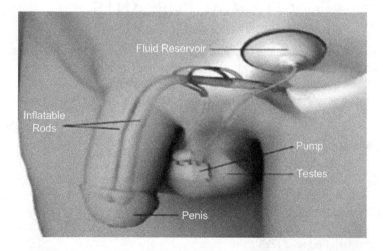

FIGURE 5.24   Penile implants.

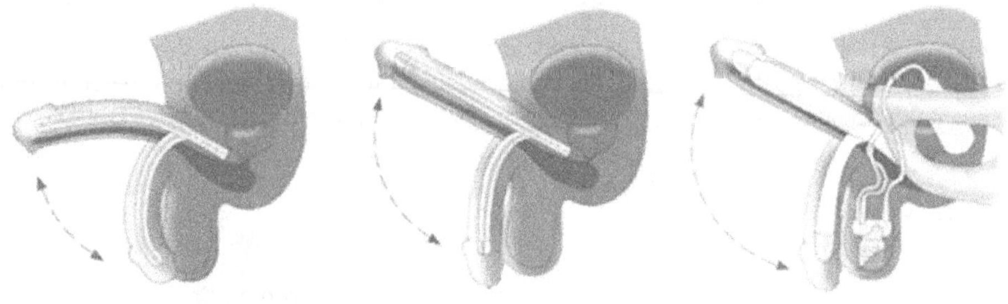

SOFT PENILE IMPLANT   MALLEABLE PENILE   INFLATABLE PENILE
                        IMPLANT   IMPLANT

FIGURE 5.25   Types of penile implant (diagram from Zephyr Surgical Instruments).

small amounts of metal in the form of rear tip extenders, connectors or springs within the scrotal pump valves (Figure 5.25).

Penile prosthesis modifications were tried using single tubing connectors, a lock-out valve in a fluid reservoir or a pump to prevent autoinflation. The life expectancy of penile implants varies from 15 to 20 years with the currently available improved implants. Impregnated coatings and hydrophilic or anti-adherence surface coatings reduce infections, the most dreaded complication.

The common issues encountered with these implants are infection, failure of the device, penis size shortening and local injury. Rarely hematoma, floppy glans, urethral injury and vascular, bladder and bowel injury can occur.

Contraindications

- Situational ED during a disturbed situation
- Any infection – urinary tract infection or pulmonary infection
- Uncontrolled diabetes mellitus

CERVICAL IMPLANTS

Cervical and spine implants are medical implants used by orthopedicians to stabilize the spine or reduce stress on the nerve(s) due to decompression; they are especially useful in treating cervical degenerative disc disease (CDDD). Cervical total disc replacement aims at restoring or preserving the physiological motion of the spine. The development of a spinal fusion is enhanced by permitting temporary stabilization.

Dynamic Cervical Implant (DCI) [32]

DCI was originally developed as a U-shaped titanium stabilizing device used in treating cervical spine degeneration and later modified. It is designed to provide pain relief and also limits excessive flexion and extension and cervical rotation as well as lateral bending of the cervical spine. DCI acts as a shock absorbent, thus guarding the adjacent segments from excessive stress and accelerated degeneration in the cervical spine. The anterior edge of DCI's runcinate teeth maintains the stability of the operated segment, secures anchorage, and prevents implant migration or dropping off, as well as having axial elasticity.

Implanted anteriorly into the cervical disc space from C3 to C7, DCI may be helpful in hernia of the cervical disc, cervical canal stenosis and cervical degenerative disc disease.

Contraindications of DCI

- Any systemic, spinal or localized infections – acute or chronic
- Uncontrolled metabolic diseases, obese patients, pregnant patients, hypersensitivity to the implant material
- Osteoporosis, significant osteopenia, vertebral fractures and/or tumors and at any cervical level that has absence of motion on preoperative flexion/extension radiographs

Spinal implants are used in the treatment of back pain, fractures and deformities like scoliosis, kyphosis, degenerative disorders of the disc, etc. They facilitate the fusion of two vertebrae, replacing the damaged discs. They not only correct deformities, but also strengthen and improve spine stability.

Anterior Cervical Implants

1. Cages have bone grafts or bone growth stimulating factors and will facilitate vertebral fusion leading to better stability of the spine.
2. Spacers are solid material, used to restore or correct spine alignment.
3. Cervical bone plates enhance the cervical spine sturdiness post-surgery, promoting vertebral fusion and supporting the healing spine.
4. Artificial cervical discs help in better segmental movement between vertebrae and are used to treat degenerative disease.

Posterior Cervical Implants

These include the plates (or rods), screws, clamps, hooks and wires, all improving the cervical spine stability immediately after surgery, providing spine stability during healing and maintaining cervical spine alignment.

Complications or adverse effects include unfastening of any or all of the implant components, any malfunctioning, implant migration, hypersensitivity reaction, postoperative change in spinal curvature, loss of correction, height/reduction of implant, infection, persistent CSF leakage, meningitis, loss of neurological function including paralysis, cauda equina syndrome, neurological deficits, reflex deficits, non-union, delayed union, mal-union, loss of or increase in spinal mobility or function and inability to perform the activities of daily living.

LARYNGEAL IMPLANTS

Laryngeal implants are devices surgically inserted in the larynx permanently for correcting glottic insufficiency associated with the paralysis of the recurrent laryngeal nerve. They are indicated for vocal fold medialization and for closing a glottic insufficiency or an urgent indication when it may lead to fatal aspiration complication. Such an implant injection may improve phonation by producing size augmentation of the displaced or deformed vocal fold. The two main laryngeal implantation products are as follows. [33]

Injectable Implants

Injection laryngoplasty uses highly viscous substances for attaining vocal fold medialization. Owing to the use of highly viscous substances, a high-pressure administration device is mandatory and the needle must be of a sufficient gauge. Polydimethylsiloxane particles may be injected into the paraglottic space, leading to localization, producing permanent augmentation in the lamina propria of the vocal fold without causing foreign body granuloma formation. Bovine collagen, extensively used in aesthetic facial surgery, is used even for injection laryngoplasty. A special preparation with the cross-linked collagen fibers significantly slows the resorption process. In some, mandatory allergy testing may be performed prior to use to rule out the presence of pre-formed antibodies against collagen. Hyaluronic acid is an alternative to collagen due to its characteristic similarities and rapid resorption. It is embedded in hydrogels to improve durability for three to six months. In cases of recurrent laryngeal nerve palsy where interim voice improvement is necessary until recovery, it is appropriate for temporary laryngoplasty injection [34].

Solid Implants

With the solid ingredients, solid implants are placed in the paraglottic space thus making a window in the larynx.

Silastic Implant

Biocompatibility is excellent; the extrusion rate seems similar to other medical implants. Cheaper material and customization feasibility make silastic implants a favorite for thyroplasty.

Pre-Formed Devices

This system is made of hydroxyl apatite, which is highly biocompatible. Unfortunately, due to osseointegration of hydroxyl apatite, it is generally impossible to remove these after implantation.

Laryngeal Stents

- Montgomery T-tube – a T-shaped silicone tube with two long legs to be put into the trachea and the subglottic larynx while the short leg is positioned in the tracheostomy site. These are expensive and require specialized tools for implantation, yet are the most widely used. They can cause granuloma formation at the cranial and caudal end; if placed close to the glottic level, subglottic damage can occur, and if kept at the transglottic level, there is risk of aspiration. The "double-cannula-technique" is a modified version that has replaced almost completely other types of laryngeal stents.
- Titanium vocal fold medialization implant (TVFMI) – popular for its ease of use, affordable cost and insertion which can be done using standard instruments.

Human larynx stents can be utilized in postoperative stabilization in case of laryngotracheal stenosis, stenting of damaged larynx and to preserve or reconstruct a post-oncological resected larynx [35]. Risks associated with laryngeal implants such as vocal fold medialization devices include infection, extrusion/migration of the device, airway compromise, adverse tissue reaction or granular tissue formation, poor voice quality, device breakage, revision surgery, etc.

References

1. Michael J. Miller. *Breast Implants and Related Methods of Breast-Modifying Surgery. The Breast, 2-Volume Set, Expert Consult Online and Print* (Fourth Edition), 2009.

2. Garry S Brody. *Silicone Breast Implant Safety and Efficacy.* https://emedicine.medscape.com/article/1275451-print

3. *Breast Implants.* FDA. https://www.fda.gov/medical-devices/breast-implants/types-breast-implants

4. https://www.fda.gov/medical-devices/implants-and-prosthetics/cerebral-spinal-fluid-csf-shunt-systems

5. *What is a Cochlear Implant?.* FDA. https://www.fda.gov/medical-devices/cochlear-implants/what-cochlear-implant

6. MV Kirtane, Gauri Mankekar, Nishita Mohandas, Rajesh Patadia. Cochlear implants. *Int J Otorhinolaryngol Clin.* 2010 May–August;2(2):133–137.

7. Deep et al. Cochlear implantation: An overview. *J Neurol Surg B.* 2019;80:169–177.

8. Douglas A. Miller, Carol A. Sammeth. *Middle Ear Implants: An Alternative to Conventional Amplification.* Feb 2022; Chap11. https://r.search.yahoo.com/_ylt=AwrPpZz6b8BioxIYdQS7HAx.;_ylu=Y29sbwNzZzM EcG9zAzEEdnRpZAMEc2VjA3Ny/RV=2/RE=1656807546/RO=10/RU=https%3a%2f%2fwww.researchgate .net%2fpublication%2f358785829_Middle_Ear_Implants_An_Alternative_to_Conventional_Amplification/ RK=2/RS=V52PrJVCnxf1QXjWCKvJyem5Oo8-

9. David S. Haynes, Jadrien A. Young, George B. Wanna, and Michael E. Glasscock III. Middle ear implantable hearing devices: An overview. *Trends Amplif.* 2009 Sept;13(3):206–214.

10. Committee on Practice Bulletins-Gynecology. Long-acting reversible contraception work group. practice bulletin no. 186: long-acting reversible contraception: implants and intrauterine devices. Obstet Gynecol. 2017 Nov;130(5):e251–e269. doi: 10.1097/AOG.0000000000002400. PMID: 29064972.

11. https://www.cdc.gov/reproductivehealth/contraception/index.htm

12. T. Wang See, T. Kim, D. Zhu. Hernia mesh and hernia repair: A review. *Engi Regen.* 2020;1:19–33

13. https://www.fda.gov/medical-devices/implants-and-prosthetics/hernia-surgical-mesh-implants

14. https://www.drugwatch.com/hernia-mesh/

15. https://www.fda.gov/medical-devices/metal-metal-hip-implants/general-information-about-hip-implants

16. C.Y. Hu, TR. Yoon. Recent updates for biomaterials used in total hip arthroplasty. *Biomater Res.* 2018;22:33. doi: 10.1186/s40824-018-0144-8

17. https://www.drugwatch.com/transvaginal-mesh/

18. AS Chung, OA Suarez, KA McCammon. AdVance male sling. *Transl Androl Urol.* 2017;6(4):674–681. doi: 10.21037/tau.2017.07.29

19. *Urogynecologic Surgical Mesh: Update on the Safety and Effectiveness of Transvaginal Placement for Pelvic Organ Prolapse.* FDA. Center for Devices and Radiological Health; July 2011.

20. AK Dash and GC Cudworth II. Therapeutic applications of implantable drug delivery systems. *J Pharmacol Toxicol Methods.* 1998;40(1):1–12. doi: 10.1016/S1056-8719(98)00027-6

21. Zaki AJ Mohammad, et al. Implantable drug delivery systems: A review. *Int J Pharm Tech Res.* 2012;4(1):280–292.

22. Juliana C Quarterman, Sean M Geary, Aliasger K Salem. Evolution of drug-eluting biomedical implants for sustained drug delivery. *Eur J Pharmaceut Biopharmaceut.* 2021 Feb;159:21–35. doi: 10.1016/j.ejpb.2020.12.005.

23. https://www.nhlbi.nih.gov/health-topics/defibrillators

24. P Mathew, A Kanmanthareddy. Prosthetic heart valve. In: *StatPearls.* Treasure Island: StatPearls Publishing; 2021 Jan. Available from: https://www.ncbi.nlm.nih.gov/books/NBK536987/

25. AT Chuang, CE Margo. Greenberg PB retinal implants: a systematic review. Br J Ophthalmol. 2014;98:852–856.

26. TC Lin, HM Chang, et al. Retinal prostheses in degenerative retinal diseases. *J Chin Med Assoc.* 2015 Sep; 78(9): 501–505. doi: 10.1016/j.jcma.2015.05.010.

27. G Iyer, B Srinivasan, S Agarwal, D Talele, E Rishi, P Rishi, et al. Keratoprosthesis: Current global scenario and a broad Indian perspective. *Indian J Ophthalmol.* 2018;66:620–629.

28. Borja Salvador-Culla, Paraskevi E. Kolovou. Keratoprosthesis: A review of recent advances in the field. *J Funct Biomater.* 2016:7;13. doi:10.3390/jfb7020013

29. *Dental implants, Prosthodontics (textbook).* https://ebooks.care4dental.com/ebooks/BookDetails-227 -Textbook_of_Prosthodontics_(pdf)

30. Brian Le, Arthur L. Burnett. Evolution of penile prosthetic devices. *Korean J Urol.* 2015;56:179–186. doi: 10.4111/kju.2015.56.3.179 pISSN 2005-6737

31. Greear GM, Ghali FM, Hsieh TC. Semirigid penile prosthesis: technique and review of literature. *J Vis Surg.* 2020;6:17. doi: 10.21037/jovs.2019.11.07

32. Junfeng Zeng, Yuchen Duan, Hao Liu, Beiyu Wang, Quan Gong, Yi Yang, Hua Chen, Xin Rong. Dynamic cervical implant (DCI) in treating cervical degenerative disc disease: a systematic review and meta-analysis. *Int J Clin Exp Med.* 2017;10(6):8700–8708.

33. C. Sittel. Larynx: implants and stents. *GMS Curr Top Otorhinolaryngol Head Neck Surg.* 2009;8:Doc04. doi: 10.3205/cto000056. Epub 2011 Mar 10. PMID: 22073097; PMCID: PMC3199813.

34. GE Arnold. Vocal rehabilitation of paralytic dysphonia. *Arch Otolaryngol.* 1962;76:358–368.

35. RB Bell, DS Verschueren, EJ Dierks. Management of laryngeal trauma. *Oral Maxillofac Surg Clin North Am.* 2008;20(3):415–430. doi: 10.1016/j.coms.2008.03.004.

Pediatric Medical Devices

6

K. P. G. Uma Anitha, Gayathri Segaran, and Mythili Sathiavelu

Pediatric medical devices cover a broad array of indications and risk profiles, and have helped to reduce disease burden and improve quality of life for numerous children. However, many of the devices used in pediatrics are not intended for or tested on children. Several barriers have been identified that pose difficulties in bringing pediatric medical devices to the market. These include a small market and small sample size; unique design considerations; regulatory complexities; lack of infrastructure for research, development, and evaluation; and low return on investment (Espinoza, 2019). In the last decade, only 24% of class III life-saving devices approved by the US Food and Drug Administration (FDA) were for pediatric use—and most of those were for children over 12. Of these, less than 4% were labeled for pediatric patients ages zero to two years old, and the number of approved devices is even lower for neonatal patients. For these young patients, adult medical devices are often manipulated by pediatric specialists in order to provide stop-gap solutions. However, these repurposed devices are not always able to fulfill the unique needs of children's biology and growth patterns (Weber, 2021).

INCUBATORS AND RADIANT WARMERS

Incubators and radiant warmers are used in maintaining the body temperature of newborn neonate infants. This is done so that the energy required for metabolic heat production is minimized. The output of heat from these devices is regulated by servocontrol to keep the skin temperature constant at a site on the abdomen where a thermistor probe is attached. In the incubators, the air temperature can also be controlled as an alternative to the skin temperature as servocontrol. Increased ambient humidity, heat shields, and cloths had been used to decrease the evaporative or nonevaporative heat loss of the infants in the incubators under certain conditions. Double-walled incubators, with a second inner layer of Plexiglas, reduce radiant heat loss. They can also reduce total heat loss, but only when air temperature is controlled rather than skin temperature.

A neonatal incubator is an enclosed device where a premature infant is kept in a sterile and controlled environment for observation and care. The biological parameters are constantly monitored to check the

DOI: 10.1201/9781003220671-6

safety of the babies. To observe the vital signs of premature infants continuously, sensors and electrodes are required, which are kept in contact with the infant, with the vital signs being displayed on a monitor. Any abnormal indication in the parameters of the device will be indicated by an alarm system.

The minimal oxygen consumption in a radiant warmer is the same or perhaps slightly higher than it is for the same infant in an incubator. The partition of body heat loss is different with the radiant warmers when compared with the incubators. Radiant warmers usually increase the convective and evaporative loss of heat and insensible water loss and eliminate the radiant heat loss or change it to a net gain. A thin polyethylene film heat shield could be used with a radiant warmer to reduce the loss of heat by convection and evaporation. The major advantage of the radiant warmers is the accessibility they provide to critically ill infants without disturbing the thermal environment. Their major disadvantage is the increase in insensible water loss the radiant warmers produce. Most infants can be cared for more safely either in an incubator or radiant warmer bed (Bell, 1983),

An incubator is a device in which an infant can be kept at the appropriate temperature and humidity, with the right ventilation to facilitate respiration, in an atmosphere with a known and controlled gaseous mixture of oxygen and helium. A densimometer is used to determine the composition of the gaseous mixture within the chamber and to ascertain that this composition of gases remains constant during its use. A mixture of carbon dioxide and oxygen can be used if necessary as a respiratory stimulant. The incubators were originally designed for newborn neonates of diabetic mothers, in order to tackle neonatal asphyxia, and the device has proven helpful in several instances.

Incubators are a fixture in Neonatal Intensive Care Units (NICUs). They are used in combination with other equipment and procedures to ensure that the infants who need extra support have the best possible environment and continuous monitoring. They act as a second womb designed to protect the infant and provide the optimal conditions for their development.

Reasons an Infant may Need an Incubator

Premature Birth

Babies born prematurely need additional time for their lungs and other vital organs to develop further. (Their eyes and ear drums may also be so sensitive that even normal light and sound could cause permanent damage.) Also, babies born extremely early will not have had the time to develop fat just under the skin and will need help to keep themselves warm and toasty.

Infection

Incubators reduce the chance of infection from germs and additional infection while the infant heals from an illness. Incubators also provide a protected space where it's possible to monitor the vitals of the infant 24/7 when multiple IVs for medication, fluids, etc., are needed.

Breathing Issues

Babies sometimes will have fluid or meconium in their lungs. This could lead to an infection and an inability to breathe well. The newborn might also have immature lungs that are not completely developed and that require monitoring and extra oxygen.

Effects of Gestational Diabetes

The baby is placed in the incubator when the mother has gestational diabetes, so that the baby can be kept warm and safe and time can be taken to monitor their blood sugars.

Jaundice

Some incubators have special lights in order to reduce jaundice, where the infant has yellowing skin and eyes. Jaundice in newborns is a common issue and can occur when babies have a high level of bilirubin, a yellow pigment that is produced during the normal breakdown of red blood cells.

Long or Traumatic Delivery

The infant may require constant monitoring and additional medical support if they have experienced trauma. The incubator also offers a safe and womb-like environment where a baby can recover from the trauma.

Low Birth Weight

When the baby is extremely small, even if not premature, the baby may not be able to stay warm without the additional help an incubator offers. Additionally, very small babies might struggle with many of the same vital functions that premature babies do like breathing and eating, and might benefit from the extra oxygen and controlled environment that an incubator offers.

Role of an Incubator

It is easy to think of an incubator as just a bed for a sick baby, but it's so much more than a place for sleeping.

Unlike a simple bassinet, an incubator provides an environment that can be adjusted to provide an ideal temperature as well as the right amount of oxygen, light, and humidity. Without this precisely controlled environment in the incubator many infants would not be able to survive, especially babies born a few months early.

Apart from temperature control, an incubator provides protection from allergens, germs, light, excessive noises, etc., that may also cause harm. An incubator also controls the humidity, allowing it to protect a baby's skin from losing more water and becoming brittle or cracking. An incubator also has equipment to track a range of things including the baby's temperature and heart rate. This monitoring helps to constantly track the baby's health status.

Incubators can be used along with medical procedures:

- Feeding through an IV
- Delivering blood or medications through an IV
- Constantly monitoring vital functions
- Ventilating
- Special lights for jaundice treatments

An incubator not only protects the baby, but also provides an ideal environment for medical professionals to monitor and to treat the infant. You may come across many different types of incubators.

Types of Incubators

There are three common types of incubators: The open incubator, the closed incubator, and the transport incubator. Each incubator is designed differently with different advantages and limitations.

Open Incubators

An open incubator is also called a radiant warmer. In an open incubator, the baby is placed on a flat surface with the radiant heat element either positioned above or offering heat from below.

The heat output is controlled automatically by the temperature of the baby's skin. In the open incubator the opening is above the baby. Due to this open air space, open incubators cannot provide the same control over humidity as closed incubators. But the open incubators can still monitor the baby's vital functions and keep the baby warm; since it is possible to touch the baby directly from above, it is easy to achieve skin-to-skin contact with the baby in an open incubator. Open incubators work very well for infants who primarily need to be temporarily warmed up and have their vital statistics measured. The control of humidity and guarding from airborne germs are not well maintained in the open incubators, so they are not ideal devices for babies requiring a more controlled environment and germ protection.

Closed Incubators

A closed incubator is a device in which the baby is completely enclosed. It has portal holes on the sides to allow IVs and human hands to treat the infant inside. It is designed to keep germs, light, and other elements away. A closed incubator is like a climate-controlled bubble. The main difference between a closed incubator and an open incubator is the way in which the heat is circulated and the temperature is controlled. A closed incubator allows warm air to be blown through a canopy that surrounds the baby. The temperature and humidity can be controlled manually from outside of the incubator or adjusted automatically, based on the skin sensors attached to the baby. The automatically adjusting incubators of this type are called servo-control incubators. Closed incubators have their own microenvironments. Therefore closed incubators are ideal for babies who need less sound, germ protection, and humidity control. Some closed incubators have two walls to help prevent heat and air loss. These are commonly called double-walled incubators.

Transport or Portable Incubators

These incubators are used to transport babies between two different locations, when a baby is transported to a different hospital—where there is access to additional care—to get services not offered at their current location. A transport incubator has a mini ventilator, an IV pump, a pulse oximeter, a cardio-respiratory monitor, and an oxygen supply. As transport incubators are small typically, they fit well in spaces that regular open and closed incubators might not.

Takeaway

Incubators are an important piece of medical equipment that provides a controlled environment for premature and ill babies. Without incubators fewer babies would be able to survive tough beginnings. Incubators are like a second womb or a safe bubble surrounding the baby. Although it can produce some anxiety to be surrounded by incubators in the NICU visiting your baby, comfort may come in knowing the hum of the electrical equipment means that the baby is getting the oxygen and heat needed. An incubator may not be a mother's arms, but it can provide safety, warmth, and important data (https://www.healthline.com/health/baby/incubator-babys).

INFANT PHOTOTHERAPY LAMPS

Phototherapy is light treatment for newborns who develop jaundice. It is performed with a special type of light but not with ultraviolet light. It is blue, and it may emit light in the blue-green spectrum with wavelengths of 430–490 nm. This therapy is given with a lamp known as a bili-light or with a bili-blanket. A shining and fluorescent light from the bili-light lamps is used on the bare skin of the newborn. Jaundice is a yellow discoloration on the skin and in the eyes of newborns due to the pigment bilirubin. Sixty percent of babies are born with jaundice. But few babies have high enough bilirubin levels at birth to cause brain damage. The reason might be an infection at birth, breast milk, or low birth weight. Phototherapy helps to get rid of the accumulated excess bilirubin by making it water-soluble. This phototherapy process allows the baby's liver to break down and remove the bilirubin from their blood through urine and stools. The particular wavelength of this light used in this therapy can break down the bilirubin into a form the baby can get rid of. The baby with jaundice is kept under a special light. The baby's eyes are covered to protect them from any damage due to light. The baby's body might lose more water through the skin, so supplemental feeding is given to the baby. In conventional and fiberoptic phototherapy, the therapy stops for about 30 minutes every 3 to 4 hours, and the baby is given to the mother for breastfeeding, changing the nappy, and cuddling (Dr. Anita Dhanorkar).

Bilirubin

Neonatal jaundice is usually a self-resolving action and is found in about 60% of normal newborns; it typically ends between 72 and 96 hours after birth.[1] Jaundice or hyperbilirubinemia is due to an increase in the bilirubin concentration, beyond the normal levels, and is evident with yellow pigment in the skin, conjunctiva, and mucous membranes. It is estimated that about 60% of newborns have jaundice in the first few days after birth. Six percent of newborns may develop hyperbilirubinemia (> 220 mumol/L), which can potentially cause bilirubin encephalopathy or kernicterus, a severe neonatal disease. In healthy individuals, the concentration of bilirubin in blood plasma is negligible (< 17 µmol/L), but there is an increase in the individual with jaundice (> 30 µmol/L). The concentration of bilirubin in the newborn increases immediately after birth due to high hemoglobin turnover, as it is unable to eliminate bilirubin quickly. This is seen in approximately 60% of term infants and in 80% of preterm infants.[2] If not treated, it leads to serious brain damage. Therefore, it is important to have an early diagnosis. Treatment usually is light therapy, and in severe cases blood transfusion (Kumar, 2011).

In the past, the preferred method for detecting hyperbilirubinemia in newborns was serum bilirubin (SB). SB in neonates is usually based on visual evaluation by physicians. The collection of blood by skin puncture exposes the neonate to trauma and the risk of infection. For predicting serum bilirubin levels new noninvasive devices avoid skin punctures in newborns. One such device that has been studied extensively is the jaundice meter. It is a portable light-weight instrument that uses reflectance measurements on the skin which determine the yellowness in the skin, namely transcutaneous bilirubin (TcB). Though the TcB amount correlates with the serum bilirubin (SB) levels, it is difficult to accurately predict the serum bilirubin levels due to many factors.

The transcutaneous bilirubinometer provides a digital assessment of skin pigmentation by xenon reflectance. It is possible to derive an estimated amount of plasma bilirubin from the number displayed by the meter, and it is the most commonly suggested method for identifying plasma bilirubin (Lorne Holland, Kenneth Blick).

Neonatal jaundice occurs in nearly 80% of preterm babies. The management of neonates with jaundice requires the measurement of total serum bilirubin (TSB). Total serum bilirubin (TSB) is determined by analyzing plasma or serum samples by spectro-photometric methods, which requires the drawing of blood which causes pain to the neonate. There are a wide range of intra- and inter-laboratory variables in the performance of bilirubin analyzers. These disadvantages have led to a search for a noninvasive and reliable technique for the estimation of TSB. A large number of studies have demonstrated the possibility of prediction of serum bilirubin in neonates by measuring the yellowness of the skin in the jaundiced neonate using transcutaneous bilirubinometers.

The transcutaneous bilirubinometer has a different detailed operating procedure, but the basic principle remains the same. The optic head of the meter is gently pressed against the neonate's skin (usually the forehead or upper part of the sternum). For correct measurement, the optic head should make full contact with the skin and there should be no gaps between the head and the skin. This should be achieved by gentle pressure.

The commonly used sites are the forehead and the upper end of the sternum. The meter readings for each site should be compared with the actual TSB before a particular site is chosen. The correlation coefficients for other sites such as the lower limbs are poor. Hyperemia at the test site may affect the results. Measurements against bruises, birthmarks, and subcutaneous hematoma should be avoided.

Clinical Utility of Transcutaneous Bilirubinometers

Often a pediatrician is interested in corroborating his clinical estimate of the icterus with the actual serum bilirubin level. Any such technique should ideally be accurate, noninvasive, and valid. A large number of studies have tested the agreement between transcutaneous bilirubinometer results and TSB. Most studies have found fair to excellent correlation between the two. Transcutaneous bilirubinometers can serve as a screening tool, especially where the services of a neonatologist are not available. However, this cannot serve as a substitute for TSB estimations.

PEDIATRIC VEIN FINDERS

Venipuncture is the practice of drawing blood by penetrating the vein with a needle. It is an invasive procedure which causes the child distress, pain, and even unavoidable extreme reactions. Peripheral venous cannulation and venipuncture are frequently necessary in pediatric neonates and are the most stressful and painful situations. Obtaining these in infants and toddlers can be challenging even for trained nurses and pediatricians. About 60% of children report distress during venipuncture. Performing IV placement with as few attempts as possible is advocated, due to the physical and emotional distress for children, which can negatively affect eventual subsequent procedures. Moreover, more than one attempt to achieve this procedure is required in about one-third of children. Some conditions may exacerbate venipuncture's difficulties, such as increased subcutaneous tissues in newborns, the requirement for frequent venous cannulation due to chronic disease, obesity, dark skin color, and malnourishment. Failure in IV placement can be predicted by a specific score, known as the difficult intravenous access (DIVA) score. Due to this disadvantage near-infrared light technology is routinely used, which gives an advantage to venipuncture in a pediatric blood center setting (Conversano, E., Cozzi, G) nerve injury involving the lateral antebrachial cutaneous nerve (LACN), which can lead to the so-called 'causalgia' or complex regional pain syndrome (CRPS) (Ramos).

Recently, a technological development has provided trans-illuminating devices, using near-infrared light-emitting diodes (NIR-LED) for visualizing superficial veins with hemoglobin absorbing the light emitted, which forms an image on the skin surface.

In recent years, specific tools have been developed and employed to enhance the success in venipuncture in pediatrics. One of the techniques is based on NIR technology. The skin is exposed to near-infrared light by machinery which is absorbed by the blood, and reflected by the surrounding tissue. The machinery captures the information, and then processes it digitally through a computer and projects a digital real-time image of the patient's vein pattern on the skin directly (Cuper NJ).

From the high-level architecture (HLA) perspective, a NIR spectroscope comprises two elements: (i) a NIR light source and (ii) a NIR-sensitive camera which is capable of capturing the surface of the skin illuminated by the light source, which is then further processed and displayed for clinical usage [1–3].

Hemoglobin is a heterotetramer which has subunits of alpha- and beta-globin (the protein part) that are bound to a heme prosthetic group (iron-containing compound). As to its major function, it is able to transport oxygen (O_2)-rich blood (oxyhemoglobin) from the lungs to the peripheral tissues and carbon dioxide (CO_2)-rich blood (deoxyhemoglobin) along the opposite route [9]. The imaging, through the use of trans-illuminating devices, allows a deeper look below the skin with the best wavelength range for better contrast between the skin and veins.

This technique gives a clear visualization of the subcutaneous vein pattern as a consequence of the different optical properties of the tissues and human blood. The difference is due to the fact that veins are rich in deoxygenated hemoglobin, a molecule which almost completely absorbs the NIR light, in contrast to the arteries, which contain oxygenated hemoglobin. Due to this, the vein pattern appears highlighted in comparison with the surrounding tissue, which is the striking quality of any NIR imaging device.

PEDIATRIC NEBULIZERS

Nebulizers have been available since the beginning of the twentieth century. Nebulization to generate medical aerosols from a drug solution is a commonly used method. To deliver a drug by nebulization, the drug must first be dispersed in a liquid medium. The drug particles in the drug are subjected to a dispersing force contained within the aerosol droplets, which are then inhaled (Mohammed Ali). Nebulizers are devices used in delivering a drug from a reservoir solution with a facemask or mouthpiece. Nebulization transforms a drug solution into a fine mist which can be inhaled. This method delivers a high dose of a drug and can be achieved usually by inhaling devices. The fine mist produced is inhaled by the child during inspiration through a close-fitting face mask, tracheostomy mask, or mouth piece. Nebulization therapy might be part of acute care for a child with respiratory distress or can be used for a chronically ill child with a long-term respiratory condition.

Inhaled medications are the mainstay of treatment for many children with pulmonary diseases. This type of therapy is given to patients who receive different types of respiratory support. Improvements in the survival and development of new technology have changed the prognosis of many pediatric pulmonary conditions. This heterogeneous population includes pediatric patients with asthma, pediatric patients with respiratory distress requiring invasive mechanical ventilation or noninvasive ventilation (NIV) support, pediatric patients requiring transnasal support in the form of high-flow nasal cannula (HFNC), and spontaneously breathing tracheostomized pediatric patients.

Many aerosol delivery devices are also available to deliver inhaled aerosols to children. Nebulizers are pressurized metered-dose inhalers (pMDIs). There are also soft mist inhalers and dry powder inhalers for different drugs.

There are two types of nebulizers: (i) jet (or pneumatic) small-volume nebulizers and (ii) ultrasonic nebulizers. Jet nebulizers are based on the venturi principle, whereas ultrasonic nebulizers use the converse piezoelectric effect to convert alternating current to high-frequency acoustic energy. The major features of both types of nebulizer are the duration of treatment at each time of use, particle size distributions produced, and aerosol drug output.

The formulation of the drug solution is usually designed to optimize drug solubility and stability; small changes in formulation may also affect inhaled mass, particle size distribution, and treatment time. The differences between nebulizer brands probably have a greater impact than differences in formulation. There are several advantages to jet nebulization, including the fact that effective use requires only simple, tidal breathing, and that dose modification and dose compounding are possible.

PULMONARY DRUG DELIVERY

Jet Nebulizers

The working principle of jet nebulizers is based on the Bernoulli principle. Jet nebulizers use compressed air or oxygen which is passed through a narrow orifice creating a low-pressure area at the adjacent liquid feed tube at 6–8 L/minute. This evacuates the solution, with the drug being drawn up from the fluid reservoir and scattered in the gas stream through fine droplets. There are fine ligaments in this tube, and the impact of the solution on these ligaments generates droplets. Baffles trap the larger droplets. Jet Nebulizer uses compressed gas to make an aerosol (tiny particles of medication in the air).

Ultrasonic Nebulizers

Ultrasonic nebulizers use a piezoelectric crystal, vibrating at a high frequency (usually 1–3 MHz), to generate a fountain of liquid in the mobilizing chamber to create the aerosols and do not require gas flow. The vibrations are transmitted to the drug solution through a buffer to form a fountain of liquid in the nebulization chamber. Ultrasonic nebulizers produce a more uniform sized particle than jet nebulizers, but are not widely used due to the cost. They make aerosols through high-frequency vibrations. The particle size is larger than the particle size with a jet nebulizer.

MESH NEBULIZERS

In mesh nebulizers, the liquid passes through a very fine mesh to form the aerosol. This kind of nebulizer creates the smallest particles. It's also the most expensive.

Nebulizers are good devices for small children or infants with asthmatic medication. They are also helpful in children with trouble using an asthmatic inhaler or when in need of a large dose of an inhaled medication. Nebulization therapy is often called breathing treatment. Nebulizers can be used with a variety of medications, both in controlling asthma and for any relief. These include:

Corticosteroids used in treating inflammation

- Flunisolide
- Budesonide
- Triamcinolone
- Fluticasone

Bronchodilators to open airways

- Formoterol
- Salmeterol
- Levalbuterol

Nebulizers have different parts: A mask or mouthpiece, nebulizer cup, air compressor, compressor tubing, and medication (either unit dose vials or bottles with measuring devices.

PEDIATRIC STETHOSCOPES

Pediatric stethoscopes are similar to adult stethoscopes, except for a small difference in the size and shape of the chest piece which allows for more accurate auscultation, and they are available in child-friendly shapes and colors.

Digital stethoscopes (DS) and computerized breath sound analysis have been used in assessing normal and abnormal breathing sounds in children. This technique involves using recordings to obtain the power spectrum profiles using the Fourier transform, providing information in addition to what is available to the human ear. Neonates experience a high burden of respiratory problems, with a limited number of predictive models and therapeutic advances for bronchopulmonary dysplasia. DS and computerized analysis are a novel tool to study neonatal breathing sounds (Lindsay Zhou).

Auscultation with a large stethoscope head places undue force on the chest or abdomen of a tiny baby. Auscultation and the associated pressure applied by the auscultator may be an unpleasant experience for extremely low-birthweight infants. Care should be taken to use the smallest stethoscope possible and to apply minimum pressure when examining low-birthweight infants.

Large nursing-style stethoscopes are often used on extremely premature infants, whereas a smaller neonatal stethoscope is used for the term neonate. Stethoscope heads were weighed using precision scales, and a ratio of stethoscope head weight to baby weight was calculated (SHBW ratio). The crude ratio does not take into account the added effect of the clinician pressing the stethoscope onto the chest. The weight of a large stethoscope head is 41 g and that of a small stethoscope head is 28 g. The SHBW ratio was 1:15 for the large stethoscope head (D S Urquhart, V P Balasubramaniam Lindsay Zhou, Faezeh Marzbanrad).

INFANT STETHOSCOPE

This stethoscope is similar to the pediatric and neonate stethoscope; the only difference lies in its diameter. In an infant stethoscope, the chest piece is roughly 2.6 cm which gives accurate auscultations. The non-latex device prevents allergic reactions; this device is ideal for infants. It is used to listen to the heart sounds and other vital organs to diagnose and assess the patients.

NEONATAL STETHOSCOPE

This stethoscope is used for diagnosing newborn neonates and physical assessment. The device head with the smallest diameter has very accurate auscultations, without any noise interference from the environment. The devices are made of a non-latex material that avoids allergic reactions along with a non-chill ring. The smaller size helps in accurate diagnosis in a relatively short period that requires no adjustments.

It looks like a regular stethoscope, but the distinguishing factor is the color and size of the chest piece. With its small chest piece that enables accurate placement, and alluring colors which make it look like a toy. This would intrigue children who were usually frightened of large stethoscopes. Such a stethoscope is used to assess and diagnose sick children (D S Urquhart, and V P Balasubramaniam).

SPHYGMOMANOMETER

Hypertension in children and adults has increased in prevalence mainly due to obesity in this particular population. The appropriate measurement of BP is a prerequisite in adults and in children for the diagnosis of hypertension and to avoid misdiagnosis. The noninvasive methods for measuring BP are the auscultatory method using conventional mercury or aneroid devices and the automated method using electronic devices.

The mercury sphygmomanometer is a standard device. It is widely used in situations in which blood pressure is not the primary variable of interest when comparing the results with other studies having used the same instrument. Automated oscillometric devices are used for measuring blood pressure, especially when the differences in BP between groups of people are more important than absolute levels. The devices are not subjected to observers and set are in particular mode suitable for children. This device is especially useful in the absence of an observer and the accuracy of device were considered.

The word 'sphygmomanometer' was derived from the Greek word sphygmos, meaning the beating of the heart or the pulse, and manometer, a device for measuring pressure. The device was introduced by an Italian physician, Scipione Riva-Rocci (1896). Then, an American physiologist, Joseph Erlanger (1874–1965), studied the principles of sphygmomanometry and devised a recording sphygmomanometer.

A sphygmomanometer, or sphygmometer, is an instrument for measuring arterial blood pressure, and it consists of an inflatable cuff, an inflating bulb, and a gauge showing the blood pressure.

There are two types of sphygmomanometers, a mercury column and a gauge with a dial face. The sphygmomanometer most frequently used consists of a gauge attached to a rubber cuff which is wrapped around the upper arm and is inflated to constrict the arteries. A blood pressure reading for an adult might vary depending on age and many other factors. Children and adults with smaller or larger than average sized arms may need special-sized pressure cuffs.

This device is more precise and needs to be operated by a trained person.

Mercury manometer: This is a mercury-based unit and has a manually inflatable cuff attached by a tubing system to the unit that is calibrated in millimeters of mercury. When measuring the blood pressure, the unit is kept upright on a flat surface and the gauge is read at eye level. Unit breakage may lead to a dangerous mercury contamination.

There is another type of mercury sphygmomanometer which is called a RandomZero sphygmomanometer.

This instrument was devised to overcome the observer biases in the standard mercury device. The device has a reservoir that contains mercury, but the observer will not be aware of readings registered. This amount is visible at the end of the reading (Matthew W. Gillman, Nancy R. Cook).

Aneroid/mechanical manometer: An aneroid unit, it is free of mercury and consists of a cuff that can be applied with one hand for self-testing, a stethoscope that is attached, and a valve that inflates and deflates automatically, with the data displayed on an easy-to-read gauge that functions in any position. The unit is sensitive and if dropped requires recalibration. This type is in common use but should be checked against a mercury manometer if they are suspected to be out of calibration.

Digital or automated oscillometric manometer: This is an electronic device which operates easily and practically in a noisy environment. This device is comprised of a cuff which can be applied with one hand for self-testing and a valve that is automatically inflated and deflated. The reading is digitally displayed, and a stethoscope is not needed. This device is useful for the hearing-impaired, and for automatic input into instruments for storage or graphical display. Some more expensive models also remember and print out recordings.

The digital manometer uses the oscillometric principle of measuring blood pressure.

The device measures the mean arterial pressure and uses algorithms for calculating the systolic and diastolic values. It does not actually measure the blood pressure, but derives the readings. The digital manometers require little training and involve attention only to the subject and environmental factors, application of the right cuff, and correct use of the machine controls (Gillman and Cook, 1995).

There is no need for an observer, and it is easy to use for small children as there is no need for auscultation. The disadvantage of the device is that it is very expensive. The movement of the child's arm also causes artifactual readings during the measurement. The first readings and the different models of the devices show various measurement algorithms and so could measure different quantities.

The most appropriate method for measuring blood pressure in children is auscultation. Measurements derived by the oscillometric devices that exceed the 90th percentile should be repeated by auscultation. The suitable cuff size with an inflatable bladder width that has at least 40% of arm circumference at a point midway between the olecranon and the acromion. For an optimal cuff, the bladder length of the cuff should be about 80% to 100% of the circumference of the arm. It is important that the bladder width-to-length ratio should be at least 1:2. Blood pressure is check to a great degree, either with a cuff that is very small, or with a cuff that is too large. When a cuff is very small, the next larger cuff size should be used, even if it appears large. When appropriate cuffs are used, the cuff-size effect is obviated.

PEDIATRIC THERMOMETERS

The investigation and in treating the pediatric patients are actually determined by body temperature. It's difficult to find a quick and convenient method for parents and health care workers to measure body temperature accurately. The main goal of measurement of the body temperature is to estimate the core temperature, which is the temperature of the blood that bathes the temperature-regulating center in the hypothalamus. There exists a gradient between the body site where the temperature is measured and the hypothalamus. In contrast to popular dogma, the gradient is not constant. The rectal temperature is not reliable as it is higher than the axillary temperature. It is difficult to choose a body site to use as a reference standard for comparing readings obtained by different instruments or at different sites (Joan L Robinson, MD).

Axillary digital thermometers (ADTs) and non-contact (infrared) forehead thermometers (NCIFTs) are commonly used in pediatric settings, where an incorrect body temperature measurement may delay treatment or lead to incorrect diagnoses and therapies (Franconi et al., 2018). Several studies comparing ADT or NCIFT with other methods have found conflicting results. To investigate whether ADT and NCIFT can be used interchangeably, a comparative observational study was conducted involving 205 children aged 0 to 14 years who were consecutively admitted to the pediatric emergency department.

The most commonly used devices for measuring body temperature are infrared thermometers, glass mercury thermometers, and chemical point thermometers (Li et al., 2013). Though glass thermometers have decreased in use in pediatric patients recently, due to their accurate measuring of the temperature and low cost they are still widely used for patients who are suspected of a high temperature (Sibbald, 2003). Although some have been replaced by electronic and infrared thermometers, glass thermometers are still used widely (Barbarak Kuhn, 2002). In most places, pediatrics currently use glass thermometers to measure body temperature (Zhang et al., 2014; Wang, 2009).

While measuring a patient's body temperature, it is necessary to determine the core body temperature, which is defined as the temperature of the core tissue of the body. The core body temperature is measured noninvasively using axillary thermometry, oral thermometry, tympanic membrane thermometry, cutaneous infrared thermometry, or rectal thermometry (El-Rashdi and Barry, 2006).

TYPES OF THERMOMETERS

Glass mercury thermometers were once a staple in most medicine cabinets. But currently, mercury thermometers are not recommended as they can break and allow the mercury to vaporize and be inhaled.

Digital thermometers: Digital thermometers are the most accurate and quick to measure temperature. These thermometers use electronic heat sensors for recording body temperature. They are used in the rectum (rectal), mouth (oral), or armpit (axillary). Temperatures taken in the armpit are typically the least accurate of the three.

Digital ear thermometers (tympanic membrane): Digital thermometers use an infrared scanner for measuring temperature in the ear canal. But earwax or a curved ear canal can interfere with the accuracy of an ear thermometer temperature.

Temporal artery thermometers: Temporal thermometers use an infrared scanner for measuring the temperature of the temporal artery of the forehead. This thermometer can be used when a child is asleep.

Infrared (IFR) tympanic thermometers: Infrared (IFR) tympanic thermometers may be considered ideal, measuring both practical and core temperatures, but ear wax and conditions such as otitis media may compromise the readings (Ataş Berksoy, 2018).

PULSE OXIMETRY

Oxygen saturation (SpO_2) is an indirect index of oxygen supply-to-demand balance (Takuo Aoyagi 1970, Aoyagi T, Miyasaka K. 2002, Makajima et al., 1975). When a person's oxygenation status shows a reduced partial pressure of oxygen, decreased oxygen saturation in arterial blood and in this case, it should be called hypoxemia. Hypoxemia in children is associated with an increase in mortality and can be complicated, in the cases of pneumonia, bronchiolitis, asthma, and sepsis [5]. Hypoxemia among children with pneumonia contributes to diagnosis, is crucial in patient management, and helps in determining prognosis (Hess DR, Branson RD).

The World Health Organization (WHO) recommends an oxygen saturation threshold value of 90%, measured by pulse oximetry, as the cut-off point for oxygen administration in populations living at 2,500 m asl or less. In clinical practice, the 'normal' SpO_2 at sea level has been estimated to be between 95% and 100%; however, several authors consider that values of 95% and 96% are abnormal [3]. In altitudes above 3,000 m asl, where oxygen saturation values are lower than at sea level, the 90% cut-off point could be less useful (Schoenberg et al., 1999, Andrade, V., Andrade, F., Riofrio).

Pulse oximetry is a readily available and noninvasive method for measuring the pulse oxygen saturation (Spo_2) which can be obtained by placing a small probe on the finger, toe, or in the ear lobe of children. In infants and in neonates, the probe may also be placed on the feet, palms, cheeks, arms, tongue, nose, or nasal septum. A portable small pulse oximetry probe is used in children, for premature neonates.

The basic technology used in pulse oximetry is the photoplethysmographic (PPG) waveform. The PPG waveform is an amplified and highly filtered light absorbed by local tissue over time. A pulse oximeter has two light-emitting diodes that transmit two wavelengths of light on one side, and a photodetector on the other side. Red light is transmitted at 660 nm and NIR light is transmitted at 940 nm through the intervening tissue (skin, arteries, capillaries, veins, bone, and fat), with the light which is not absorbed in its pathway detected by the photodetector on the opposite side (Nasr and James, 2019).

The pulse oximeter is a vital device in the care of infants and children with cardiopulmonary disease (Salyer, 2003).

There is a change in the absorption of light relative to the amount of oxygenated and deoxygenated hemoglobin when the quantity of blood in the tissue changes. Measuring the changes in the absorption of light allows the estimation of the heart rate and the arterial oxygen saturation. The oximeter should distinguish between the absorption and the pulsatile changes in absorption which are caused by the changes in blood volume with each heartbeat. The background absorption changes when there is a change in the shape or position of the tissues through which the light passes, which can cause false readings.

The pulse oximeter has the ability to monitor the functional oxygen saturation of hemoglobin in the arterial blood (SaO_2 continuously and transcutaneously). To recognize the setting, in which pulse oximeter readings of SpO_2 may result in false estimates of the true SaO_2, an understanding of two basic principles of pulse oximetry is required (i) how oxyhemoglobin (O_2Hb) is distinguished from deoxyhemoglobin (HHb) and (ii) how the SpO_2 is calculated only from the arterial compartment of blood.

Pulse oximetry is based on the principle that O_2Hb and HHb absorb red and NIR light differently. There are significant differences in the absorption of O_2Hb and HHb at red and NIR light because these two wavelengths penetrate tissues well, whereas blue, green, yellow, and far-IR light are significantly absorbed by non-vascular tissues and water. O_2Hb absorbs a higher amount of IR light and a lower amount of red light than the HHb. The highly oxygenated blood with higher concentrations of O_2Hb appears bright red to the eye because it scatters more red light than the HHb. The HHb absorbs more red light and appears less red. The light that is transmitted through the finger is then detected by a photodiode on the opposite arm of the probe. The relative amounts of red and IR light absorbed are used by the pulse oximeter to ultimately determine the proportion of Hb bound to oxygen.

Pediatric Hearing Aids

Hearing sounds and words helps children learn to talk and to understand. Children with hearing loss may develop trouble in speech, language, and social skills. They may also have trouble learning in school and may have difficulty in communication. There are many effects of hearing loss on development.

There are different types of hearing aids. The behind-the-ear (BTE) hearing aid is the most commonly used for young children because it can attach to different earmold types; the earmold can also be easily replaced as the child grows, the earmold can be easily handled, it works with many types of hearing loss, and the earmolds are soft and safe for small ears in children.

American Speech-Language-Hearing Association (ASHA)

All hearing aids have a microphone to pick up sound, a processor that analyzes the sound (filtering out unwanted sounds like excess wind noise, for example, while amplifying desired sounds), and a receiver that delivers the amplified sound deep inside the ear. A battery powers the unit, and it can be rechargeable. Hearing aids made especially for infants and kids work very similarly to adult hearing aids with a few differences: Pediatric hearing aids are manufactured to be more durable than adult models. Pediatric hearing aids are more compatible with other assistive devices. For kids, this is especially important to facilitate communication and learning (Dr. Mandy Mroz).

Types of Hearing Aids

There are several types of hearing aids. Some hearing aids are worn on the body, and others fit behind the ear or in the ear. People with bilateral hearing loss wear two hearing aids.

Types of hearing aids include:
- **Behind-the-ear (BTE) hearing aids.** There are two main parts in a BTE hearing aid. It has a tiny hard plastic case which is behind the ear which holds the electronics that make up the actual hearing aid. This is connected to a plastic piece called an earmold that fits inside the outer part of the ear. Sound travels from the hearing aid through the earmold and into the ear. BTEs are used by people of all ages to treat mild to profound hearing loss.
- **In-the-ear (ITE) hearing aids.** These fit inside the outer ear. ITEs help in mild to severe hearing problems. Some ITEs have a telecoil installed. A telecoil is a small magnetic coil that allows the wearer to receive the sound through the circuitry in the hearing aid, rather than through a microphone. Telecoils make it easier to hear. They also help in hearing special sound systems, called induction loop systems.

- **Canal hearing aids.** These are directly in the ear canal, and there are two different types. An in-the-canal (ITC) hearing aid is made to fit the size and shape of a person's ear canal, and the completely-in-canal (CIC) hearing aid is slightly different from the ITC. It is slightly hidden in the ear canal. Both canal hearing aids are used to treat mild to severe hearing loss.

References

Andrade, V., Andrade, F., Riofrio, P. et al. Pulse oximetry curves in healthy children living at moderate altitude: A cross-sectional study from the Ecuadorian Andes. *BMC Pediatr* 2020;20:440. https://doi.org/10.1186/s12887-020-02334-z

Aoyagi T, Miyasaka K. Pulse oximetry: Its invention, contribution to medicine and future tasks. *Anesth Analg* 2002;94(1 Suppl):S1–S3.

Ataş Berksoy E, Bağ, Ö, Yazici, S, Çelik, T. Use of noncontact infrared thermography to measure temperature in children in a triage room. *Medicine* 2018 Feb;97(5):e9737 doi: 10.1097/MD.0000000000009737

Barbarak Kuhn T. *Fundamental Skills and Concepts in Patient Care*. Philadelphia: Lippincott Williams &Wilkins; 2002.

Dr. Mandy Mroz is the president of Healthy Hearing. As an audiologist American Speech-Language-Hearing Association (ASHA). *Making Effective Communication: A Human Right, Accessible and Achievable for All.*

Edward F. Bell infant incubators and radiant warmers. 1983 Oct;8(3–4):351–375. https://www.healthline.com/health/baby/incubator-baby#takeaway

El-Rashdi AS, Barry W Thermometry in paediatric practice. *Arch Dis Childhood* 2006;91:351–356.

Espinoza J, Cooper K, Afari N, Shah P, Batchu S, Bar-Cohen Y. Innovation in pediatric medical devices: Proceedings from the west coast consortium for technology & innovation in pediatrics 2019 annual stakeholder summit. *JMIR Biomed Eng* 2020;5(1):e1746.

Franconi I, La Cerra C, Marucci AR, Petrucci C, Lancia L. Digital axillary and non-contact infrared thermometers for children. *Clin Nurs Res* 2018 Feb;27(2):180–190. doi: 10.1177/1054773816676538. Epub 2016 Nov 8. PMID: 28699399.

Gillman MW, Cook NR. Blood pressure measurement in childhood epidemiological studies. *Circulation* 1995 Aug 15;92(4):1049–1057.

Hess DR, Branson RD. Noninvasive respiratory monitoring equipment. In: Branson RD, Hess DR, Chatburn RL, editors. *Respiratory Care Equipment*. Philadelphia: JP Lippincott; 1995:193.

Holland L, Blick K, Suckling RJ, Liang IA, Kirk JM. Transcutaneous bilirubinometry as a screening tool for neonatal jaundice. Implementing and validating transcutaneous bilirubinometry for neonates. 1995. https://www.newbornwhocc.org/pdf/tran.pdf

Kumar P, Chawla D, Deorari A. Light-emitting diode phototherapy for unconjugated hyperbilirubinaemia in neonates. *Cochrane Database Syst Rev* 2011 Dec;(12):CD007969. [PMC free article] [PubMed] [Google Scholar]

Li Y-W, Zhou L-S, Li X Accuracy of tactile assessment of fever in children by caregivers: A systematic review and meta-analysis. *Ind Pediatr* 2017a;54:215–221.

Li Y-W, Zhou L-S, Li, X. Accuracy of tactile assessment of fever in children by caregivers: A systematic review and meta-analysis. *Ind Pediatr* 2017b;54(91):351–356.

Li Z, Zhang L, Su Y Comparison of measurement time and effect of non-contact infrared thermometer and mercury thermometers. *Chin Nurs Manage* 2013;S1:158–159.

Makajima S, Hirai Y, Takase H, et al. Performances of new pulse wave earpiece oximeter. *Respir Circ* 1975;23:41–45.

Medical Author: Dr. Anita Dhanorkar, BHMS Medical Reviewer: Pallavi Suyog Uttekar, MD Medically Reviewed on 11/3/2020

Medically Reviewed by Dan Brennan, MD on March 26, 2020. https://www.webmd.com/asthma/guide/home-nebulizer-therapy

Nasr VG, James A. DiNardo pulse oximetry. *Pediatr Rev* 2019 Nov;40(11):605–608. doi: 10.1542/pir.2018-0123

Robinson JL, MD. Body temperature measurement in paediatrics: Which gadget should we believe? *Paediatr Child Health* 2004 Sept;9(7): 457–459, doi: 10.1093/pch/9.7.457

Salyer JW. Neonatal and Pediatric Pulse Oximetry, MBA RRT-NPS FAARC. *Resp Care* 2003 April;48(4)

Schoenberg R, Sands DZ, Safran C. Making ICU alarms meaningful: A comparison of traditional vs. trend-based algorithms. In Proceedings of the AMIA Symposium, 1999, 379–383. Available at http://www.amia.org/pubs/symposia/D005686.PDF (accessed 2/1/03).

Sibbald B. City bans medical devices that contain mercury. *Can Med Assoc J* 2003;168:78.

Sphygmomanometer (Internet communication, 20 October 2007 at http://en.wikipedia.org/wiki/Sphygmomano meter)

Sphygmomanometer (Internet communication, 20 October 2007 at http://www.answers.com/topic/sphygmomanometer)

There are two main types of photo therapies given to newborns: Medical Author: Dr. Anita Dhanorkar, BHMS Medical Reviewer: Pallavi Snyog Uttekar, MDMedically Reviewed on 11/3/

Urquhart DS, Balasubramaniam VP. Stethoscope head to body weight ratios in the extremely preterm infant, ADC Fetal and Neonatal. *BMJ J* n.d.

Wang Y. Guidelines for diagnosis and treatment of acute fever in children aged 0–5 years in China (interpretation version): Definition of fever and measurement of body temperature. *Chin J Evid-Based Pediatr* 2009;1:60–64.

Weber C. Solving unmet needs with innovative pediatric medical devices. *IEEE Pulse* 2021 Jan–Feb;12(1):24–27, doi: 10.1109/MPULS.2021.3053755

Zhang L, Gong Y, Jin X. Investigation on the use of thermometer in 12 medical institutions. *Chin Nurs Manage* 2014;6:648–650

Zhou L, Marzbanrad F, Fattahi D, King A, Malhotra A. The digital stethoscope and computerised sound analysis: A novel method for examining neonatal breath sounds. *J Paediatr Child Health* 2020; (S2 pahe):33.

Medical Device Use for Cardiovascular Diseases

7

Sameer Khasbage, Sayan Kumar Das,
Surjit Singh, and Shobhan Babu Varthya

INTRODUCTION

Cardiac implantable electronic devices, including pacemakers, implantable cardioverter defibrillators (ICD), biventricular pacemakers, and cardiac loop recorders, are designed to help control or monitor irregular heartbeats in people with certain heart rhythm disorders and heart failure [1]. Chronic heart failure (CHF) is a common condition characterized by symptoms of breathlessness and fatigue in the presence of cardiac dysfunction, most frequently impairment of contraction of the left ventricle (left ventricular systolic dysfunction). The management of CHF due to left ventricular systolic dysfunction is well supported by evidence from clinical trials and includes angiotensin-converting enzyme inhibitors, beta-receptor antagonists, aldosterone receptor antagonists, and newer agents such as ivabradine and neprilysin inhibitors. In addition, device therapy, especially pacemaker therapy, principally ICDs and cardiac resynchronization therapy (CRT), has become a key part of the armamentarium used to control the condition. Implantable electronic cardiac devices have revolutionized therapy within cardiology and are recommended in both national [3] and international guidelines to treat bradycardia, tachy-arrhythmia, and chronic heart failure secondary to left ventricular systolic dysfunction [2, 3]. The therapeutic use of cardiac pacing traditionally falls within the field of electrophysiology, but increasingly, heart failure physicians are taking the lead on implant decisions and the monitoring of CHF patients with these devices. Over time, through observational, preclinical, and clinical studies, the pacemaker has developed from an externally powered device, to a fully implantable, automated device with battery longevity of more than eight years capable of transmitting data wirelessly for remote follow-up. While early pacemakers were electronic metronomes, modern iterations have added complex hardware and software around that basic function to allow for extremely complex and sophisticated programmability [4, 5]. Here we provide an overview of current practice in device management with a focus on cardiovascular diseases, their intended use, and adverse events related to them.

DOI: 10.1201/9781003220671-7

DEFIBRILLATORS

John McWilliam, in 1899, hypothesized ventricular fibrillation (VF) to be a cause of death in humans following which, in 1933, William Kouwenhoven conclusively established that electrically induced ventricular fibrillation could be reversed with an appropriate counter-shock. Claude Beck developed an alternating current defibrillator for internal defibrillation which saw its first clinical use on a 14-year-old boy suffering a VF during an operation in 1947 [6]. Cardiac arrest is one of the most common causes of death across the world. In cardiovascular events, where there is an absence of synchronized myocardial contractions, defibrillation uses electrical impulses as a therapeutic modality for the termination of this non-perfusing rhythm and is an important component of cardiopulmonary resuscitations [7]. Electrical stimulation of a sufficient strength raises the transmembrane potential to the activation threshold leading to the depolarization of the myocardial cells which in turn leads to the disruption of the on-going dysrhythmia. After the termination of the abnormal rhythm, the sinoatrial node restores the normal sinus rhythm [8]. The indication for defibrillation is limited to ventricular fibrillation and pulseless ventricular tachycardia whereas it is to be avoided in patients with asystole and pulseless electrical activity. Conscious patients with a pulse or sinus rhythm are absolute contraindications for defibrillation. In contrast to defibrillation, cardioversion is aimed at terminating perfusing arrythmias and making way for the restarting of the normal sinus rhythm [7]. Defibrillators can be classified primarily into two types, namely, manual and automated. Intended to be used in conjunction with electrocardiogram, the manual defibrillators require medical expertise where a trained health professional diagnoses the rhythm following which the voltage and timing are determined [9]. The automated defibrillators require minimal medical expertise for their usage and can be further subclassified into automated external defibrillators (AED), ICD, and wearable cardioverter defibrillators (WCD).

Automated External Defibrillators (AED)

Indicated for use in case of a sudden cardia arrest (Figure 7.1A and B) where early defibrillation in combination with CPR in the first few minutes of an arrest can be a life-saving intervention, automated cardiac defibrillators are portable devices which are designed for emergency use by untrained or briefly trained non-medical personnel. The AED system houses electrodes which can detect and interpret electrocardiograms as well as deliver a tailored electrical shock without requiring the expertise of a medical professional.

They can be classified into two types based on accessibility, namely, public access AED which are intended for use by non-medical personnel and are commonly available at public places such as airports

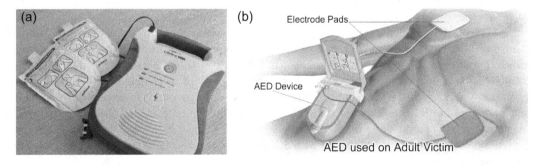

FIGURE 7.1   (a) Automated external defibrillators (AED). (b) BruceBlaus, CC BY-SA 4.0 (https://creativecommons.org/licenses/by-sa/4.0), via Wikimedia Commons.

and community centers, and professional use AEDs which are intended to be used by first responders who have received AED-related training.

Based on the automaticity of the device, AEDs can also be classified as semi-automated or fully automated. Semi-automated AEDs analyze rhythm to determine the need for an electrical shock but prompt the user for the discharge of the shock, whereas a fully automated AED analyzes the rhythm and delivers the shock without requiring user intervention [10]. Although relatively safe, AED use can be associated with a few adverse events which can be patient related, user related, or both. Patients might incur skin burns at the site of contact with electrodes, myocardial necrosis, and even precipitation of other arrhythmic conditions including asystole. Users need to pay close attention to immediate environmental conditions as there is a high possibility of accidentally shocking oneself during use [11].

Implantable Cardioverter Defibrillator (ICD)

Capable of amending most life-threatening arrhythmias (Figure 7.2), the ICD is a fully automated implantable device that can perform both cardioversion and defibrillation. Hence, they play a pivotal role in prophylaxis as well as the management of patients who harbor a risk of developing Ventricular Fibrillation (VF) and Ventricular Tachycardia (VT) resulting in sudden cardiac death [12]. The pulse generator housing the battery is generally placed subcutaneously just below the clavicle on the left side of the chest whereas the leads extending out from the generator are placed in the left ventricle. Risks associated with ICD insertion include bleeding from the site of insertion, damage to local blood vessels, traumatic rupture of myocardium, and displacement of the leads from the intended site facilitating the need for further surgical procedures for reinsertion. Restrictions post-insertion mainly are directed towards avoiding exposure to strong electromagnetic fields as they may disrupt the ICD resulting in it malfunctioning [13].

Wearable Cardioverter Defibrillator (WCD)

Indicated for patients at risk of developing sudden cardiac death, wearable cardioverter devices are an alternative to ICDs or where the implantation of ICDs is not feasible or is contraindicated, for example, in patients with active infections. These wearable external devices are capable of detection and defibrillation and can be worn for years as a prophylactic measure against sudden cardiac death.

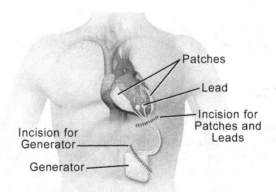

**Implantable Cardioverter
Defibrillator Leads on the Heart**

FIGURE 7.2 Internal cardioverter defibrillator. BruceBlaus, CC BY-SA 4.0 (https://creativecommons.org/licenses/by-sa/4.0), via Wikimedia Commons.

While four monitoring and three defibrillating electrodes are built into the chest harness, the defibrillation unit is attached to a belt around the waist. Placed circumferentially around the chest, the monitoring electrodes serve as two surface electrocardiogram leads whereas the defibrillation electrodes are positioned in accordance with providing an apex to posterior defibrillation [14].

CARDIAC ABLATION CATHETERS

Catheter ablation is used to treat certain types of arrhythmias, or irregular heartbeats, that cannot be controlled by medicine or where there is a high risk for ventricular fibrillation (v-fib), sudden cardiac arrest, or atrial fibrillation. Ablation requires cardiac catheterization to place flexible tubes, or catheters, inside the heart to make scars. A series of catheters are passed through the blood vessel, guided by fluoroscopy, to the correct location in the heart. A cardiac ablation catheter emits either radiofrequency waves, or extremely cold temperatures, or laser through the catheter to create a scar called the ablation line. The scar forms a barrier preventing the transmission of electrical impulses from the damaged heart tissues to the surrounding healthy tissue. This stops abnormal electrical signals from traveling to the rest of the heart and causing arrhythmias. Catheter ablation carries risk of bleeding, infection, vascular damage, myocardial damage, arrhythmias, blood clots and radiation induced cancer [15, 16].

Woven Dacron Catheters

Woven Dacron catheters exhibit bioflexibility as a result of their proprietary polyurethane woven shaft construction. Bioflexibility allows the catheter to soften at body temperature and conform to endocardium for excellent contact and stability. The Dacron catheters have the advantage of stiffness, which helps maintain catheter shape with enough softness at body temperature Mapping accuracy is enhanced through the combination of bioflexibility, stable positioning, and high-resolution electrograms [17].

Synthetic Catheters

Synthetic catheters cannot be manipulated or change shape within the body, so they are less desirable. The synthetic catheters are cheaper and offer smaller sizes (2 to 3 French) [18].

Ablation Catheters

Sixty-four-pole roving catheters: This mapping (mini basket) catheter has an 8 F bidirectional deflectable shaft and a basket electrode array (usual mapping diameter 18 mm) with 8 splines, each spline containing 8 small (0.4 mm^2), low-impedance electrodes (total 64 electrodes). The interelectrode spacing along the spline is 2.5 mm (center-to-center). Mapping can be performed with the basket in variable degrees of deployment (diameter ranging from 3 mm to 22 mm). The location of each of the 64 electrodes is identified by a combination of a magnetic sensor in the distal region of the catheter and impedance sensing on each of the 64 basket electrodes. The location of each basket electrode is obtained whether the basket is fully or only partially deployed [12, 13].

STENTS

Intracoronary stents represented a major advance in interventional cardiology. Percutaneous transluminal coronary angioplasty to deform or ablate obstructive coronary atherosclerotic narrowing is performed increasingly with inflatable balloons, excisional and rotational atherectomy devices, stents, and lasers. Progress has been made since the introduction of this technology with respect to procedural success as well as the increasing complexity of coronary lesions treated. Early coronary re-occlusion as well as late restenosis, however, remain limitations of Percutaneous transluminal coronary angioplasty (PTCA). Recently, high-dose systemic antiplatelet drug therapy has been shown to limit early complications after PTCA by ≈35%; however, bleeding complications have ensued [19].

Bare metal stents (BMSs): Bare metal stents became the therapeutic choice over angioplasty, intimal hyperplasia, and secondary restenosis with good tolerability in patients. Here, we aim to show that stents are effective and more tolerable than earlier procedures. The original bare metal stents were composed of a 316 L stainless steel alloy composed of iron, nickel, and chromium. The advent of bare metal stents significantly reduced periprocedural complications, but bare metal stents did not have an overly profound impact on restenosis rates. Additionally, stent thrombosis emerged as an important and potentially fatal complication [19, 20].

Tubular wire: Flexible tube (catheter) into an artery. Sometimes the catheter will be placed in your arm or wrist, or in your upper leg (groin) area [21].

Tubular mesh: A stent (defined as a tubular metal mesh) is a scaffolding device used to hold tissue in place in a specific stretched or taut position. Tubular mesh stents consist of wires wound together in a meshwork, forming a tube. Finally, slotted tube stents are made from tubes of metal from which a stent design is laser cut. Any number of stent designs can be created within a coil, tubular mesh, or slotted tube framework [22]. Cardiovascular stents are small, expandable metal mesh tubes typically placed inside a coronary artery to open and support narrowed or weakened arteries. This loss of arterial function is most often caused by atherosclerosis and its subsequent residue [23].

Slotted tube: Slotted tube stents are made from tubes of metal from which a stent design is laser cut. The first human implant was in 1996. The radial strength of the slotted tube is optimized by an orthogonal locking mechanism, and there is virtually no shortening after expansion. This particular stent was found to display a very low elastic recoil percentage (2.35% under 0.2 bar pressure) among 23 tested stents. In addition, the late minimal lumen diameter of the stent is similar to the initial dilated diameter [24].

Drug-eluting stents (DES): Even though stents are well tolerated and effective, the incidence of restenosis remains a major concern. Therefore drug-eluting stents were introduced to prevent restenosis. Among the various drug eluting stents, stents with anti-proliferative agents significantly reduced restenosis rates to <5%. Earlier patients with calcified intimal thickening and fibrosed vessels required angioplasty as the treatment opportunity however, with the introduction of DES, these subsets of population were also treated with stents [20].

Biodegradable polymer-coated drug-eluting stents: Safety concerns and biocompatibility became more important drivers of polymer selection with next-generation products. As a result, efforts were geared to reducing polymer-induced hypersensitivity. An early porcine model looking at five biodegradable and three permanent polymers in the absence of an anti-proliferative drug showed that both polymer types can cause significant vessel inflammation and neointimal thickening.

Zotarolimus-eluting stent: Endeavor (Medtronic Inc.), a 91 μm CoCr strut with a phosphorylcholine biocompatible polymer that eluted zotarolimus over a two-week period, was the first commercially available zotarolimus-eluting stent (ZES). Polylactic acid/polyglycolic acid copolymer showed the least amount of fibrocellular proliferation, and its subunits polyglycolic acid (PGA) and polylactic acid (PLA, also known as PLLA) are some of the bioabsorbable polymers being utilized in bioabsorbable products (Figure 7.3).

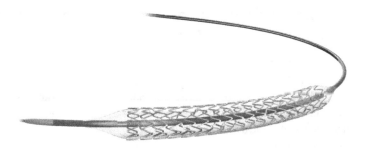

FIGURE 7.3   Drug-eluting stent. Jack McLure, CC BY-SA 4.0 (https://creativecommons.org/licenses/by-sa /4.0), via Wikimedia Commons.

Biodegradable scaffolds: Bioabsorbable stent platforms potentially represent the next generation of technology, and the idea is intuitively attractive for many reasons. Poly-L-lactic acid (PLLA) has previously been used in numerous medical devices and demonstrated predictable degradation kinetics and good safety in previous coronary applications. It is the basis for the bioresorbable vascular scaffold (BVS) stent (Abbott Vascular, Abbott Park, IL, USA) [20].

Polymer-free drug-eluting stents: Polymer-free drug-eluting stents are based on different technologies for drug binding and release without the use of polymer coatings [25]. To tackle the issue of polymer-associated inflammation seen with early-generation devices, newer-generation DESs leveraged either more biocompatible polymer or polymer-free elution technologies. To date, a number of polymer-free DESs have been developed, and three such devices have both Conformité Européene (CE) mark approval for use in Europe [25, 26]. First-generation DP-DES were developed to reduce the risk of in-stent restenosis and target lesion revascularization associated with BMS. Despite these promising results, first-generation DP-DES were shown to have an increased risk of very late (>12 months) stent thrombosis compared with BMS. The pathophysiology of stent thrombosis has been attributed to various factors, such as polymer-induced hypersensitivity reaction, stent malposition, incomplete strut re-reendothelialization, and accelerated neo-atherosclerosis. To address this issue, a new generation of DP-DES was developed, with improvements in anti-proliferative drugs, polymer coatings, and strut thickness. The introduction of second-generation DP-DES reduced the risk of very late stent thrombosis associated with the preceding generation of devices. Nevertheless, the potential thrombogenic nature of the polymer coating in second-generation DP-DES remains a concern, and suggestions have been made to extend the duration of dual antiplatelet therapy (DAPT) in patients receiving DP-DES. PF-DES were designed to achieve similar advantages of BMS (reduced risk of stent thrombosis) and DP-DES (reduced risk of target lesion revascularization). These devices consist of a microporous metallic stent platform and an inorganic coating that can be loaded with an anti-proliferative drug. The theoretical benefit of PF-DES is the elimination of the need for a polymer coating, which acts as a potential chronic inflammatory stimulus. However, the main challenge for PF-DES has been the attainment of a sufficient level of anti-proliferative drug in the inorganic coating to ensure the inhibition of neointimal hyperplasia and in-stent restenosis [27] (Figure 7.4).

Shape memory stents: Smart materials have intrinsic properties that change in a controlled fashion in response to external stimuli. Currently, the only smart materials with a significant clinical impact in cardiovascular implant design are shape memory alloys, particularly Nitinol. Recent prodigious progress in material science has resulted in the development of sophisticated shape memory polymers. In this chapter, we review the literature and outline the characteristics, advantages, and disadvantages of shape memory alloys and shape memory polymers which are relevant to clinical cardiovascular applications [27].

A shape memory polymer (SMP) stent may enhance flexibility, compliance, and drug elution compared to its current metallic counterparts. Thermally activated SMP is a unique class of polymeric materials that can maintain a secondary shape and then recover a pre-determined primary shape when sufficiently heated. SMP has been shown to have promising applications in intravascular medical devices for thrombectomy, aneurysm embolization, and as vascular stents. It is fabricated from thermoplastic polyurethane.

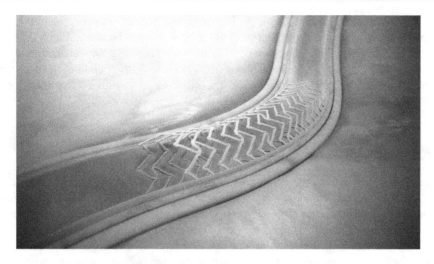

FIGURE 7.4   Biodegradable scaffolds. https://www.scientificanimations.com/, CC BY-SA 4.0 (https://creative-commons.org/licenses/by-sa/4.0), via Wikimedia Commons.

A solid SMP tube formed by dip coating a stainless steel pin was laser-etched to create the mesh pattern of the finished stent. At a physiological flow rate, the stent did not fully expand at the maximum laser power (8.6 W) due to convective cooling. However, under zero flow, simulating the technique of endovascular flow occlusion, complete laser actuation was achieved in the mock artery at a laser power of ~8 W [28].

CARDIAC PACEMAKERS

Over the past 60 years since the first human pacemaker implant, significant improvements have been made to the devices themselves and to the lead systems. The improved battery materials made it possible to produce smaller devices with greater longevity and a wide range of technologies enabling communication between the device and the operator. Lead wires are the weaker part of the cardiac pacing system; improvements in conductor materials and hybrid insulation have been shown to improve reliability. With the recent development of leadless pacing systems, the failures of implantable leads can be prevented. These enhancements have allowed more widespread use of heart stimulation or cardiac pacing in veterinary applications since the first canine implant reported in 1967 [29]. We briefly discuss certain cardiac pacemakers such as battery-powered wearable pacemakers, an implantable pulse generator (IPG), and endocardial leads with IPG with biocompatible polymers and biostable metals.

BATTERY-POWERED, WEARABLE PACEMAKER

The first pacemakers of the 1950s were bulky external devices that relied on mains power. A patient had no choice but to live tethered to the wall socket, and a power cut could be fatal. In response to this problem, an American, Earl Bakken, developed the first wearable battery-powered cardiac pacemaker [30]. Battery-powered, wearable pacemakers are also in the category of external pacemakers. External, patient portable, battery-powered pulse generators are designed to provide a wide range of choices in pacing rate, current amplitude, and mode of action. Common features are that they are small in size (approx. 11.7 × 7.4

× 3.1 cm), are light in weight (approx. 3.0 g), can be strapped to the patient's chest or limbs, are designed to accept, directly or by adapters, all or almost all electrodes likely to be utilized with them, are readily serviced for battery changes or cleaning, are capable of gas autoclaving for sterilization or contamination control, and are of increasingly dependable reliability. These units operate in the asynchronous and R-wave inhibited modes over a wide range of rates. Their low trigger sensitivity may allow for their use in atrial as well as ventricular noncompetitive pacing [31].

Drawbacks

The most common complications are related specifically to particulars of application such as thrombophlebitis. Operating complications are inherent in the situation, as external fails to achieve required therapeutic benefits due to interference in external power supply like the external electrodes are temporarily connected the pulse generators are subject to disruption and interference because they are exposed and mobile. They are handled, mishandled, and serviced by various personnel or even patients. The major problems are an increased incidence of external damage, wetting, wire shorting, poor external electrode contact, gross electrode displacement or internal electrode malposition, battery depletion, and the increased risk of AC interference or induced fibrillation [32, 33].

AN IMPLANTABLE PULSE GENERATOR

Artificial pacemakers are electronic devices that stimulate the heart with electrical impulses to maintain or restore a normal rhythm in people with slow heart rhythms. Temporary pacemakers are intended for short-term use during hospitalization. They are used because the arrhythmia is expected to be temporary and eventually resolve, or because the person requires temporary treatment until a permanent pacemaker can be placed. Permanent pacemakers are intended for long-term use. The pacemaker is most commonly implanted into soft tissue beneath the skin in an area below the clavicle, which is known as prepectoral implantation. The pacemaker leads are typically inserted into a major vein and advanced until the leads are secured within the proper regions of heart muscle. The other ends of the leads are attached to the pulse generator [34]. Leadless pacemakers are generally implanted through a leg vein and placed directly in the heart muscle without the need for a separate pulse generator. People who have a permanent pacemaker will require periodic surveillance of the implanted device. The status of the pacemaker will be regularly checked to provide information regarding the type of heart rhythm, the functioning of the pacemaker leads, the frequency of utilization of the pacemaker, the battery life, and the presence of any abnormal heart rhythms. The pulse generators are usually powered by lithium batteries that function for an average of five to eight years before they need to be replaced. When the batteries start to wear out, they do so in a very slow and predictable fashion, allowing sufficient time to be detected and pulse-generator replacement planned. Replacing the pulse generator usually requires a simple procedure in which a skin incision is made over the old incision, the old generator is removed, and a new generator is implanted and joined with the existing leads, assuming the existing leads are functioning normally [35].

Drawbacks

The pacemaker leads are usually used indefinitely, unless a specific problem occurs (e.g., the lead loses contact with the heart, the lead breaks, or the lead is not functioning properly). In such circumstances, the lead may require replacement. Often, the old lead is left in place but disconnected from the pulse generator and capped, and a new lead is inserted. Removal of an old lead is feasible but difficult in most cases, because of the formation of scar tissue binding the lead to the blood vessels and heart muscle. Lead removal is usually necessary if the system becomes infected.

Avoiding electromagnetic interference: Although contemporary pacemakers are less susceptible to interference than older models, electromagnetic energy can interfere in some cases.

Cellular phones: People with a pacemaker or a defibrillator should know that items with strong magnetic fields (e.g., cellular phones with magnets for wireless charging, magnetic accessories such as certain "smart watches") can affect the function of the device if they are very close (less than six inches) to their device. Cell phones without strong magnets are unlikely to cause problems with pacemakers or defibrillators.

Anti-theft systems: Electromagnetic anti-theft security systems are often found in or near the workplace, at airports, in stores, at courthouses, or in other high-security areas. Although interference with a pacemaker is possible, it is unlikely that any clinically significant interference would occur with the transient exposure associated with walking through such a field. Based upon several studies and observations, experts advise that patients with pacemakers should be aware of the location of anti-theft systems and move through them at a normal pace and avoid leaning on or standing close to an anti-theft system.

Metal detectors at airports: Similar to anti-theft systems, metal detectors at airports can potentially interfere with pacemakers, although this is unlikely. Such exposure has been shown to cause interference in some cases and may be related to the duration of exposure and/or distance between the security system and the pacemaker. Metal detectors will likely be triggered by the presence of a pacemaker, and therefore at places such as airports, it will be important for individuals with pacemakers to carry an identification card for their pacemaker, and airport personnel will likely prefer to do a manual search.

External electrical equipment: External electrical fields do not seem to cause a problem for most people with a pacemaker. However, in workplaces that contain welding equipment or strong motor-generator systems, because interference can inhibit pacing, it is recommended that a person with an implanted cardiac device remain at least two feet from external electrical equipment.

Diagnostic or therapeutic procedures: Certain types of surgery and procedures may interfere with pacemakers. Most importantly, the use of electrocautery can inhibit pacemaker function. Magnetic resonance imaging (MRI) uses a strong magnetic field that is pulsed on and off at a rapid rate. In the past, this procedure was a relative contraindication for patients with a pacemaker. However, with the introduction of specialized pacemakers that are "MRI safe," MRI scans can be performed. Even patients with a standard pacemaker (i.e., not designated "MRI safe") can often undergo MRI scans with careful monitoring and other appropriate precautions. Other contraindications include transcutaneous electrical nerve/muscle stimulators (TENS), a method of pain control; diathermy, which heats body tissues with high-frequency electromagnetic radiation or microwaves; extracorporeal shock wave lithotripsy, the use of sound waves to break up gallstones and kidney stones; therapeutic radiation for cancer or tumors, which can cause permanent pacemaker damage; and any surgery in which electrocautery is being used. The risks are greatest when the electrocautery is being performed close to the pulse generator [36–38].

ENDOCARDIAL LEADS (PASSIVE FIXATION LEADS AND ACTIVE FIXATION LEADS)

Lead fixation technology (either active or passive fixation) plays a crucial role in boosting the efficiency of cardiovascular implantable electronic devices (CIEDs) including ICDs, pacemakers, and CRT devices [39,40]. Active fixation pacing leads are more commonly used, as they are associated with easy fixation, reliability, and repositioning, possible deployment in alternative pacing sites with optimal pacing and sensing thresholds, lower rates of dislodgement, chronic removability, and easy extraction [40–42]. Passive fixation technology is, on the contrary, associated with drawbacks such as a lack of reliable, unmoving LV lead retention in the proximal or middle segments of coronary veins. Although passive fixation leads are stable in the atrial appendage, active fixation leads are necessary to prevent dislodgement in patients with prior cardiac surgery. The lead dislodgement may result in an increase in pacing thresholds, failure to capture, or failure to sense [43].

LEADLESS CARDIAC PACEMAKERS (LCP)

An LCP is a small (volume 0.8 cm^3) single-chamber PM that is implanted directly into the RV by a special catheter and introducer sheath via transfemoral access. Therefore, it does not require the subcutaneous pocket or transvenous lead. The first LCP was Nanostim (St Jude Medical), implanted worldwide between 2013 and 2016. The device was recalled in 2016, due to battery failures, but the concept of LCPs has been widely accepted [44–46]. At present, the only type of LCP available on the market is the Micra transcatheter pacing system. The pacing mode is similar to transvenous PMs, so an LCP may be used as an alternative device. However, the system is limited to the RV component, meaning that an LCP may be indicated only for patients requiring single-chamber pacing, e.g., permanent atrial fibrillation (AF) with bradycardia or for those with low expected stimulation percentage [44, 47]. The potential benefits of LCPs must be confronted with the limited data on the long-term follow-up, and also the procedure of device replacement or retrieval is still debated. One worldwide experience of 40 successful device retrievals revealed that it may be feasible and safe if performed with a special sheath and a snare catheter and introduced via femoral access. The most common reasons for extraction included elevated pacing threshold, endovascular infection, and indications for a system upgrade to a transvenous device. If it is necessary to replace the battery, a new LCP may be implanted next to old devices without the extraction of previous ones; however, current clinical experience is very limited [48, 49].

Contraindications to leadless pacemaker implantation are few but may include mechanical tricuspid valve, pre-existing pacemaker or defibrillator leads, inferior vena cava filter, unfavorable venous anatomy, morbid obesity preventing telemetry communication, concern for the loss of AV synchrony resulting in a pacemaker syndrome, and severe pulmonary hypertension [44].

Indications: Permanent atrial fibrillation with atrioventricular (AV) block or significant pauses, sinus rhythm with intermittent advanced heart block in patients of limited life span or very low levels of physical activity, sinus bradycardia with infrequent pauses, syncope with electrophysiologic study findings concerning for increased risk of heart block [44].

PROSTHETIC (ARTIFICIAL) HEART VALVES

A heart contains four valves (tricuspid, pulmonary, mitral, and aortic valves) which open and close as blood passes through the heart. Blood enters the heart in the right atrium and passes through the tricuspid valve to the right ventricle. From there, blood is pumped through the pulmonary valve to enter the lungs. After being oxygenated, blood passes to the left atrium, where is it pumped through the mitral valve to the left ventricle. The left ventricle pumps blood to the aorta through the aortic valve [50]. There are many potential causes of heart valve damage, such as birth defects, age-related changes, and effects from other disorders, such as rheumatic fever and infections causing endocarditis. High blood pressure and heart failure can enlarge the heart and arteries, and scar tissue can form after a heart attack or injury [51]. The three main types of artificial heart valves are mechanical, biological (bioprosthetic/tissue), and tissue-engineered valves.

Mechanical Valves

Mechanical valves come in three main types – caged ball, tilting-disc, and bileaflet – with various modifications on these designs. Caged ball valves are no longer implanted. Bileaflet valves are the most common type of mechanical valve implanted in patients today [52] (Figure 7.5A–C).

Caged Ball Valves

The first artificial heart valve was the caged ball valve, a type of ball check valve, in which a ball is housed inside a cage. When the heart contracts and the blood pressure in the chamber of the heart exceeds the pressure on the outside of the chamber, the ball is pushed against the cage and allows blood to flow. When the heart finishes contracting, the pressure inside the chamber drops and the ball moves back against the base of the valve forming a seal. In 1952, Charles A. Hufnagel implanted caged ball heart valves into ten patients (six of whom survived the operation), marking the first success in prosthetic heart valves. A similar valve was invented by Miles "Lowell" Edwards and Albert Starr in 1960, commonly referred to as the Starr-Edwards silastic ball valve. This consisted of a silicone ball enclosed in a methyl metacrylate cage welded to a ring. The Starr-Edwards valve was first implanted in a human on August 25, 1960, and was discontinued by Edwards Lifesciences in 2007. Caged ball valves are strongly associated with blood clot formation, so people who have one require a high degree of anticoagulation, usually with a target international normalised ratio (INR) of 3.0–4.5 [53].

Tilting-Disc Valves

Introduced in 1969, the first clinically available tilting-disc valve was the Bjork-Shiley valve. Tilting-disc valves, a type of swing check valve, are made of a metal ring covered by an expanded polytetrafluoroethylene (ePTFE) fabric. The metal ring holds, by means of two metal supports, a disc that opens when the heart beats to let blood flow through, then closes again to prevent blood flowing backwards. The disc is usually made of an extremely hard carbon material (pyrolytic carbon), enabling the valve to function for years without wearing out [54].

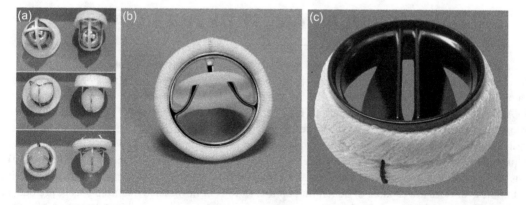

FIGURE 7.5   (a) Caged ball valve. Dr. Mirko Junge, CC BY 3.0 (https://creativecommons.org/licenses/by/3.0), via Wikimedia Commons. (b) Chitra valve. Phulwari28, CC BY-SA 3.0 (https://creativecommons.org/licenses/by-sa/3.0), via Wikimedia Commons. (C) Aortic bileaflet prosthetic valve. Stif Komar, CC BY-SA 3.0 (https://creativecommons.org/licenses/by-sa/3.0), via Wikimedia Commons.

Bileaflet Valves

Introduced in 1979, bileaflet valves are made of two semicircular leaflets that revolve around struts attached to the valve housing. With a larger opening than caged ball or tilting-disc valves, they carry a lower risk of blood clots. They are, however, vulnerable to blood backflow [55].

The major advantage of mechanical valves over bioprosthetic valves is their greater durability. Made from metal and/or pyrolytic carbon, they can last 20–30 years [56].

Disadvantages: Increased risk of blood clots; people with mechanical valves need to take anticoagulants, such as warfarin, for the rest of their lives [56]. Also, they cause mechanical hemolytic anemia and cavitation [57].

Bioprosthetic Tissue Valves

Bioprosthetic valves are usually made from animal tissue (heterograft/xenograft) attached to a metal or polymer support. Bovine (cow) tissue is most commonly used, but some are made from porcine (pig) tissue. The tissue is treated to prevent rejection and calcification [58, 59]. Alternatives to animal tissue valves are sometimes used, where valves are used from human donors, as in aortic homografts and pulmonary autografts. An aortic homograft is an aortic valve from a human donor, retrieved either after their death or from a heart that is removed to be replaced during a heart transplant. A pulmonary autograft, also known as the Ross procedure, is where the aortic valve is removed and replaced with the patient's own pulmonary valve. A pulmonary homograft is then used to replace the patient's own pulmonary valve. This procedure was first performed in 1967 and is used primarily in children, as it allows the patient's own pulmonary valve (now in the aortic position) to grow with the child [52]. Advantages: Bioprosthetic valves are less likely than mechanical valves to cause blood clots, so do not require lifelong anticoagulation. As a result, people with bioprosthetic valves have a lower risk of bleeding than those with mechanical valves. Disadvantages: Implants typically last 10–20 years, therefore, multiple implantation may be required during the patient's lifetime. [52].

Functional requirements of artificial heart valves: Minimal regurgitation, minimal transvalvular pressure gradient, non-thrombogenic, self-repairing [60].

VENTRICULAR ASSIST DEVICES (VADS)

The traditional treatment for medically refractory HF has been heart transplantation. Many patients with advanced HF are not eligible for heart transplantation due to existing comorbidities or advanced age. A major advancement in the treatment of HF has been the emergence of the left ventricular assist device (LVAD) both as a bridge to transplantation (BTT) and as destination therapy (DT). The LVAD has revolutionized and improved the care of the sickest HF patients. The first use of a ventricular assist device is attributed to Michael DeBakey to support a patient in post-cardiotomy shock. Ventricular assist devices are intended to supplement or totally replace the cardiac output required to support systemic circulation. This goal is achieved by removing blood (preload) from the left ventricle and ejecting it into the proximal aorta. These devices are capable of generating up to 8 to 10 L of flow based on pump speed, preload, and blood pressure [61–63]. A mechanical circulatory support pump may be positioned extracorporeally or intracorporeally as a biventricular assist device (BiVAD), a right ventricular assist device (RVAD), or more commonly as an LVAD. Moreover, the pump characteristic further sub-stratifies it into a pulsatile or non-pulsatile device [64].

Ventricular assist devices aid in decreasing load on the heart while maintaining cardiac output and blood supply to organs. Broadly VAD can be categorized into the following types depending upon the necessity and duration of circulatory support:

- **Bridge to recovery** – only temporary support for days to weeks during which time reversibility of ventricular insult may occur followed by weaning and removal of the device. This includes patients with acute cardiogenic or post-cardiotomy shock, acute inflammatory cardiomyopathies, and myocardial infarction.
- **Bridge to transplantation** – these patients meet the criteria but need additional circulatory support while awaiting transplantation.
- **Destination therapy** – reserved for patients who are not candidates for transplantation yet require the use of a VAD as a final therapy until death [65].

Components

VADs used in the outpatient setting are implanted devices placed through a median sternotomy typically during cardiopulmonary bypass. The VAD is connected to the heart by an inflow cannula that decompresses the ventricular cavity and an outflow cannula that returns blood to either the ascending aorta or the main pulmonary artery. The pumping chamber of the VAD is implanted sub-diaphragmatically to a pre-peritoneal or intra-abdominal position or may be situated in a paracorporeal position outside the body [66].

Different Generations

First-Generation LVAD: Paracorporeal Ventricular Assist Device

The first LVAD that retained the native heart (Abbott Laboratories) was a pneumatically powered pump placed outside the body (paracorporeal) and connected to cannulas that pulled blood by vacuum from the LV into a reservoir and returned it to the aorta in a pulsatile but asynchronous manner by pneumatic power. It could be used for single or biventricular support, but there were no clinical trials conducted with this device.

Second-Generation LVADs

The pulsatile HeartMate XVE: The size of the device limited its use to patients with larger body size. It also heralded the transition from pneumatic to electrical power, which necessitated a percutaneous driveline to transmit the energy from an external battery power source to the pump via the driveline. This design dramatically reduced the size of the portable drive unit compared with the paracorporeal ventricular assist device and allowed freedom of activity. The success of this device was first demonstrated in patients receiving BTT and led to sufficient equipoise in the field to conduct the first prospective randomized trial in the field (Randomized Evaluation of Mechanical Assistance for the Treatment of Congestive Heart Failure Study) comparing the HeartMate vented electric LVAD to optimized medical therapy alone in patients not considered candidates for heart transplant. However, the device had significant problems with bearing wear and durability, with a very significant percentage of patients requiring device replacement [67, 68]. The Medtronic HeartWare™ HVAD™ System includes a VAD that helps the heart pump and increases the amount of blood that flows through the body in patients with advanced heart failure. The system is designed to help patients with end-stage heart failure when one of the heart's natural pumps (a ventricle) does not perform well. Without treatment, these patients have very low survival. In 2017, the US Food and Drug Administration (FDA) approved the HVAD System for patients with advanced heart failure who are not candidates for heart transplants (called "destination therapy"). The HVAD System is also available as a bridge to heart transplant in eligible patients. In 2018 the FDA approved a less invasive implant procedure for the HVAD Pump, making it the only LVAD approved in the US for implant via a thoracotomy. A thoracotomy involves two small incisions between the patient's ribs, and this implant approach has been shown to lead to shorter hospital stays [69].

HeartWare HVAD System: HeartWare HVAD (Medtronic Corp), which was the first LVAD to be entirely contained within the pericardial space, eliminated the need for a pump pocket. The HVAD uses a centrifugal rather than axial flow design as well as partial magnetic levitation to suspend the rotor, eliminating the presence of bearings in the bloodstream [70, 71]. The system can pump enough blood every minute to decrease heart failure symptoms. A physician programs the system to deliver the proper amount of flow for the body's needs. It was first approved in Europe in 2009. Medtronic has stopped the distribution and sale of the HVAD System as of June 3, 2021, and has notified physicians to cease new implants of the Medtronic HVAD System and transition to an alternative commercial LVAD for all future implants. Prophylactic explant of the HVAD System is not recommended at this time [72, 73].

Complications and adverse events: Stroke, gastrointestinal bleeding, mucosal arteriovenous malformations, and LVAD thrombosis. Failure to stabilize the exit site may result in poor tissue incorporation and ascending infection. While treatment with targeted short-term antibiotic therapy may be effective, it is common to require either long-term antibiotic therapy or surgical debridement for control. Deep-tissue infections related to the pump or the surgical implantation are often more difficult to treat and may lack definitive therapy [66].

CONCLUSION

Cardiovascular medical devices revolutionized medical management in cardiovascular diseases. Cardiovascular diseases, like coronary artery blocks, conduction abnormities, or valvar diseases are now treated using various devices like stents, defibrillators or cardiac ablation therapy, and prosthetic values respectively.

References

1. Types of cardiac devices [Internet]. [cited 2021 Oct 3]. Available from: https://nyulangone.org/conditions/cardiac-device-management-in-adults/types
2. Gierula J, Kearney MT, Witte KK. Devices in heart failure; diagnosis, detection and disease modification. *Br Med Bull*. 2018 Mar 1;125(1):91–102.
3. History | Dualchamber pacemakers for symptomatic bradycardia due to sick sinus syndrome and/or atrioventricular block | Guidance | NICE [Internet]. NICE; [cited 2021 Oct 3]. Available from: https://www.nice.org.uk/guidance/TA88/history
4. Brignole M, Auricchio A, Baron-Esquivias G, Bordachar P, Boriani G, Breithardt O-A, et al. ESC Guidelines on cardiac pacing and cardiac resynchronization therapy: the Task Force on cardiac pacing and resynchronization therapy of the European Society of Cardiology (ESC). Developed in collaboration with the European Heart Rhythm Association (EHRA). *Eur Heart J*. 2013 Aug;34(29):2281–329.
5. Casaclang-Verzosa G, Gersh BJ, Tsang TSM. Structural and functional remodeling of the left atrium: clinical and therapeutic implications for atrial fibrillation. *J Am Coll Cardiol*. 2008 Jan 1;51(1):1–11.
6. Ball CM, Featherstone PJ. Early history of defibrillation. *Anaesth Intensive Care*. 2019 Mar 1;47(2):112–5.
7. Ong MEH, Lim SH, Venkataraman A. Defibrillation and cardioversion. In: Tintinalli JE, Stapczynski JS, Ma OJ, Yealy DM, Meckler GD, Cline DM, editors. *Tintinalli's Emergency Medicine: A Comprehensive Study Guide* [Internet]. 8th ed. New York: McGraw-Hill Education; 2016 [cited 2021 Oct 2]. Available from: accessmedicine.mhmedical.com/content.aspx?aid=1121502347
8. Mechanisms of defibrillation [Internet]. [cited 2021 Oct 2]. Available from: https://www.ncbi.nlm.nih.gov/pmc/articles/PMC3984906/
9. defibrillator_manual.pdf [Internet]. [cited 2021 Oct 2]. Available from: https://www.who.int/medical_devices/innovation/defibrillator_manual.pdf

10. Health C for D and R. Automated External Defibrillators (AEDs). FDA [Internet]. 2021 Jun 24 [cited 2021 Oct 2]; Available from: https://www.fda.gov/medical-devices/cardiovascular-devices/automated-external-defibrillators-aeds

11. Defibrillation [Internet]. Healthgrades. 2014 [cited 2021 Oct 2]. Available from: https://www.healthgrades.com/right-care/heart-health/defibrillation

12. Slater AD, Singer I, Stavens CS, Zee-Cheng C, Ganzel BL, Kupersmith J, et al. Treatment of malignant ventricular arrhythmias with the automatic implantable cardioverter defibrillator. *Ann Surg.* 1989 May;209(5):635–41.

13. Implantable Cardioverter Defibrillator (ICD) Insertion [Internet]. [cited 2021 Oct 2]. Available from: https://www.hopkinsmedicine.org/health/treatment-tests-and-therapies/implantable-cardioverter-defibrillator-icd-insertion

14. Sandhu U, Rajyaguru C, Cheung CC, Morin DP, Lee BK. The wearable cardioverter-defibrillator vest: Indications and ongoing questions. *Prog Cardiovasc Dis.* 2019 Jun;62(3):256–64.

15. Catheter ablation | NHLBI, NIH [Internet]. [cited 2021 Oct 3]. Available from: https://www.nhlbi.nih.gov/health-topics/catheter-ablation

16. Ghzally Y, Ahmed I, Gerasimon G. Catheter ablation. In: *StatPearls* [Internet]. Treasure Island: StatPearls Publishing; 2021 [cited 2021 Oct 3]. Available from: http://www.ncbi.nlm.nih.gov/books/NBK470203/

17. WOVEN™ Fixed Curve Diagnostic Catheter [Internet]. www.bostonscientific.com. [cited 2021 Oct 3]. Available from: https://www.bostonscientific.com/en-US/products/catheters--diagnostic/woven-catheters.html

18. Ghzally Y, Ahmed I, Gerasimon G. Catheter ablation. In: *StatPearls* [Internet]. Treasure Island: StatPearls Publishing; 2021 [cited 2021 Oct 3]. Available from: http://www.ncbi.nlm.nih.gov/books/NBK470203/

19. van der Giessen WJ, Lincoff AM, Schwartz RS, van Beusekom HMM, Serruys PW, Holmes DR, et al. Marked inflammatory sequelae to implantation of biodegradable and nonbiodegradable polymers in porcine coronary arteries. *Circulation.* 1996 Oct 1;94(7):1690–7.

20. Nikam N, Steinberg TB, Steinberg DH. Advances in stent technologies and their effect on clinical efficacy and safety. *Med Devices Auckl NZ.* 2014 Jun 3;7:165–78.

21. Angioplasty and stent placement: heart: MedlinePlus medical encyclopedia [Internet]. [cited 2021 Oct 3]. Available from: https://medlineplus.gov/ency/article/007473.htm

22. Butany J, Carmichael K, Leong SW, Collins MJ. Coronary artery stents: Identification and evaluation. *J Clin Pathol.* 2005 Aug 1;58(8):795–804.

23. Metal Mesh: An overview. *ScienceDirect Topics* [Internet]. [cited 2021 Oct 3]. Available from: https://www.sciencedirect.com/topics/engineering/metal-mesh

24. Schmidt T, Abbott JD. Coronary stents: History, design, and construction. *J Clin Med.* 2018 May 29;7(6):126.

25. Chiarito M, Sardella G, Colombo A, Briguori C, Testa L, Bedogni F, et al. Safety and efficacy of polymer-free drug-eluting stents. *Circ Cardiovasc Interv.* 2019 Feb 1;12(2):e007311.

26. Colleran R, Byrne RA. Polymer-free drug-eluting stents. *Circulation.* 2020 Jun 23;141(25):2064–6.

27. Wu JJ, Way JAH, Kritharides L, Brieger D. Polymer-free versus durable polymer drug-eluting stents in patients with coronary artery disease: A meta-analysis. *Ann Med Surg.* 2018 Dec 11;38:13–21.

28. Baer GM, Small W, Wilson TS, Benett WJ, Matthews DL, Hartman J, et al. Fabrication and in vitro deployment of a laser-activated shape memory polymer vascular stent. *Biomed Eng OnLine.* 2007 Nov 27;6:43.

29. DeForge WF. Cardiac pacemakers: A basic review of the history and current technology. *J Vet Cardiol.* 2019 Apr;22:40–50.

30. Pacemaker.pdf [Internet]. [cited 2021 Oct 1]. Available from: https://www.uwa.edu.au/science/-/media/Faculties/Science/Docs/Pacemaker.pdf

31. Rogel S, Hasin Y. Increased excitability of the heart induced by electrical stimulation in the absolute refractory period. *Chest.* 1971 Dec;60(6):578–82.

32. Whalen RE, Starmer CF. Electric shock hazards in clinical cardiology. *Mod Concepts Cardiovasc Dis.* 1967 Feb;36(2):7–12.

33. Parker B, Furman S, Escher DJ. Input signals to pacemakers in a hospital environment. *Ann N Y Acad Sci.* 1969 Oct 30;167(2):823–34.

34. Gimbel JR, Cox JW. Electronic article surveillance systems and interactions with implantable cardiac devices: risk of adverse interactions in public and commercial spaces. *Mayo Clin Proc.* 2007 Mar;82(3):318–22.

35. Solan AN, Solan MJ, Bednarz G, Goodkin MB. Treatment of patients with cardiac pacemakers and implantable cardioverter-defibrillators during radiotherapy. *Int J Radiat Oncol Biol Phys.* 2004 Jul 1;59(3):897–904.

36. Cohen JD, Costa HS, Russo RJ. Determining the risks of magnetic resonance imaging at 1.5 tesla for patients with pacemakers and implantable cardioverter defibrillators. *Am J Cardiol.* 2012 Dec 1;110(11):1631–6.

37. Kusumoto FM, Schoenfeld MH, Barrett C, Edgerton JR, Ellenbogen KA, Gold MR, et al. ACC/AHA/HRS guideline on the evaluation and management of patients with bradycardia and cardiac conduction delay: Executive summary: A report of the American College of Cardiology/American Heart Association Task Force on clinical practice guidelines, and the heart rhythm society. *J Am Coll Cardiol*. 2019 Aug 20;74(7):932–87.

38. Olshansky B. Pacemakers (beyond the basics). Available from: https://www.uptodate.com/contents/pacemakers-beyond-the-basics

39. A long-term, prospective, cohort study on the performance of right ventricular pacing leads: comparison of active-fixation with passive-fixation leads. *Scientific Reports* [Internet]. [cited 2021 Oct 2]. Available from: https://www.nature.com/articles/srep07662

40. Rajappan K. Permanent pacemaker implantation technique: part II. *Heart Br Card Soc*. 2009 Feb;95(4):334–42.

41. Sadamatsu K. Complication of pacemaker implantation: An atrial lead perforation [Internet]. *Modern Pacemakers: Present and Future*. IntechOpen; 2011 [cited 2021 Oct 2]. Available from: https://www.intechopen.com/chapters/13788

42. Cano O, Osca J, Sancho-Tello M-J, Olagüe J, Castro JE, Salvador A. Failure of the active-fixation mechanism during removal of active-fixation pacing leads. *Pacing Clin Electrophysiol PACE*. 2011 Oct;34(10):1217–24.

43. Gul EE, Kayrak M. Common pacemaker problems: Lead and pocket complications [Internet]. *Modern Pacemakers: Present and Future*. IntechOpen; 2011 [cited 2021 Oct 2]. Available from: https://www.intechopen.com/chapters/13786

44. Lee JZ, Mulpuru SK, Shen WK. Leadless pacemaker: Performance and complications. *Trends Cardiovasc Med*. 2018 Feb 1;28(2):130–41.

45. Wiles BM, Roberts PR. Design and evaluation of the micra transcatheter pacing system for bradyarrhythmia management. *Future Cardiol*. 2019 Jan;15(1):9–15.

46. Sperzel J, Hamm C, Hain A. Nanostim: Leadless pacemaker. *Herzschrittmachertherapie Elektrophysiologie*. 2018 Dec;29(4):327–333.

47. Groner A, Grippe K. The leadless pacemaker: An innovative design to enhance pacemaking capabilities. *J Am Acad Physician Assist*. 2019 Jun;32(6):48–50.

48. Steinwender C, Lercher P, Schukro C, Blessberger H, Prenner G, Andreas M, et al. State of the art: leadless ventricular pacing: A national expert consensus of the Austrian Society of Cardiology. *J Interv Card Electrophysiol*. 2020 Jan;57(1):27–37.

49. Afzal MR, Daoud EG, Cunnane R, Mulpuru SK, Koay A, Hussain A, et al. Techniques for successful early retrieval of the Micra transcatheter pacing system: A worldwide experience. *Heart Rhythm*. 2018 Jun;15(6):841–6.

50. Heart Valve Replacement: Which Type Is Best for You? [Internet]. Cleveland Clinic. 2018 [cited 2021 Oct 2]. Available from: https://health.clevelandclinic.org/heart-valve-replacement-which-type-is-best-for-you/

51. Muraru D, Anwar AM, Song J-K. Heart valve disease: tricuspid valve disease [Internet]. *The EACVI Textbook of Echocardiography*. Oxford University Press; [cited 2021 Oct 2]. Available from: https://oxfordmedicine.com/view/10.1093/med/9780198726012.001.0001/med-9780198726012-chapter-37

52. Bloomfield P. Choice of heart valve prosthesis. *Heart*. 2002 Jun 1;87(6):583–9.

53. Matthews AM. The development of the Starr-Edwards heart valve. *Tex Heart Inst J*. 1998;25(4):282–93.

54. Sun JCJ, Davidson MJ, Lamy A, Eikelboom JW. Antithrombotic management of patients with prosthetic heart valves: current evidence and future trends. *Lancet Lond Engl*. 2009 Aug 15;374(9689):565–76.

55. Prosthetic heart valves. *Circulation* [Internet]. [cited 2021 Oct 2]. Available from: https://www.ahajournals.org/doi/10.1161/circulationaha.108.778886

56. Tillquist MN, Maddox TM. Cardiac crossroads: deciding between mechanical or bioprosthetic heart valve replacement. *Patient Prefer Adherence*. 2011 Feb 17;5:91–9.

57. Johansen P Mechanical heart valve cavitation. *Expert Rev Med Devices*. 2004 Sep;1(1):95–104.

58. Pibarot P, Dumesnil JG. Prosthetic heart valves: selection of the optimal prosthesis and long-term management. *Circulation*. 2009 Feb 24;119(7):1034–48.

59. Hickey GL, Grant SW, Bridgewater B, Kendall S, Bryan AJ, Kuo J, et al. A comparison of outcomes between bovine pericardial and porcine valves in 38,040 patients in England and Wales over 10 years. *Eur J Cardio-Thorac Surg Off J Eur Assoc Cardio-Thorac Surg*. 2015 Jun;47(6):1067–74.

60. Tissue-engineered heart valves: A call for mechanistic studies. *Tissue Engineering Part B: Reviews* [Internet]. [cited 2021 Oct 2]. Available from: https://www.liebertpub.com/doi/10.1089/ten.teb.2017.0425

61. Uriel N, Drakos SG. Advances in mechanical circulatory support. *Curr Opin Cardiol*. 2016 May;31(3):275–6.

62. Lim HS, Howell N, Ranasinghe A. The physiology of continuous-flow left ventricular assist devices. *J Card Fail*. 2017 Feb;23(2):169–80.

63. Patel CB, Cowger JA, Zuckermann A. A contemporary review of mechanical circulatory support. *J Heart Lung Transplant Off Publ Int Soc Heart Transplant*. 2014 Jul;33(7):667–74.

64. Chaanine AH, Pinney SP. Mechanical circulatory support as a bridge to heart transplantation. In: Eisen H, editor. *Heart Failure* [Internet]. London: Springer; 2017 [cited 2021 Oct 2]. p. 639–63. Available from: http://link.springer.com/10.1007/978-1-4471-4219-5_27

65. Wilson SR, Givertz MM, Stewart GC, Mudge GH. Ventricular assist devices the challenges of outpatient management. *J Am Coll Cardiol.* 2009 Oct 27;54(18):1647–59.

66. Miller LW, Rogers JG. Evolution of left ventricular assist device therapy for advanced heart failure: A review. *JAMA Cardiol.* 2018 Jul 1;3(7):650.

67. Frazier OH, Rose EA, Oz MC, Dembitsky W, McCarthy P, Radovancevic B, et al. Multicenter clinical evaluation of the HeartMate vented electric left ventricular assist system in patients awaiting heart transplantation. *J Thorac Cardiovasc Surg.* 2001 Dec;122(6):1186–95.

68. Rose EA, Gelijns AC, Moskowitz AJ, Heitjan DF, Stevenson LW, Dembitsky W, et al. Long-term use of a left ventricular assist device for end-stage heart failure. *N Engl J Med.* 2001 Nov 15;345(20):1435–43.

69. Publishing B. FDA approves heartmate II for destination therapy [Internet]. *Cardiovascular News.* 2010 [cited 2021 Oct 2]. Available from: https://cardiovascularnews.com/fda-approves-heartmate-ii-for-destination-therapy/

70. Aaronson KD, Slaughter MS, Miller LW, McGee EC, Cotts WG, Acker MA, et al. Use of an intrapericardial, continuous-flow, centrifugal pump in patients awaiting heart transplantation. *Circulation.* 2012 Jun 26;125(25):3191–200.

71. Slaughter MS, Pagani FD, McGee EC, Birks EJ, Cotts WG, Gregoric I, et al. HeartWare ventricular assist system for bridge to transplant: combined results of the bridge to transplant and continued access protocol trial. *J Heart Lung Transplant Off Publ Int Soc Heart Transplant.* 2013 Jul;32(7):675–83.

72. Medtronic heartware HVAD system approved for destination therapy [Internet]. [cited 2021 Oct 2]. Available from: https://www.meddeviceonline.com/doc/medtronic-heartware-hvad-system-approved-for-destination-therapy-0001

73. Lavare cycle: Medtronic HVAD system. Medtronic [Internet]. [cited 2021 Oct 2]. Available from: https://www.medtronic.com/us-en/healthcare-professionals/products/cardiac-rhythm/ventricular-assist-devices/hvad-system/lavare-cycle.html

Neurological Devices

8

Shalini Pattabiraman, Harini Sriram, Basanta Manjari Naik, and Indumathy Jagadeeswaran

INTRODUCTION

Medical technologies that interface with the central and peripheral nervous system for use in diagnostics, preventive therapies, and symptomatic treatments are classified as neurological devices. In recent years, neurological medical devices (neuro-technologies) are emerging as a promising technology in diagnostic and symptomatic treatments, with the potential to prevent disease progression in future [1]. Given the higher incidence and the nature of neurological conditions being treated, such as stroke, epilepsy, Parkinson's disease, Alzheimer's disease, traumatic brain injury (TBI), brain tumor, and pain, these neurological medical devices can have a significant impact in improving public health and overall disease burden worldwide. The higher prevalence of neurological disorders, increased aging population, rapid technical advancements, and increased demand for more non-invasive devices, besides other factors, have drawn huge investments by private players in neurological devices and their research and development (R&D) [1]. The Food and Drug Administration (FDA) has approved several safe and effective neurological devices that have brought optimism and a substantial impact on mental and physical neurological impairments in patients [2]. Based on their degree of risk, the FDA (21 CFR part 882, 2016) [3] has categorized medical devices into class I (lowest risk), class II (moderate risk), and class III (high risk) neurological devices. Within the FDA, the Center for Devices and Radiological Health (CDRH) is committed to increasing access to safe and effective medical devices for US patients (FDA, 2015a) [4], and the Division of Neurological and Physical Medicine Devices (DNPMD) acts as the primary regulatory body that reviews the clinical trials and marketing applications involving medical device neuro-technologies [2]. Here in this chapter, we have discussed the medical neurological devices based on their clinical application in three main categories: Neurodiagnostic and neurosurgical devices, neurointerventional devices, and neurostimulation devices, with an emphasis on their advantages and limitations (Figure 8.1).

NEURODIAGNOSTIC AND NEUROSURGICAL DEVICES

Electroencephalogram

Electroencephalogram (EEG) is a recording of electrical activity produced by the neurons within a human brain using an electrophysiological technique. The neurons in the human brain produce signals called

DOI: 10.1201/9781003220671-8

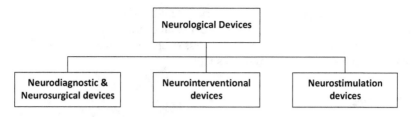

FIGURE 8.1 Categories of neurological devices discussed in the present chapter.

action potential, which transmit from one nerve cell to another. This electrical activity is very small and is measured in microvolts by EEG [5].

Working Principle

The electrodes are placed on the scalp at different points, and each electrode is connected to a differential amplifier. Each amplifier has two inputs, one connected to the active electrode and the other connected to a common reference electrode [6]. EEG works on the principle of differential amplification, or the difference in voltage between the active electrode and the reference electrode. The differences in these electric potentials are characterized as the EEG waveforms [7].

In analog EEG, these signals are printed on a paper as deflections of a pen whereas in digital EEG, these signals are digitized using an analog-to-digital converter. The rate at which this analog-to-digital conversion of signals occurs is referred to as the sampling rate. The digital EEG signals can be filtered and stored electronically [5, 7].

Clinical Applications [5–7]

- To evaluate conditions which involve dynamic cerebral function such as seizures, unusual spells, and epilepsy.
- To monitor the depth of anesthesia during surgical procedures.
- To differentiate organic encephalopathy or delirium from other psychiatric problems.
- It functions as a supplementary test for brain death.
- To localize the damaged tissue in the brain.
- In subjects with coma, it can be used to come up with a prognosis.
- To determine when to wean the patients off anti-epileptic medications.
- In carotid endarterectomy, it can be used to indicate cerebral perfusion.
- To monitor secondary brain damage during conditions such as subarachnoid hemorrhage.

Limitations [5, 7]

- Poor spatial resolution.
- Very sensitive towards certain post-synaptic potentials.
- The signal can be smeared by skull, cerebrospinal fluid, or meninges resulting in confusion regarding the intracranial source.
- The inverse problem, it is impossible to map an EEG signal to a specific intracranial source mathematically.
- Other general electrical activity in the body or the environment may influence the cerebral activity therefore impacting the EEG waveforms.

Polysomnogram

Polysomnogram (PSG) is a procedure used to record, analyze, and interpret physiological signals collected from different parts of the human body during sleep [8]. It is a multidimensional approach used to record stages of sleep, rapid eye movement, electrical activity of muscle tissue, breathing pattern, and electrical activity of the brain during sleep [9]. A PSG is an overnight procedure aimed at recreating a typical night's sleep of a person assessing wakefulness, sleep disturbances, stages of sleep, respiration, cardio-pulmonary functions, and body movements [10].

Working Principle

To perform a sleep study PSG utilizes electrooculogram, electromyogram, electrocardiogram, electroencephalogram, respiratory effort, oral and nasal airflow pressure, transcutaneous CO_2, and pulse oximetry to study sleep-related issues [11]. During a polysomnogram procedure the bio-electrical potentials from different parts of the body are recorded, amplified, and filtered, in order to display and analyze them. So, the equipment is a series of amplifiers that amplify these waveforms and pass them through filters, thus enabling them to be visualized at different sensitive settings [10]. The various components of a polysomnogram are:

- Electroencephalogram (records the electrical activity of brain)
- Electromyogram (records the electrical activity of muscles)
- Electrooculogram (records eye movements)
- Electrocardiogram (records cardiac functions)
- Nasal pressure transducer and thermister (monitors nasal airflow pressure and temperature)
- Chest and abdominal belts (records respiratory effort and body movements)
- Pulse oximetry (monitors oxygen saturation)

Clinical Applications [9, 11, 12]

- To diagnose sleep-related breathing disorders such as sleep apnea and sleep hypoxia
- To study nocturnal seizures and nightmares occurring with seizures
- To assess periodic limb movement disorder
- To evaluate central nervous system hypersomnias such as narcolepsy and idiopathic hypersomnia

Limitations [9, 13]

- This procedure lacks a standard protocol, which makes it difficult to compare sleep studies of one laboratory to another.
- Since this is an overnight procedure, it is considered labor intensive, expensive, and tedious.
- Home sleep studies may lack the presence of a sleep technologist who can correct technological issues which may occur during the night.
- A single overnight study may not be enough to gather sleep pattern data, thus resulting in inconsistency with the clinical findings of patients.
- Though PSG is the most widely used sleep study, it cannot determine the etiology of the apnea-hypopnea syndrome.
- PSG cannot be used to diagnose insomnia.
- Certain factors influencing sleep such as unfamiliar surroundings may cause 'first night effects' thus producing some misleading PSG data.
- It is not able to diagnose circadian rhythm sleep disorders.

Nerve Conduction Studies

Nerve conduction studies are a part of peripheral neurophysiological examination. This procedure involves the study of electrical activity of the peripheral nerves which helps to assess their function, conduction, and axon integrity. These studies provide diagnostic, descriptive, and prognostic information about the peripheral nerves [14].

Working Principle

The procedure involves the application of a depolarized square wave electrical pulse on the skin over a peripheral nerve, which activates the sensory and the motor axons of the nerve. This electrical wave pulse further results in production of: [15]

i. A nerve action potential which can be recorded on the same nerve at a particular distance
ii. A compound muscle action potential which arises by the activation of the muscle fibers targeted by the nerve

This is achieved with the help of either surface or needle electrodes. Surface electrodes are used when study of the whole of a muscle is required, whereas needle electrodes can record only a small area of muscle or nerve. Surface stimulators are used to stimulate the nerves through the skin; this can also be done by placing a needle near the nerve or the nerve root. The different types of nerve conduction studies include motor nerve conduction studies, sensory conduction studies, and F waves [15].

Clinical Applications [13–16]

- To diagnose muscular and near muscular disorders such as herniated disk disease, Guillain Barré syndrome, carpal tunnel syndrome, Charcot-Marie-Tooth disease, sciatica nerve problems, polyneuropathy, and neuropathy
- Provides information to locate lesions in the length of a nerve
- To assess cranial nerve and spinal cord function
- To assess the nerve components such as velocity, amplitude, and shape
- To define the extent of the nerve injury or damage
- To determine if a neuropathy is due to injury to the nerve axon or the myelin sheath

Limitations [16, 17]

- It cannot be used to assess small-fiber neuropathy.
- The presence of abnormal innervation may complicate the NCS.
- A study performed during the early course of a disease might fail to record some subtle nerve changes therefore requiring repeated nerve stimulation.
- The results of these studies are highly context specific, which might require a neurophysiologist to understand the parameters combined with the clinical findings in order to interpret the results.
- The nerve conduction varies with age, so the reference values in the case of pediatrics and older age groups are not very well defined, which makes it difficult to interpret neural sensory responses.

Long-Term Electroencephalographic Monitoring (LTM)

LTM is a process of prolonged EEG in order to record seizures and disturbances of neurologic function [18]. LTM expands the limited sampling time associated with the regular EEG and is usually performed in a hospital setting [19].

Working Principle

There are three different methods of long-term EEG monitoring:

1 Prolonged analog or digital EEG
2. Prolonged analog or digital ambulatory EEG
3. Prolonged analog or digital video EEG with telemetry

This is an inpatient procedure performed in a safe environment like an epilepsy monitoring unit [19]. Patients in this unit undergo continuous EEG and video monitoring (usually 24 hours a day) and require a 3- to 5-day stay.

Clinical Applications [20–23]

- To classify the types of seizures and electro clinical syndromes
- To quantify the number and frequency of seizures, and ictal and interictal epileptiform discharges
- To verify the epileptic nature of new spells or seizures
- To diagnose epileptic paroxysmal abnormalities or events
- To differentiate between epileptic and non-epileptic seizures
- To perform presurgical evaluation of medically refractory epilepsy
- To localize the epileptogenic region of the brain
- To detect non-convulsive seizures in ICU patients
- To assess the level of sedation and detect silent neurological events
- To detect ischemia

Limitations [23]

- It is a labor-intensive and tedious procedure.
- Usually, patients in the ICU require some simultaneous tests such as MRI, which can hinder continuous monitoring.
- The displacement of electrodes and artifacts cause issues in the generation of consistent data.
- The data generated is very large which makes it very challenging to analyze and interpret it.

Intraoperative Neurophysiological Monitoring (IONM)

Intraoperative neurophysiological monitoring (IONM) is an electrophysiological technique used during surgeries to evaluate neural structure integrity and consciousness [24]. It is an emerging and most promising field, which has been utilized in attempts to minimize neurological morbidity from operative manipulations. IONM is a multimodal monitoring platform which warns the surgical team about possible iatrogenic injury to nerve tissues during surgical manipulations, and hence it prevents surgery-induced neurological deficit. It functions as an effort to avert the neurological complications arising during surgeries [25]. It helps to prevent or significantly minimize any irreversible damage to the neurological structure and thus avoids postoperative neurological deficit. The IONM equipment/ device is a multi-channel (32–64) device with the signal acquisition and stimulator delivery system needed to monitor all the modalities necessary for the type of surgery being performed. It monitors neural tissues and the localization of the neural structures [24].

There are different techniques used for IONM, and each of these techniques monitors a specific neural pathway [24].

- Evoked potentials
- Electroencephalography
- Electromyography

Evoked Potentials

The electrophysiological triggered responses of the nervous system, when an external stimulus of known intensity, duration, and frequency is applied, are called an evoked potential [26]. Various stimuli are used to elicit evoked potential, but the most common ones are visual, auditory, motor, and somatosensory [24, 26]. Evoked potential are modalities of intraoperative neuromonitoring techniques which are used to monitor a specific neural pathway [24].

Clinical Applications [24–26]

- Provides information on the peripheral and central nervous system pathways.
- Provides data which can be used to delineate the sensory system lesions that are clinically misleading based on physical findings.
- Used to locate the lesions on the nervous systems anatomically, thus helping to monitor the progression.

The most used evoked potential techniques are discussed below.

Somatosensory Evoked Potential (SSEP)
This technique involves stimulation of the peripheral nerve, and the signal transmission is recorded through the dorsal column in the spinal cord, medial lemniscus, thalamus, and into the somatosensory cortex [26]. It monitors the dorsal column-medial lemniscus pathway [24]. The amplitude and the latency of the waveforms generated are monitored to assess the intraoperative changes [27]. These techniques are used in spine and spinal cord surgeries, brain and brain stem surgeries, cerebrovascular surgeries, pelvic fracture surgery, thorax-abdominal aortic aneurysm repair, brachial plexus and lumbosacral plexus surgery, carotid endarterectomy, and thyroid surgery [24].

Motor Evoked Potential (MEP)
This technique monitors the motor pathway, by stimulating the motor cortex transcranially through the scalp [26]. The transcranial electrical stimulation excites corticospinal projections at various levels at the neuromuscular junction [24]. The electrical wave generated transmits down the spinal cord and synapses, thus causing depolarization and muscle contraction [27]. Based on the electrode placement and the intensity of the stimulation the evoked potentials can be recorded at various sites on the brain, superficial white mater, deep white matter, and the pyramidal decussation. The pyramidal tract transports the generated MEPs. This technique is used during stereotactic surgery on the brain stem, and thalamus and cerebral cortex, cervical surgery, and all the other surgeries where SSEPs are used [24].

Visual Evoked Potential (VEP)
This technique is used to monitor the optic pathway in response to a light stimulus. The retina converts the visual stimuli into nerve signals, which are transported to the brain via the optical pathway – retina to optic nerve, optic chiasma via the optic tract, lateral geniculate body, optic radiation, and then to the visual cortex occipital lobe. This technique is used during optic nerve surgery, orbital surgery, and pituitary gland surgery [24].

Brainstem Auditory Evoked Potential (BAEP)
This technique is used to monitor the auditory pathway in the brainstem in response to sound stimuli. The signal travels through the cochlear hair cells to the auditory cortex through the vestibulocochlear nerve, lateral lemniscus, inferior colliculus, and medial geniculate body [24]. The resulting potential or waveform has seven peaks generated from the different structures along the pathway which in turn help in the identification of the site of damage [26]. This technique is used during acoustic neuroma resection, vestibular nerve resection, vascular loop decompression, vestibular schwannomas, facial nerve decompression, brainstem tumor resection, auditory brainstem implant, posterior fossa procedure, localization of the cortex through cortical stimulation, and the assessment of ischemia at the cochlea and eighth nerve [24].

Limitations [26]

- The general anesthetics like volatile agents may cause alterations in the generated potentials.
- Each type of evoked potential technique is specific to monitoring one pathway, so a combination of EP techniques might be required when multiple pathways are at risk during surgeries.
- The electrical potentials generated are very small and can be interfered by other electrical instruments present in the operating theaters.
- In the case of SSEPs and BAEPs, there is an extra time requirement to average the signal (enhance the signal to noise ratio).
- If needle electrodes are used, they can be inserted only after the anesthesia since they can be painful. Needle electrodes can cause infection and sometimes, they can also lead to needle stick injuries.
- The corkscrew electrodes used in MEPs can cause localized bleeding.

Quantitative Sensory Testing

Quantitative sensory testing is a non-invasive and non-aversive procedure to quantify and monitor the sensory function in patients with neurologic symptoms [28–30]. It determines the sensory threshold in response to a calibrated sensory stimulus [31]. The most common sensory modalities used in clinical practice as stimuli for QST are light touch, vibration, thermal stimuli (hot & cold), and pain stimuli. [29, 30].

Working Principle

This procedure is defined by the stimuli properties such as modality, intensity, and spatial characteristics. It analyzes the quality of the response signal produced and quantifies the intensity of the evoked signal. Computerized systems with stimulators are used to evoke and determine the sensory threshold. Various algorithms have been developed for the assessment of the threshold [32]. The two general schemes used are:

The Method of Limits
In this method the intensity of the stimuli is either increased or decreased until the subject can indicate or feel the stimulus, and thus the stimulus is stopped using a feedback control like a button press. The threshold values are determined as the mean of the values obtained by a series of stimuli responses. This method is dependent on the motor abilities of the subject, reaction time, and rate of change of stimuli [30, 32].

The Method of Levels
In this method a set of stimuli of known intensity and modality are applied to the skin and for each stimulus, the subject response (whether the stimulus is felt or not) is recorded. It is often called a 'forced choice' algorithm. Depending on the subject's response to the stimulus, the intensity of the subsequent stimulus is either increased or decreased. This method doesn't depend on the reaction time of the subject but it is time-consuming [30, 32].

Clinical Applications [28, 29, 31, 32]

- To quantify sensory deficits.
- The large myelinated nerve fibers are evaluated using light touch and vibration stimuli.
- The small myelinated and unmyelinated sensory nerve fibers are evaluated using thermal stimuli.
- Thermal hyperalgesia and hypoesthesia are studied using the pain modality.
- The QST data can be used in parametric statistical analysis which enables the screening of large populations in clinical trials.
- To identify diffuse polyneuropathy in patients who are exposed to industrial toxins.
- To detect peripheral neuropathy early in patients undergoing chemotherapy.
- To study the afferent pain pathway from the periphery to the brain which is used to predict the postoperative pain score.

Limitations [29]

- It cannot be used to localize sensory nerve function deficit or loss.
- Dysfunction of the central nervous system or the peripheral nerves can lead to abnormalities in the QST data.
- The results can change due to distraction, boredom, mental fatigue, and drowsiness since it is a psychophysical test.
- It is patient dependent and can produce false abnormal results if the patient is biased towards an abnormal result or is cognitively impaired.

Repetitive Nerve Stimulation

Repetitive nerve stimulation is an electrodiagnostic test used to diagnose neuromuscular junction disorders [33]. The motor fibers within a nerve are stimulated transcutaneously at regular intervals, and impulses are generated. These impulses travel across the neuromuscular junction into the muscle, where electric potential responses are recorded [34].

Working Principle

In this technique, a series of stimuli is applied to evoke the peripheral nerve, and the compound muscle action potentials (CMAP) generated at the targeted muscle is recorded with an active surface electrode placed over the muscle and a referential electrode over the tendon of the same muscle. The waveform amplitude and the area of the muscle action potential response indicate the number of muscle fibers activated by the stimulus. This is called the synaptic efficacy of the nerve [33].

Clinical Applications [35]

- To study neuromuscular transmission
- To diagnose the neuromuscular junction disorders – presynaptic (Lambert-Eaton myasthenia syndrome), synaptic (cholinesterase inhibitor toxicity), and post-synaptic (myasthenia gravis)

Limitations [33–35]

- Limb and muscle movement might alter the recording electrode placement thus producing inaccurate results.

- The limb temperature can also impede the amplitude, latencies, and conduction velocities resulting in inaccurate results.
- Immobilization of the recording electrode and tested muscle is limited.

Electromyography

Electromyography (EMG) is an electrodiagnostic technique used to measure the electrical activity of the muscles in response to a nerve stimulus. Based on the stimulus applied, the muscles contract which can be voluntary or involuntary [36]. The functional unit of a muscle contraction is a motor unit. Each motor unit consists of a single motor neuron and multiple muscle fibers. When the motor nerves are stimulated, the action potentials are generated, and they reach a depolarization threshold, in turn causing the muscle fibers to contract. This depolarization spreads across the membrane of the muscle, and the muscle action potential generated is measured as voltage. The motor unit action potential is the summation of the individual action potential of the muscle fibers present in that motor unit. Thus, an EMG signal is the algebraic summation of the motor unit action potentials generated in the area where the electrode is placed [37].

Working Principle

During the test, one or more electrodes are inserted into the Muscle. The electrical activity generated is recorded in an oscilloscope, and an audio amplifier is used to amplify and hear the activity. The electrical activity of the muscle is measured during rest, slight contraction, and forced contraction. When the muscle is resting, usually there is no electrical activity. Then the subject may be asked to contract the muscle; this stimulation generates the required action potential thus providing information about the integrity of the muscle in response to the nerve stimulation [37, 38].

There are two types of electromyography [38]:

1. Clinical (Diagnostic)

Diagnostic or clinical EMG is used to study the duration and the amplitude of the motor unit action potential. It is used to diagnose neuromuscular pathology and also detects spontaneous discharges from the relaxed muscle.

2. Kinesiological

Kinesiological EMG is used to study the link between muscular function and movements of the body segments, thus evaluating the timing of the muscle activity with respect to the body movements.

The electrodes used for kinesiological EMG are further classified as:

a. Surface Electrodes

These are non-invasive and directly applied on the skin. There are two types of surface electrodes:

i) Active surface electrodes: These have a built-in amplifier which helps to decrease the movement artifacts and increases the signal to noise ratio. They don't require gels.
ii) Passive surface electrodes: These don't have a built-in amplifier, thus requiring skin preparation and the application of gel. Once the signal is amplified, many movement artifacts are also amplified and the signal to noise ratio is decreased.

Surface electrodes are easily reproducible and good for movement application. But they can only be used on surface muscles, and there is a high chance of potential disturbance from the adjacent muscles [37].

b. Fine Wire Electrodes

These are also called needle electrodes, since they are inserted into the muscle using a needle. Since they are inserted into the specific muscle, they have can be used to test deep muscles and small muscles. But since the needle insertion can cause discomfort, it can lead to tightness in the muscle which can interfere with the results. The fine wire electrodes also need to be stimulated after the needle is inserted which can increase the discomfort [37].

Clinical Applications [37]

- To diagnose neuromuscular disorders
- To distinguish myopathy from neurogenic muscle weakness
- To identify chronic denervation and fasciculation in a normal muscle
- To detect the distribution of neurogenic abnormalities
- To differentiate focal nerve, plexus, and radicular pathology
- To identify the pathophysiology of peripheral neuropathy
- To diagnose motor neuron disease

Limitations [37, 38]

- In obese subjects, the examination of certain muscles is challenging.
- Low pain tolerance in subjects can limit the testing.
- Needle insertion may be harmful for subjects prone to infections or those with a weakened immune system.
- Certain skin problems such as lymphedema limit the use of needles.
- Examination of the muscles near lungs poses a threat of puncturing the pleura.

Single Fiber EMG (SFEMG)

SFEMG is a selective technique which is used to record the activity of a specific muscle fiber. The needle electrode used for this technique has a very small recording surface making this a selective test. A contracted needle or a facial concentric needle electrode is used to generate the signals. The time interval between the generation of two action potentials of the same motor unit is called a 'jitter' [39]. Jitter is the most sensitive electrophysiological measure of the safety factor of neuromuscular transmission [33]. The jitter measurement is expressed as mean consecutive difference (MCD) [39].

Clinical Applications [40]

- To study the neuromuscular transmission disorders
- To quantify the density of muscle fibers in a motor unit

Limitations [36, 40]

- The single fiber electrodes are expensive and cannot be reused.
- Pathological conditions such as reinnervation and immature nerve endings may produce false jitter values.
- The test is highly sensitive.

3D Rotational Angiography

This is an innovative technique used to visualize cardiac structures. It is a three-dimensional reconstruction of the images from direct angiography with supplemental two-dimensional fluoroscopy [41].

Working Principle

The principle is the same as that of a CT scan; the images obtained are reconstructed into 3D images. The X-ray system is rotated over the patient to capture the images of interest. A contrast medium is injected into the left atrium in order to differentiate the cardiac structures. The esophagus is opacified using a barium paste before the images are acquired. The rotational angiographic images of the left atrium, pulmonary vein, and esophagus will be captured and segmented with fluoroscopy on the computer system [41].

Clinical Applications [41, 42]

- To visualize cardiac structures with depth perception and volume appreciation
- To depict the internal carotid artery multidimensionally
- For the placement of stent graft in iliac aneurysm
- In peripheral angioplasty and stenting
- To detect stenosis of the inferior mesenteric artery
- To detect the misalignment of intravascular stents

Limitations [41, 42]

- The use of contrast limits its use for subjects with renal insufficiency.
- This technique is sensitive to patient movements.
- To get adequate results, proper isocentering is essential.
- It does not display any electrogram data.

Computed Tomographic Angiography

CTA is a non-invasive method used to visualize the vasculature with the help of an iodinated contrast medium. The contrast medium is injected through an IV line, and the area of interest is opacified. Then the X-ray (CT) is used to scan and obtain cross-sectional images of the blood vessels and tissues [43].

Clinical Applications [43–45]

- To visualize the vasculature before surgeries for better planning
- To perform endovascular procedures such as transcatheter aortic valve replacement and endovascular repair
- To evaluate in-stent restenosis in iliac and femoral arteries
- To evaluate subjects with aortoiliac, aortofemoral, or axillofemoral bypass grafts
- To detect intracranial aneurysms and intracranial stenosis

Limitations [44]

- The use of contrast limits its use on subjects with renal insufficiency.
- It exposes the subjects to radiation.
- Some of the scanners may have limited view field.
- Subjects with dental implants or fillings produce beam hardening artifacts.
- Certain physiological data such as the floe direction and velocity is missing.

Diagnostic Cerebral Angiography

Diagnostic cerebral angiography is a technique used to visualize the cerebral vasculature with the help of a contrast medium. It provides detailed images of the arteries and veins in the brain which are too small to be visualized with any other imaging technique [46, 47].

Working Principle

A mild sedative is administered to the subject in order to help them relax and not move during the procedure. A flow directed microcatheter is inserted into the blood vessels through the femoral artery (usually in the groin area) and is carefully navigated through the carotid or vertebral vessels. When the catheter is in the desired position, the contrast dye is injected. The dye flows and the images are captured for analysis [47].

Clinical Applications [46, 47]

- To diagnose cerebral aneurysms, fatty plaques, blood clots, vasculitis, or other vasculature abnormalities
- To evaluate the arteries of the head and neck before surgeries
- To find a clot which may or may not have caused a stroke
- To diagnose dural arteriovenous fistulas
- To identify narrowing of arteries or leakage

Limitations [46]

- The contrast dye can be allergenic, and cannot be used with renal insufficient subjects.
- The insertion of catheter may cause a blood clot or bleeding, leading to loss of blood flow to legs or lower extremities.
- The navigation of the catheter might damage an artery or arterial wall.

Magnetic Resonance (MR) Perfusion

MR perfusion is a non-invasive imaging technique used to measure a cerebral perfusion while assessing cerebral blood flow, cerebral blood volume, and transit time [48].

Working Principle

The perfusion MRI can be performed with or without the use of exogenous contrast agent. The different modalities of this technique are [49, 50]:

1. Dynamic Susceptibility Contrast (DSC-MRI)

This technique is used only in the brain for the diagnosis of cerebral ischemia and brain tumors. It involves the injection of a magnetic resonance contrast through IV, and the signal loss is recorded during the navigation of the dye through the bolus across the tissue.

2. Dynamic Contrast Enhanced (DCE-MRI)

In this technique, the magnetic resonance images are captured before, during, and after the bolus injection of the contrast dye.

3. Arterial Spin Labeling (ASL-MRI)

This technique is used to quantitatively analyze the cerebral blood flow, using the magnetically labeled blood as an endogenous tracer. It is completely non-invasive.

Clinical Applications [48]

- To diagnose cerebrovascular diseases and other brain disorders
- To evaluate tissues after acute stroke
- To assess tumors histologically
- To evaluate neurodegenerative disorders
- To visualize extra-axonal tumors
- To identify the location and extent of tumors

Limitations [48]

- The DSC-MRI technique is artifact susceptible and user dependent.
- The DCE-MRI technique has complex image acquisition and lacks user-friendly pharmacokinetic model post-processing software.
- The ASL-MRI technique involves longer scanning time or longer acquisition time.

Transcranial Doppler

Transcranial Doppler (TCD) is an ultrasound technique which is used to study cerebrovascular hemodynamics. It is a rapid, non-invasive, and inexpensive tool to obtain some real time data about the blood flow characteristics within the basal arteries in the brain [51].

The carotid Doppler technique is used to evaluate atherosclerosis of the carotid artery. It measures the thickness of the tunica media, and thus helps in studying the plaque morphology related to the risk of stroke [52].

Working Principle

The examination is performed using a 2 MHz frequency ultrasound probe [53]. The ultrasound examination of a vessel by TCD is called insonation. The probe is placed at various areas of the skull where there is a lack of bone covering, also called acoustic windows. There are four main types of acoustic windows, with each window used to examine different arteries [53]. A complete TCD examination includes the data from all four acoustic windows [51, 52].

The four acoustic windows used for TCD examination are:

1. The Trans Temporal Window

This is used to insonate the middle cerebral artery (MCA), the anterior cerebral artery (ACA), the posterior cerebral artery (PCA), and the terminal portion of the internal carotid artery (TICA), prior to its bifurcation [53, 54].

2. The Trans Orbital Window

This is used to insonate the ophthalmic artery (OA) and the internal carotid artery at the siphon level [53, 54].

3. The Trans Oraminal Window

This is also called the suboccipital window and is used to insonate the distal vertebral arteries (VA) and the basal artery (BA) [53, 54].

4. The Submandibular Window

This is used to insonate the distal portions of the extra cranial internal carotid artery [53, 54].

Clinical Applications [52–56]

- To diagnose focal vascular stenosis.
- To detect stenosis and occlusion of the carotid siphon and intracranial vertebral arteries.
- To detect acute ischemic stroke.
- Repeated TCD studies are used to track arterial occlusion before and after thrombolysis.
- To provide real time data on blood flow and velocity in the intracranial collateral channels activated in acute and chronic steno-occlusive cerebrovascular diseases.
- As a screening tool and preventive measure to prevent stroke in children with sickle cell anemia.
- To detect circulating cerebral micro emboli (solid and gaseous).
- To visualize the blood flow pattern resulting in cerebral circulatory arrest and brain death.
- To monitor vasospasm after subarachnoid hemorrhage.

Limitations [53, 54, 56]

- Its accuracy depends on the knowledge and experience of the interpreter.
- It has a limited ability to detect the distal branches of the intracranial vessels.

Gait Analysis

Gait analysis is a technique which is used to study the parameters of the human gait. It involves a complete physical examination of the hip, knee, and ankle joints, and any abnormal neurologic signs that cause gait abnormalities, and examination of muscle spasticity, muscle weakness, muscle or joint contractors, and extrapyramidal motions. The abnormalities of the lumbar spine, pelvis, or lower extremities are determined radiologically [57]. A detailed gait analysis, other than the observational gait analysis, is performed in a motion analysis laboratory [57–59]. It uses EMG to study muscle activity, the dynamic range of motion is measured BY kinematics, kinetics is used to study the force acting on the moving body, the energy expenditure is measured by energetics, and the foot pressure is measured using foot transducers [57–59].

Clinical Applications [58, 59]

- To evaluate development disabilities in children
- To study the effect of total joint arthroplasty on the gait
- To evaluate gait in subjects with lower extremity amputation or to assess the upper extremity function in those with upper extremity amputation
- To evaluate sport activities using high-speed cameras and a high-resolution video system
- To study the effect of anterior ligament injuries and reconstruction on gait

Ocular Physiology

Eyes receive and process the energy from the light, producing action potential in nerve cells, and those action potentials are relayed to the brain through the optic nerve also called the cranial nerve II. The light is focused and transmitted to the retina with the help of the cornea, iris, ciliary body, and lens. The choroid, aqueous humor, vitreous humor, and lacrimal system maintain the ocular pressure, physiological balance, and ocular tissue nourishment [60].

Optic Nerve Testing

An ophthalmoscope is used to observe the optic disc, retinal vessels, and fovea. A pupil swing light test is performed by moving the light back and forth from one eye to another. A visual acuity test is performed by asking the subject to read letters on a standardized chart placed 20 feet away. A visual fields test is performed by confrontation [60].

Clinical Applications [60]

- To diagnose papilledema – disc swelling, hemorrhages, and exudates
- To diagnose diseases of the retina and optic nerve such as macular degeneration, scotoma, optic atrophy, retrobulbar neuropathy, central retinal artery occlusion, central retinal vein occlusion, proliferative diabetic retinopathy, cytomegalovirus retinitis, and levers hereditary optic atrophy
- To detect lesions of the optic chiasma
- To study visual field defects
- To monitor visual illusions or hallucinations
- To diagnose visual agnosias

Skin Biopsy

Skin biopsy is a safe, painless technique used to study the small nerve fibers. It is performed with the help of a disposable punch on the desired site, after local anesthesia. The site does not need any stitches and heals on its own within a week. The obtained skin specimens are fixed, cryo-protected, and processed immunohistologically to examine the innervation of the epidermis, dermis, and sweat glands [61–63].

Clinical Applications [61–63]

- To monitor peripheral neuropathy
- To detect autonomic neuropathy by assessment of the denervation of sweat glands
- To detect demyelinating neuropathies

Muscle Biopsy

Muscle biopsy is an invasive procedure used to evaluate and diagnose neuromuscular diseases. Electromyography is used to identify the affected muscle. Local anesthesia is used; the skin in the affected areas is incised using a scalpel. The subcutaneous layer and the layer of fascia are carefully removed to expose the muscle. Then the group of fibers is gently separated from the belly of the muscle. The separated muscle fibers are surrounded with sutures before cutting the fiber ends. The muscle tissue is excised based on the planned testing or the nature of the underlying disease. Bleeding at the surgical site is stopped, the fascia is closed, and the subcutaneous tissue is sutured and the skin is closed with the help of a gauge or bandage. The healing process takes time, and follow-up visits are scheduled in order to observe the site for infection or bleeding. The muscle specimen obtained is carefully cryopreserved and transported to the pathology laboratory for immunohistological studies [64, 65].

Clinical Applications [64, 65]

- To study neurogenic atrophy and muscle weakness
- To observe the myopathic changes in an underlying muscle disease
- To study the disease-specific changes in the muscle

Nerve Biopsy

Nerve biopsy is an invasive technique used to evaluate peripheral neuropathies. The sural nerve is easily accessible and sensory in nature, which makes it the most preferred nerve for biopsies. [86] The procedure is carried out under local anesthesia, and an incision will be made along the saphenous vein on the affected area. The fascia will be dissected to expose the nerve and vein. Nerve ligation causes an acute pain even under anesthesia. The proximal piece of the segment is frozen without fixation. The distal segment is fixed using formalin and then incubated for epoxy resin embedding [66, 67].

Clinical Applications [64, 66]

- To detect pathological immunoglobulin deposits
- In differential diagnosis of hereditary neuropathies
- To identify pathological features of a suspected genetic condition
- To gain insight into inflammatory neuropathies
- To make a therapeutic decision when vasculitis, granulomatous inflammation, amyloidosis, or atypical chronic inflammatory demyelinating polyradiculoneuropathy (CIDP) is suspected

Neurointerventional Devices

Neurothrombectomy Devices

These are the set of devices used for the removal of thrombus/clot in conditions of acute ischemic stroke due to the occlusion of large cerebral vessels refractory to medical treatments like IV recombinant tissue plasminogen activator (rtPA). They help in the revascularization of the ischemic zone without any risk of intracranial hemorrhage [68, 69].

The various devices used for thrombectomy are

 i. Clot retrievers (MERCI clot retriever)
 ii. Aspirator/suction device (catheter or continuous flush catheters)
 iii. Snare-like devices (endovascular snares) for the disruption of clot
 iv. Ultrasonic and laser devices for the disruption of clot

Clinical Applications [69, 70]

- Can be used in cases refractory to medical treatment (pharmacologic thrombolysis) and in cases where thrombi are more resistant to fibrinolytics
- Avoid/minimize the risk of intracerebral hemorrhage induced by pharmacologic thrombolysis
- Can be used beyond the short timeframe to which rtPA is limited
- Might help in the rapid recanalization of occluded vessels compared to the use of pharmacological agents (thrombolytics)

Limitations [69, 70]

- The procedure needs intubation and heavy sedation or anesthesia and hence there are risks associated with it.
- Proper training and expertise are needed to use the devices for thrombectomy from cerebral vessels.
- Might have technical difficulty in navigating the mechanical devices into the intracranial vessel which can cause injury to the neurovasculature resulting in conditions like vessel dissection, perforation, or rupture.
- While dislodging thrombus, it may subsequently embolize into other unaffected vessels leading to new ischemic zones in the brain.

Neurovascular Stenting Devices

These devices are used for the stent-assisted cooling treatment of unruptured brain aneurysms, especially wide-neck, intracranial, and saccular aneurysms, arising from variously sized blood vessels. It is a minimally invasive technique [71–73].

Clinical Applications [71–73]

It is used for severe stenosis of the cerebral artery, and unruptured brain aneurysms.

Limitations [71, 73]

- Avoid use of neurovascular stents for SAC in patients who are not candidates for systemic anticoagulation and/or not able to receive anti-platelet medications as use of the devices requires peri-procedural anticoagulation and/or anti-platelet therapy.
- Thrombosis in or around the stent may result in serious harm, including ischemic stroke and death.
- A proper size of neurovascular stent should be selected for SAC
- Only the delivery microcatheters compatible with the appropriate neurovascular stents can be used, according to the neurovascular stent manufacturer.
- Carefully use micro-guidewires and microcatheters within and around the implanted stent; might cause vessel injury or rupture of the brain aneurysm.
- Carefully observe embolization coil(s) when they are manipulated within a brain aneurysm and avoid coil prolapse through stent struts. Ensure that the specific coil models and sizes chosen are indicated for the embolization of brain aneurysms.
- The type of brain aneurysm treated (i.e., ruptured, unruptured); the anatomical location and target vessel dimensions; the size of the brain aneurysm; the size of the device/s used.
- Appropriate patient selection as a candidate for treatment with a neurovascular stent is difficult.

These risk factors include patient age, presence of patient symptoms (e.g., cranial nerve deficit), a family history of brain aneurysm(s) or subarachnoid hemorrhage (SAH), prior SAH, gender, ethnicity, tobacco use, hypertension, brain aneurysm location, morphology, size, and changes over time of size and morphology.

Cerebral Cooling Device System

This is a technique to induce therapeutic hypothermia for improving the survival of critically ill neurological patients. These devices are used for cooling of the central nervous system, especially the brain, thereby providing neuroprotection and antiepileptogenic to an injured central nervous system. It can be categorized into non-invasive and invasive head cooling systems [74, 75].

Working Principle [74, 75]

The cerebral cooling devices (either non-invasive or invasive) reduce the brain temperature and hence slow down the brain metabolism in order to protect the neural cells from getting permanently damaged in any acute and severe brain injury. It is also a neuroprotective method in case of cardiac arrest/ failure and brain ischemia.

i. Non-invasive head cooling systems: These are surface cooling systems.
ii. Intranasal devices are used to facilitate heat loss from the upper airways by a conduction method with the help of naso-pharyngeal balloons, and by a convection method, where gas or fluid is allowed to flow through the part of the device kept in the upper airways.
iii. Head cooling is achieved by heat loss through the skull bones by a conduction and convection method. In the conduction method, the heat loss is achieved using both active and passive methods, with help of liquid cooling helmets and gel caps, respectively. In the convection method, the heat loss is achieved by fanning the head region with cold air using hoods or caps.
iv. Liquid cooling helmets containing circulating water (coolant) are used which transfer heat from the head first by conduction through the helmet and then by convection through the circulating coolant and hence are able to maintain a constant low temperature in the head region compared to the body temperature.
v. Carotid artery cooling devices are like neck bands which reduce the temperature of the carotid blood supply, and hence cool the brain.
vi. Intracranial cooling device: A part of the cooling device (embedded heat-collecting portion) is placed in a recess formed after craniotomy and the other part of the cooling device is placed nearby the dura mater to give the cooling of the desired degree. A heat-dissipating external plate is in thermal contact with the internal plate, and can be selectively sized according to a specific purpose.

Clinical Applications [75]

- Traumatic brain injury (TBI)
- Prophylactic treatment for epilepsy (acquired and posttraumatic)
- Neuroprotection in cardiac arrest

Limitations [74, 75]

- Possibility of tissue freezing and necrosis if scalp temperature is reduced too much.
- Cooling devices might alter arterial blood flow dynamics from laminar to turbulent flow which may result in blood hypercoagulability. So adequate brain imaging techniques like echo color Doppler or near infrared spectroscopy (NIRS) and other non-invasive monitoring of the cerebral blood flow are needed for the early detection of ischemia.
- Passive devices like non-circulating cooling caps contain frozen gel which might thaw and need to be refrozen periodically.
- Shivering is the most common effect of hypothermia, especially with surface cooling devices. Hence, the body, intracerebral, bladder, and tympanic temperature should be continuously monitored along with neurovital parameters like heart rate, arterial pressure, intracranial pressure (ICP), and cerebral perfusion pressure (CPP).
- The helmet/cap needs to be in close contact with the scalp for optimum heat removal.
- Automatic temperature control devices are more effective and need less labor compared to manual mode operated ones.

- Personal cooling garments also can be used.
- Neonatal head cooling devices are specifically designed and sized for neonates.
- Magnetic resonance spectroscopy (MRS) is needed for measuring brain temperature non-invasively (precision of approximately ±0.5°C in 1 mL voxels) during conductive head cooling which is very expensive.

Cerebral Angiography

Cerebral angiography is a diagnostic procedure used to examine blood vessels in the brain. This is otherwise known as intra-arterial digital subtraction angiography (IADSA). This is a minimally invasive technique where a radio opaque contrast material is injected through a catheter and X-ray imaging is done to view the various abnormalities such as aneurysms and atherosclerosis plaque in cerebral arteries. This technique can show a detailed, clear picture of blood vessels in the brain and hence rules out any need for surgery. If surgery is required, then it can be used as a guide to perform the surgeries more accurately [47, 76, 77].

Working Procedure [47, 76]

This procedure usually done without anesthetizing the patient. Some patients might need to be sedated, and in children it is done under general anesthesia. Heartbeat and blood pressure monitoring is done during the procedure. A thin catheter is inserted into an artery in the arm or leg through a small incision in the skin. Using X-ray guidance, the catheter is navigated to the area being examined. Once there, contrast material is injected through the tube and images are captured using ionizing radiation (X-rays). Today the images are acquired electronically, rather than with X-ray films, and the images can electronically manipulated so that the overlying bone of the skull does not obscure the vessels so that it is clearly seen. This technique is known as intra-arterial digital subtraction angiography (IADSA). Renal functions are assessed by measuring serum urea and creatinine. During the procedure, introducing the catheter might be painful and the contrast material, while spreading all over the body, gives a flushing or warm sensation as it is a vasodilator.

Clinical Advantages [47, 76]

- This procedure is used to evaluate arteries of the head and neck before surgery.
- It can detect or confirm abnormalities within the blood vessels in the brain, like an aneurysm (secular dilatation of an artery due to weakness of the arterial wall), atherosclerosis (a narrowing of the arteries by atheromatous plaque, arteriovenous malformation), vasculitis (an inflammation of the blood vessels, narrowing them), a brain tumor or a blood clot obstructing the blood flow, vascular dissection (a tear in the wall of an artery), or a stroke.
- It can provide additional information on abnormalities seen on MRI or CT of the head.
- It helps in preparing for the surgical treatments of removal of a brain tumor, or any vessel abnormality.
- It may also help in the diagnosis of the cause of symptoms like severe headaches, slurred speech, dizziness, blurred or double vision, weakness or numbness, or loss of co-ordination or balance.

Limitations [47, 76, 77]

- There is a risk of an allergic reaction to iodine contrast material; however, it is extremely rare. In such a situation non-iodine contrast material can be used.
- Pregnancy, any recent illnesses, medical conditions, allergies, etc., should be ruled out prior to procedure.

- Nursing mothers should avoid breastfeeding for 24 hours after contrast material injection.
- Diabetes or kidney disease should be ruled out. So renal function tests are advised prior to the procedure.
- As it is a minimally invasive procedure where a catheter is placed inside a blood vessel, it has some risks. These risks include damage to the blood vessel, bleeding and bruising at the puncture site, and infection for which precautions can be taken.
- Rarely there is a risk of blood clot around the tip of the catheter or the dislodging of an atheromatous plaque from a vessel wall by the catheter which might block the feeding artery creating a risk of stroke; however it is uncommon.
- Other rare risks include the risk of radiation exposure, puncture of the artery by catheter causing internal bleeding.
- Radiation exposure can be minimized by placing a lead drape under the pelvis to protect ovaries and testes from radiation hazards. Modern X-ray systems have very controlled X-ray beams and dose control methods to minimize stray (scatter) radiation.
- Post-procedure side effects include weakness or numbness of the limb used for catheterization, slurred speech, visual disturbances, dizziness, chest pain, difficulty breathing, rash, or any local signs of infection at the catheter site.
- Patients with impaired kidney function and who have a previous history of allergic reactions to iodine-containing contrast materials are the limitations for cerebral angiography.

Flow Disruption

Flow disruption is a modern neurointervention technique used for endovascular neurosurgery, particularly for vascular reconstruction. Flow disruption is a technique of disrupting the blood flow to a secular intracranial aneurysm. The devices used for endosaccular flow disruption are called flow disruptors, used mainly for the treatment of saccular, wide-neck, bifurcated intracranial aneurysms. Novel stent-like bridging devices and semi flow diverting stents are used with coiling techniques to increase the efficacy. Coils and flow diverting stents are used in the treatment of large wide-neck and fusiform intracranial aneurysms. But these can be less effective for aneurysms located at arterial bifurcations. Recently, newer devices have come up with better flow modulation. These devices are packed with nitinol-based material that blocks the blood flow to the aneurysm and hence gives time for the aneurysm to heal [59, 78–80].

Clinical Advantages [78–81]

- The treatment of ruptured and unruptured aneurysms, mostly wide-neck (dome-to-neck ratio of less than 2 mm or a neck diameter equal to or greater than 4 mm) cerebral aneurysms, poses unique technical challenges for endovascular coil embolization.
- Useful for the treatment of wide-neck, giant aneurysms where coiling is a little challenging as it has a tendency to herniate the coils into the parent vessel and also in situations where it is difficult to determine the neck and parent vessel interface.

Limitations [78–81]

- Higher incidence of thromboembolism
- Failure of placement at appropriate site
- Delayed parenchymal hemorrhage (rare but serious complication)
- Subarachnoid hemorrhage
- Transient ischemic attack

Neurostimulation Devices

Deep Brain Stimulation

Deep brain stimulation (DBS) involves implanting electrodes within certain areas of your brain. These electrodes produce electrical impulses that regulate abnormal impulses. Or the electrical impulses can affect certain cells and chemicals within the brain. The degree of stimulation is controlled by a pacemaker-like device placed under the skin in the chest which is connected through a subcutaneous wire to the implant in the brain. DBS is a minimally invasive surgery and is considered to be safe. It is a surgical intervention used to treat several conditions including movement disorders and dystonia, Parkinson's disease, epilepsy, addiction, depression, multiple sclerosis, and obsessive-compulsive disorder [82–84].

Clinical Advantages [82–84]

- DBS does not cause permanent damage to brain regions unlike other surgeries.
- Can be performed on one or both sides of the brain, depending on symptoms.
- The effects are reversible and can be customized individually for each patient's clinical status.
- Stimulation settings can be modified to diminish potential side effects and improve effectiveness over time.
- The device can provide uninterrupted control of symptoms for almost 24 hours a day.
- The stimulator can also be turned off if DBS causes excessive side effects.

Limitations [82–84]

Surgery is associated with mild bleeding in brain tissue, stroke, infection, seizure, pain, and swelling at the implantation site.

Repetitive Transcranial Magnetic Stimulator (rTMS)

Transcranial magnetic stimulation (TMS) is a non-invasive procedure which is used therapeutically for the stimulation of neurons in the brain, thereby improving symptoms. It takes about 30–60 minutes for one session [85, 86].

Working Principle [85, 86]

The device creates a magnetic field by which it stimulates the nerve cells and treats diseases like depression. It is called rTMS because it delivers repetitive pulsed magnetic fields of required magnitude through an electromagnetic coil placed on the cortex to stimulate nerve action potentials. In an rTMS treatment session, the patient sits on a recliner. A special electromagnetic coil is placed on the scalp over the brain area to be stimulated.

Clinical Applications [85, 86]

Treatment of the symptoms of major depressive disorder (MDD) in patients who have not achieved enough effect from medications, psychotherapy, and/or electroconvulsive therapy. Repetitive TMS is a non-invasive form of brain stimulation used for depression.

Advantages [85, 87]

- This is a painless procedure as it delivers a magnetic pulse that stimulates nerve cells and is considered to be safe and well-tolerated.

- It's thought to activate regions of the brain that have decreased activity in depression.
- Doesn't require sedation or anesthesia, surgery or implantation of electrodes unlike vagus nerve stimulation or deep brain stimulation and electroconvulsive therapy (ECT).
- It doesn't cause seizures unlike electroconvulsive therapy.
- rTMS can specifically stimulate the target brain areas unlike ECT.

Limitations [85, 87]

- Cannot be the first line of treatment.
- Not painful but might create scalp discomfort at the stimulation site like knocking or tapping on the head.
- Common side effects include mild to moderate headache, light headedness, tingling sensation in the face, jaw, or scalp, spasms and twitching of facial muscle, and temporary hearing problems due to loud magnet noise.
- Serious side effects like seizures, mania, and hearing loss are rare and can be prevented by taking precautions like adequate ear protection and ruling out prior history of seizure and bipolar disorder.
- Patients with any implanted medical devices or metals (stents, aneurysm clips or coils, other implanted stimulators like deep brain and vagus nerve stimulators, implanted pacemakers or medication pumps, cochlear implants, implants for monitoring brain activity, any other magnetic implants) are not recommended for rTMS.
- Prior history or family history of seizures or epilepsy, bipolar disorder, psychosis and substance abuse, brain damage due to injury or brain tumor, stroke, and frequent complaints of severe headaches are some contraindications for the use of rTMS.

Electroconvulsive Therapy

ECT involves placing electrodes on strategic areas of the brain and generating an electric current that essentially causes a seizure to occur in the brain. It is done under general anesthesia and muscle relaxant. ECT is usually reserved for the treatment of severe depression refractory to other medical conditions such as schizophrenia, bipolar and schizoaffective disorders. It diffusely stimulates all the brain areas without a specific target area. It can be used both inpatient and outpatient. ECT is usually given 2 to 3 times weekly for 3 to 4 weeks for a total of 6 to 12 treatments. A pre-defined treatment protocol is used for inpatients while for outpatient treatment a treatment course (up to 250 stimulation sessions) can be created which will be delivered as a series of treatment sessions [88, 89].

Working Principle [88, 89]

A transcranial electrical stimulator is used for delivering DC output current up to 2 mA to directly stimulate the brain, changing the cortical neuron excitability. This is used therapeutically for the treatment of various diseases like major depressive episodes, addiction/craving, lower limb neuropathic pain, fibromyalgia, and recovery of motor functions after stroke and brain injuries.

Clinical Applications [88, 90]

- ECT seems to cause changes in brain chemistry that can quickly reverse symptoms of certain mental disorders.
- ECT is indicated in severe depression, suicidal tendency, bipolar disorder, catatonic schizophrenia, and in dementia presenting with aggression and agitation.

Disadvantages [88, 90]

- Poor tolerance to medication or other forms of therapy (old adults).
- During pregnancy, when medications have a potentially damaging effect on the fetus.
- Immediately after treatment, confusion of a certain degree might be experienced which can last from a few minutes to several hours.
- Some people experience nausea, headache, jaw pain, or muscle ache after ECT.
- Some patients might have some retrograde memory loss which might improve within a month or two after completion of the treatment.
- During ECT, heart rate and blood pressure increase, and rarely there is precipitation of pre-existing heart problems.

TMS Neuronavigation

Neuronavigation systems are used to track the position of a transcranial magnetic stimulation (TMS) coil in real time with respect to the anatomical area of interest simply called the target area. By tracking this, the position and the orientation of the coil relative to the hot spot (where the magnetic field is greatest) can be changed. Recent models of TMS neuronavigation incorporate current flow modeling, which reveals that the pattern of the electric field induced by TMS is shaped by the cortex in proximity to the stimulator [91] which can also affect particular behavioral phenomena [92]. This helps to identify the target prior to therapy, and also helps in setting up a target to ensure a perfect TMS coil position in order to maximize the induced electric field in a target [85].

Working Procedure [91, 92]

The orientation of coil handle is a critical determinant of the number of neurons that are recruited by the TMS pulse stimulation. As a result of this, any change in the orientation of the coil handle can affect the cortical response to TMS. Once a hot spot (site most likely to evoke a motor evoked potential) has been found, the orientation of the coil handle can be recorded, ensuring that the coil orientation and hot spot position are kept constant throughout an experimental session. Targets can be identified in two ways, one method is by identifying a hot spot or a phosphene. Neuronavigations help in identifying this hot spot which ensures that the target will evoke the desired response when consistently stimulated in an experimental set up. An alternative method is to use a standard set of co-ordinates given by Montreal Neurological Institute (MNI) to locate a target and stimulate it by TMS. TMS navigation is used to transform a subject's MRI picture to a standardized co-ordinate and hence identifies the target area on the MNI co-ordinates, which is specific for an individual.

Clinical Applications [92]

- The neuronavigation system enables the TMS coil to be placed on the scalp co-ordinates accurately over the target area.
- It also helps in reproducing the TMS target area between two different sessions for a particular patient and across a group of patients.

References

1. *CAGR-Report-by-Market-Research-Future*. Neurological Devices.
2. Anderson, L., et al., FDA Regulation of Neurological and Physical Medicine Devices: Access to Safe and Effective Neurotechnologies for All Americans. *Neuron*, 2016. **92**(5): p. 943–948.

3. CFR Title 21 – Food and Drugs: Parts 882: Neurological devices. 29 Mar. 2022, www.accessdata.fda.gov/scripts/cdrh/cfdocs/cfcfr/CFRSearch.cfm?CFRPart=882. Accessed 3 Sep. 2022.

4. http://www.fda.gov/AboutFDA/CentersOffices/OfficeofMedicalProductsandTobacco/CDRH/ucm300639.htm., F.a.D.A.a., FDA 2015a.

5. Biasiucci, A., B. Franceschiello, and M.M. Murray, Electroencephalography. *Curr Biol*, 2019. **29**(3): p. R80–R85.

6. Britton, J.W., et al., *Electroencephalography (EEG): An Introductory Text and Atlas of Normal and Abnormal Findings in Adults, Children, and Infants*, E.K. St. Louis and L.C. Frey, Editors. 2016, American Epilepsy Society. Copyright ©2016 by American Epilepsy Society.: Chicago.

7. Clancy, R., Electroencephalography: Basic principles, clinical applications and related fields, ed 2. Ernst Niedermeyer Fernando Lopes da Silva Baltimore, Urban and Schwarzenberg, Editors, 1987, 940 pp, illustrated, $110.00. *Ann Neurol*, 1988. **24**(6): p. 799–799.

8. Patil, S.P., What every clinician should know about polysomnography. *Resp Care*, 2010. **55**(9): p. 1179–1195.

9. Markun, L.C. and A. Sampat, Clinician-focused overview and developments in polysomnography. *Curr Sleep Med Rep*, 2020. **6**(4): p. 309–321.

10. Kushida, C.A., et al., Practice parameters for the indications for polysomnography and related procedures: An update for 2005. *Sleep*, 2005. **28**(4): p. 499–521.

11. Rundo, J.V. and R. Downey, 3rd, Polysomnography. *Handb Clin Neurol*, 2019. **160**: p. 381–392.

12. Hirshkowitz, M., et al., National sleep foundation's updated sleep duration recommendations: Final report. *Sleep Health*, 2015. **1**(4): p. 233–243.

13. Atlas of sleep medicine. *AJNR Am J Neuroradiol*. 2006 Mar. **27**(3): p. 722–723.

14. Chang, M.C. and D. Park, Findings of electrodiagnostic studies in moderate to severe lumbar central spinal stenosis: Electrodiagnostic studies in lumbar central spinal stenosis. *Healthcare*, 2021. **9**(2): p. 164.

15. Mallik, A. and A.I. Weir, Nerve conduction studies: Essentials and pitfalls in practice. *J Neurol Neurosurg Psychiatry*, 2005. **76**(suppl 2): p. ii23–ii31.

16. Cucchiara, B. and R.S. Price, *Decision-Making in Adult Neurology, E-Book*. 2020, Elsevier Health Sciences.

17. Koo, Y.S., C.S. Cho, and B.J. Kim, Pitfalls in using electrophysiological studies to diagnose neuromuscular disorders. *J Clin Neurol*, 2012. **8**(1): p. 1–14.

18. Tatum, W.O.t., Long-term EEG monitoring: A clinical approach to electrophysiology. *J Clin Neurophysiol*, 2001. **18**(5): p. 442–455.

19. Lagerlund, T.D., et al., Long-term electroencephalographic monitoring for diagnosis and management of seizures. *Mayo Clin Proc*, 1996. **71**(10): p. 1000–1006.

20. Young, G.B. and J. Mantia, Chapter 7 - Continuous EEG monitoring in the intensive care unit. In *Handbook of Clinical Neurology*, E.F.M. Wijdicks and A.H. Kramer, Editors. 2017, Elsevier. p. 107–116.

21. Guideline twelve: Guidelines for long-term monitoring for epilepsy. *J Clin Neurophysiol*, 2008. **25**(3): p. 170–180.

22. Kobulashvili, T., et al., Current practices in long-term video-EEG monitoring services: A survey among partners of the E-PILEPSY pilot network of reference for refractory epilepsy and epilepsy surgery. *Seizure*, 2016. **38**: p. 38–45.

23. Kull, L.L. and R.G. Emerson, Continuous EEG monitoring in the intensive care unit: Technical and staffing considerations. *J Clin Neurophysiol*, 2005. **22**(2): p. 107–118.

24. Ghatol D, J. Widrich, Intraoperative Neurophysiological Monitoring. [Updated 2021 Aug 14]. In: *StatPearls [Internet]*. Treasure Island: StatPearls Publishing; 2021 Jan.

25. Charalampidis, A., et al., The use of intraoperative neurophysiological monitoring in spine surgery. *Global Spine J*, 2020. **10**(1 Suppl): p. 104s–114s.

26. So, V.C. and C.C. Poon, Intraoperative neuromonitoring in major vascular surgery. *Br J Anaesth*, 2016. **117** Suppl 2: p. ii13–ii25.

27. Levin, D.N., S. Strantzas, and B.E. Steinberg, Intraoperative neuromonitoring in paediatric spinal surgery. *BJA Educ*, 2019. **19**(5): p. 165–171.

28. Quantitative sensory testing. *Diabetes Care*, 1992. **15**(8): p. 1092–1094.

29. Chong, P.S. and D.P. Cros, Technology literature review: Quantitative sensory testing. *Muscle Nerve*, 2004. **29**(5): p. 734–747.

30. Shy, M.E., et al., Quantitative sensory testing: Report of the therapeutics and technology assessment subcommittee of the American Academy of Neurology. *Neurology*, 2003. **60**(6): p. 898–904.

31. Siao, P. and D.P. Cros, Quantitative sensory testing. *Phys Med Rehabil Clin N Am*, 2003. **14**(2): p. 261–286.

32. Hansson, P., M. Backonja, and D. Bouhassira, Usefulness and limitations of quantitative sensory testing: Clinical and research application in neuropathic pain states. *Pain*, 2007. **129**(3): p. 256–259.

33. Howard, J.F., Jr., Electrodiagnosis of disorders of neuromuscular transmission. *Phys Med Rehabil Clin N Am*, 2013. **24**(1): p. 169–192.

34. Verschuuren, J., E. Strijbos, and A. Vincent, Neuromuscular junction disorders. *Handb Clin Neurol*, 2016. **133**: p. 447–466.

35. Zivković, S.A. and C. Shipe, Use of repetitive nerve stimulation in the evaluation of neuromuscular junction disorders. *Am J Electroneurodiagnostic Technol*, 2005. **45**(4): p. 248–261.

36. Patel, P. and T. Pobre, Electrodiagnostic evaluation of neuromuscular junction disorder. In *StatPearls*. 2021, StatPearls Publishing. Copyright © 2021, StatPearls Publishing LLC.: Treasure Island (FL).

37. Mills, K.R., The basics of electromyography. *J Neurol Neurosurg Psychiatry*, 2005. **76**(Suppl 2): p. ii32–ii35.

38. Rawat, M., et al., Impact of electrodiagnostic (EMG/NCS) tests on clinical decision-making and patient perceived benefit in the outpatient physical therapy practice. *J Bodyw Mov Ther*, 2020. **24**(1): p. 170–174.

39. Selvan, V.A., Single-fiber EMG: A review. *Ann Indian Acad Neurol*, 2011. **14**(1): p. 64–67.

40. Bonner, F.J., Jr. and A.B. Devleschoward, AAEM minimonograph No.45: The early development of electromyography. *Muscle Nerve*, 1995. **18**(8): p. 825–833.

41. Morris, P.D., et al., When is rotational angiography superior to conventional single-plane angiography for planning coronary angioplasty? *Catheter Cardiovasc Interv*, 2016. **87**(4): p. E104–E112.

42. Ishihara, S., et al., 3D rotational angiography: Recent experience in the evaluation of cerebral aneurysms for treatment. *Interv Neuroradiol*, 2000. **6**(2): p. 85–94.

43. Baliyan, V., et al., Vascular computed tomography angiography technique and indications. *Cardiovasc Diagn Ther*, 2019. **9**(Suppl 1): p. S14–S27.

44. Dzialowski, I., et al., *Computed Tomography-Based Evaluation of Cerebrovascular Disease*. 2022, Elsevier. p. 660–675.e3.

45. Kumamaru, K.K., et al., CT angiography: Current technology and clinical use. *Radiol Clin North Am*, 2010. **48**(2): p. 213–235, vii.

46. Alakbarzade, V. and A.C. Pereira, Cerebral catheter angiography and its complications. *Pract Neurol*, 2018. **18**(5): p. 393–398.

47. Shin, J.H., Cerebral angiography: The first small step for the neurointerventionist. *Neurointervention*, 2020. **15**(2): p. 101–103.

48. Petrella, J.R. and J.M. Provenzale, MR perfusion imaging of the brain: Techniques and applications. *AJR Am J Roentgenol*, 2000. **175**(1): p. 207–219.

49. Jahng, G.H., et al., Perfusion magnetic resonance imaging: A comprehensive update on principles and techniques. *Korean J Radiol*, 2014. **15**(5): p. 554–577.

50. Essig, M., et al., Perfusion MRI: The five most frequently asked technical questions. *AJR Am J Roentgenol*, 2013. **200**(1): p. 24–34.

51. Rasulo, F.A., E. De Peri, and A. Lavinio, Transcranial Doppler ultrasonography in intensive care. *Eur J Anaesthesiol Suppl*, 2008. **42**: p. 167–173.

52. Lee, W., General principles of carotid Doppler ultrasonography. *Ultrasonography*, 2014. **33**(1): p. 11–17.

53. Kassab, M.Y., et al., Transcranial Doppler: An introduction for primary care physicians. *J Am Board Family Med*, 2007. **20**(1): p. 65–71.

54. Purkayastha, S. and F. Sorond, Transcranial Doppler ultrasound: Technique and application. *Semin Neurol*, 2012. **32**(4): p. 411–420.

55. Belisário, A.R., et al., Genetic, laboratory and clinical risk factors in the development of overt ischemic stroke in children with sickle cell disease. *Hematol Transf Cell Therapy*, 2018. **40**(2): p. 166–181.

56. D'Andrea, A., et al., Transcranial Doppler ultrasound: Physical principles and principal applications in neurocritical care unit. *J Cardiovasc Echogr*, 2016. **26**(2): p. 28–41.

57. Wallmann, H.W., Introduction to Observational Gait Analysis. *Home Health Care Manag Pract*, 2009. **22**(1): p. 66–68.

58. DeLuca, P.A., Gait analysis in the treatment of the ambulatory child with cerebral palsy. *Clin Orthop Relat Res*, 1991. **264**: p. 65–75.

59. Ataullah, A.H.M., De Jesus, O., *Gait Disturbances*. [Updated 2022 May 20]. In: StatPearls [Internet]. Treasure Island (FL): StatPearls Publishing; 2022 Jan-. Available from: https://www.ncbi.nlm.nih.gov/books/NBK560610/

60. Ludwig, P.E., Jessu, R., Czyz, C.N. Physiology, eye. [Updated 2021 Jul 22]. In: *StatPearls* [Internet]. 2021 Jan, StatPearls Publishing. Available from: https://www.ncbi.nlm.nih.gov/books/NBK470322/

61. Lauria, G., et al., EFNS guidelines on the use of skin biopsy in the diagnosis of peripheral neuropathy. *Eur J Neurol*, 2005. **12**(10): p. 747–758.

62. Harvey, N.T., J. Chan, and B.A. Wood, Skin biopsy in the diagnosis of neoplastic skin disease. *Aust Fam Physician*, 2017. **46**(5): p. 289–294.

63. Stevenson, P. and K. Rodins, Improving diagnostic accuracy of skin biopsies. *Aust J Gen Pract*, 2018. **47**(4): p. 216–220.
64. Dalakas, M.C., Muscle biopsy findings in inflammatory myopathies. *Rheum Dis Clin North Am*, 2002. **28**(4): p. 779–798, vi.
65. Joyce, N.C., B. Oskarsson, and L.W. Jin, Muscle biopsy evaluation in neuromuscular disorders. *Phys Med Rehabil Clin N Am*, 2012. **23**(3): p. 609–631.
66. Said, G., Indications and usefulness of nerve biopsy. *Archives of Neurology*, 2002. **59**(10): p. 1532.
67. Weis, J., et al., Processing of nerve biopsies: A practical guide for neuropathologists. *Clin Neuropathol*, 2012. **31**(1): p. 7–23.
68. Baker WL, Colby, J., Tongbram V, et al, *Neurothrombectomy Devices for Treatment of Acute Ischemic Stroke [Internet].* Agency for Healthcare Research and Quality; 2011 Jan. (Comparative Effectiveness Technical Briefs, No. 4.).
69. Jovin, T.G., et al., Neurothrombectomy for acute ischemic stroke across clinical trial design and technique: A single center pooled analysis. *Front Neurol*, 2020. **11**: p. 1047.
70. Mueller-Kronast, N.H., et al., Systematic evaluation of patients treated with neurothrombectomy devices for acute ischemic stroke. *Stroke*, 2017. **48**(10): p. 2760–2768.
71. Horowitz, M.B. and P.D. Purdy, The use of stents in the management of neurovascular disease: A review of historical and present status. *Neurosurgery*, 2000. **46**(6): p. 1335–1343.
72. Sakai, N. and C. Sakai, [Stent for neurovascular diseases]. *Brain Nerve*, 2009. **61**(9): p. 1023–1028.
73. Voelker, R., Neurovascular stent caution. *JAMA*, 2018. **319**(23): p. 2372.
74. Assis, F., et al., From systemic to selective brain cooling: Methods in review. *Brain Circulation*, 2019. **5**(4): p. 179.
75. Csernyus, B., et al., Recent antiepileptic and neuroprotective applications of brain cooling. *Seizure*, 2020. **82**: p. 80–90.
76. Case, D., et al., Neuroangiography: Review of Anatomy, Periprocedural Management, Technique, and Tips. *Semin Intervent Radiol*, 2020. **37**(2): p. 166–174.
77. Lin, N., et al., Safety of neuroangiography and embolization in children: Complication analysis of 697 consecutive procedures in 394 patients. *J Neurosurg Pediat*, 2015. **16**(4): p. 432–438.
78. Campos, J.K., et al., Advances in endovascular aneurysm management: Flow modulation techniques with braided mesh devices. *Stroke Vasc Neurol*, 2020. **5**(1): p. 1–13.
79. Dmytriw, A.A., et al., Endosaccular flow disruption: A new frontier in endovascular aneurysm management. *Neurosurgery*, 2020. **86**(2): p. 170–181.
80. Pierot, L., et al., Aneurysm treatment with WEB in the cumulative population of two prospective, multicenter series: 3-year follow-up. *J NeuroInterventional Surg*, 2021. **13**(4): p. 363–368.
81. Campos, J.K., et al., Advances in endovascular aneurysm management: Coiling and adjunctive devices. *Stroke Vasc Neurol*, 2020. **5**(1): p. 14–21.
82. Lozano, A.M., et al., Deep brain stimulation: Current challenges and future directions. *Nat Rev. Neurol*, 2019. **15**(3): p. 148–160.
83. Pycroft, L., J. Stein, and T. Aziz, Deep brain stimulation: An overview of history, methods, and future developments. *Brain Neurosci Adv*, 2018. **2**: p. 2398212818816017.
84. Fariba K, Gupta V., Deep brain stimulation. [Updated 2021 Jul 30]. In: *StatPearls [Internet].* StatPearls Publishing; 2021.
85. Kim, W.J., et al., Neuronavigation-guided Repetitive Transcranial Magnetic Stimulation for Aphasia. *J Vis Exp*, 2016. **111**.
86. Klomjai, W., R. Katz, and A. Lackmy-Vallée, Basic principles of transcranial magnetic stimulation (TMS) and repetitive TMS (rTMS). *Ann Phys Rehabilit Med*, 2015. **58**(4): p. 208–213.
87. Zheng, K.-Y., et al., Trends of repetitive transcranial magnetic stimulation from 2009 to 2018: A bibliometric analysis. *Front Neurosci*, 2020. **14**(106). doi: 10.3389/fnins.2020.00106.
88. Salik, I. and R. Marwaha, Electroconvulsive therapy. In *StatPearls*. 2021, StatPearls Publishing. Copyright © 2021, StatPearls Publishing LLC.: Treasure Island (FL).
89. Singh, A. and S.K. Kar, How electroconvulsive therapy works?: Understanding the neurobiological mechanisms. *Clin Psychopharmacol Neurosci*, 2017. **15**(3): p. 210–221.
90. Gazdag, G. and G.S. Ungvari, Electroconvulsive therapy: 80 Years old and still going strong. *World J Psychiatry*, 2019. **9**(1): p. 1–6.
91. Opitz, A., et al., How the brain tissue shapes the electric field induced by transcranial magnetic stimulation. *Neuroimage*, 2011. **58**(3): p. 849–859.
92. Thielscher, A., et al., The cortical site of visual suppression by transcranial magnetic stimulation. *Cereb Cortex*, 2010. **20**(2): p. 328–338.

Dental Devices

B. Karthika, Shamsul Nisa, and M. Pavani

Dental devices are used to treat dental problems and to maintain dental health. In this chapter we have discussed various dental devices for maintaining oral health. Hence by maintaining a person's oral health through various dental devices, that person's overall health will be promoted. This chapter also highlights imaging dental devices for radiological investigations in treating oral health problems.

THE DENTAL CHAIR AND ITS UNITS[1,2,3]

The dental chair has been used for the last 300 years. Prior to the 17th century, tooth extractions were often performed with the patient sitting on the floor, their head held firmly between the operator's knees. Everyday armchairs occasionally served to make dental procedures less awkward and fatiguing. But not until the early 1700s did Pierre Fauchard, French dental surgeon extraordinaire, set a new trend in comfort by consistently getting patients off the floor and onto a chair for an examination or extraction.

In early 1800s America, a rocker with a properly placed log served as a prototype for the mechanical dental chair. As time passed it became apparent that both patient and dentist could benefit from a more supportive yet flexible seat. Individual dentists designed and constructed their own dental chairs until the mid-1800s, when dental manufacturers took over, producing a wide selection of ornate chairs with varying degrees of headrest, footrest, back and seat adjustability.

In 1958, Dr. Sanford Golden and colleagues in California designed the Ritter-Euphorian or Golden, a fixed-seat reclining chair. As the first significant dental chair improvement in 50 years, it won the 1960 Industrial Design Institute's Gold Medal Award and was featured at the 1962 Seattle World's Fair as the ultimate seat from which an astronaut could explore space. But the true progenitor of the modern reclining chair, designed also in 1958 but by John Naughton of Iowa, featured a break in the seat back that allowed the dentist to sit and the patient to be in a prone position. Due to its more flexible seat design, Naughton's recliner was accepted as the standard by the dental profession. Today's dental chair maximizes patient comfort while providing the dentist with adjustability that allows "optimal access to the oral cavity."

The different brands of dental chairs are Gnatus, Anthos, Skanray, Bestodent, SK Dent, Confident, Hi-Tech, Salli, Fona, Carbon, Dynamic, Unicorn Denmart, Dabi Atlante and Denfort, etc.

Description of Operation

1. Each chair consists of a seat, a headrest, a back and armrests. The chair can be a standard traditional dental chair.

DOI: 10.1201/9781003220671-9

2. The spittoon is a container placed next to the dental chair, so you can rinse and spit during the dental procedures.
3. An aspirator is a small tube for sucking saliva that accumulates in the mouth or in small cavities. If right-handed, the suction and spittoon are placed on the left side of the chair and vice versa.
4. Pedals in dental equipment are used to activate the rotation of different instruments, such as adjusting a chair or activating water.
5. The instrument or equipment tray is an important and useful tool for every professional. The equipment tray consists of all the equipment that dentists require.

Functions of Components

Armrest

The armrest is on the right-hand side, and the lock is released by pulling up the armrest diagonally backward (in a direction that is parallel to the armrest axis) by about 1 cm. (The lock is released when the armrest is pulled to a point where resistance is felt.) Turn the armrest to 9 o'clock. (The armrest can turn by about 180 degrees.) To return the armrest to the former position, observe the opposite procedure to that of lock release. That is, turn the armrest to the normal working position, and then lock the armrest in position by pushing it down diagonally forward, which is opposite to the direction mentioned above. Make sure to confirm that the armrest is in the safe locked position before use.

Headrest

1. Height adjustment release button: Press down or pull up the headrest to the desired height.
2. Angle adjustment: Grasp the headrest release button on the headrest mechanism and move to the desired position.

Auto Switch

1. Preset control: The chair has two preset positions (Preset-1 and Preset-2). Momentarily move the auto mode stick switch to the left side; the chair will move to the Preset-1 position automatically. (Preset-2 is operated by the right side.)
2. Auto return: Momentarily move the auto mode stick switch upward; the chair will return to the initial position. (The seat is fully lowered and the backrest is in the upright position.)
3. Last position memory: Momentarily move the auto mode stick switch downward at the reclined backrest position (treatment position); the backrest will raise to the mouth rinsing position automatically. Momentarily depress the auto mode stick switch downward again, and the backrest will recline to the previous treatment position automatically.
4. Emergency stop: During an automatic procedure (preset, auto return or last position memory), depressing any side of the stick switch will cancel the automatic movement immediately.

Manual Switch

1. Seat lifting: Hold the manual mode stick switch upward until the seat is lifted up to the desired position.
2. Seat lowering: Hold the manual mode stick switch downward until the seat is lowered to the desired position.
3. Backrest reclining: Hold the manual mode stick switch to the left side until the backrest is reclined to the desired position.
4. Backrest raising: Hold the manual mode stick switch to the right side until the backrest is raised up to the desired position.

References

1. Glenner, R.A. Components of the dental unit 1974, https://jada.ada.org/article/S0002-8177(74)95022-3/pdf
2. Dental unit and chair, https://eurods.eu › Instr_Belmont_tbCOMPASS
3. Dental unit and chair operating instructions. *SP CLEO-II, Operating Instructions*, 1–48.

ELECTROMAGNETIC MICROMOTORS

In conventional macro-scale machines, linear and rotary motion, which is a characteristic feature of all machines, is most often generated by using electromagnetic actuation principles. Initial attempts at realizing electromagnetic micromotors were based on hybrid technologies. Guckel et al. used the Lithographie, Galvanoformung, Abformung (LIGA) process to fabricate high aspect ratio Ni microstructures constituting the stator and the rotor of a variable reluctance magnetic micromotor. The motor was operated by externally generated magnetic fields. In a later version hybrid wire bonding techniques were used to create coils. Wagner et al. placed rare earth permanent magnet rotors onto integrated planar coils. The first magnetically driven micromotor with fully integrated stator and coils, also based on the variable reluctance principle, was presented by Ahn et al. The motor used an electroplated 40 μm thick NiFe rotor and a 120 μm thick stator with a meander-type integrated inductive component which generates the magnetic flux. The electroplating molds were made of polyimide, which was patterned by plasma etching. The planar meander coils were manufactured by electroplating of Cu utilizing an 8 μm thick positive photoresist mold.[1,2,3] New UV-sensitive photoresists allow the exposure of thick layers of resist, i.e. layers of several 10 μm up to several 100 μm. With the advent of these resists a new technology for fabricating high aspect ratio microstructures has emerged, the so-called UV depth lithography or UV-LIGA method. This technique has been used to develop a variety of magnetic microactuators. The electrodynamic actuation principle is based on the generation of the Lorentz force on a current-carrying conductor due to a magnetic field. In case of a permanent magnet excited motor, the Lorentz force results from the interaction of the permanent magnet with the magnetic field of a coil. The direction of the generated electromagnetic force depends on the relative orientation of the flux density of the permanent magnet and the direction of the electric current. Hence, the electrodynamic motor concept enables force generation in two directions: Levitation force and propelling force. Two design options are possible: The moving coil approach (fixed magnet) and the moving magnet approach. The variable reluctance (VR) force motor principle is based on the generation of a force due to minimization of the magnetic resistance (reluctance). The reluctance force results from the interaction between surfaces of different permeability, whereby a normal force (FN) and a tangential force (FT) component can be distinguished. In principle, the normal forces are much larger than the tangential forces, which cause a linear or rotatory movement.[4,5,6] This aspect needs to be handled carefully in the design of variable reluctance micromotors, because VR-motor concepts with a single gap suffer from high additional friction caused by the drive itself. In our work, both the VR principle and the electrodynamic principle have been used to design linear and rotational microactuators.

Designs of Electromagnetic Micromotors[7,8]

There are two main challenges that have to be overcome. The first one is static friction. In micromotors, low lateral propulsive forces typically act under high contact pressure. Therefore, for effective operation a low friction coefficient has to be achieved. The second challenge is heat dissipation. The increase of current density and consequently of thermal losses may affect the efficiency of operation in some way and may require appropriate cooling measures.

1. **Linear VR stepper motor**: The linear VR micromotor with dimensions of about 10 mm × 10 mm comprises three or six stator systems located in parallel with vertical meander coils wound around the in-plane toothed soft magnetic poles, thus producing a horizontal magnetic flux. The comb shaped poles of the traveler extend in between the stator poles. The attractive normal forces are compensated due to two complementary gaps with nominal dimensions of 8 μm between stator and traveler. The tooth pitch is 100 μm resulting in steps of 33.3 μm or 16.7 μm over a traverse path of 3.5 mm. An unfavorable effect is the high temperature of about 160°C during continuous excitation of the motor at 2.5 A. Therefore, active cooling of the motor is mandatory.

2. **Rotatory VR stepper motor**: The rotatory VR micromotor is designed as an external rotor motor. The rotor consists of 6 or 12 soft magnetic pole shoes, which feature a toothed structure on the outer circumference. A helical coil of about ten turns is wrapped around each pole shoe. Two opposite coils are connected to the same electrical phase inducing a horizontal magnetic flux. The magnetic circuit is closed via the soft magnetic rotor yoke, which is also toothed, and the air gap (3 μm) between the stator and rotor. Due to the complementary configuration of the air gaps and a centrically arranged guidance the normal forces are compensated. Sequential activation of the pole arms results in a continuous rotatory movement of 21 rpm with discrete steps due to the tangential reluctance forces. The tooth pitch is 100 μm resulting in step widths of 33.3 μm or 16.7 μm which correspond to incremental rotation angles of 0.64° and 0.32° for a rotor diameter of 8 mm. An overall torque of 0.3 μN·m @ 0.9 A has been measured. Thermographic measurements revealed a maximum temperature of 60°C @ 0.9 A requiring an active cooling of the motor.

3. **Rotatory synchronous micromotor**: Synchronous micromotors are based on the electro-dynamic actuation principle. The rotatory model consists of a stator (diameter 1.0–5.5 mm) comprising double layer planar spiral microcoils and a rotor made of SU-8 molds containing permanent magnets with alternating axial magnetizations. The magnets are either polymer magnets or commercial sintered magnets. The configuration of the coils (three or six phases) and magnets allows rotation in continuous and stepping modes up to 7000 rpm. The maximum temperature of 32°C at 100 mA does not require active cooling. The measured torque varies by one order of magnitude between motors with polymer magnets.

4. **Linear synchronous micromotor**: The linear synchronous micromotors consist of stators designed as three-strand systems with 3 to 15 spiral coils per strand resulting in step widths of 100 to 533 μm over a traverse path of about 9 mm. The travelers contain permanent magnets with alternating axial magnetization. Sintered magnets as well as polymer magnets are used. The maximum thrust achieved for stepping mode is 283 μN at 100 mA.

References

1. Fan, L.S.; Tai, Y.C.; Muller, R.S. IC-processed electrostatic micromotors. *Sens. Actuators.* 1989;20:41–47.
2. Mehregany, M.; Nagarkar, P.; Senturia, S.D.; Lang, J.H. Operation of microfabricated harmonic and ordinary side-drive motors. In Proceedings of the IEEE Workshop on Micro Electro Mechanical Systems, Nappa Valley, CA, 11–14 February 1990:1–8.
3. Bart, S.F.; Lober, T.A.; Howe, R.T.; Lang, J.H.; Schlecht, M.F. Design considerations for micromachined electric actuators. *Sens. Actuators.* 1988;14:269–292.
4. Trimmer, W.S.N.; Gabriel, K.J. Design considerations for a practical electrostatic micro-motor. *Sens. Actuators.* 1987;11:189–206.
5. Busch-Vishniac, I.J. The case for magnetically driven microactuators. *Sens. Actuators A.* 1992;33:207–220.
6. Waldschik, A.; Feldmann, M.; Büttgenbach, S. Novel synchronous linear and rotary micro motors based on polymer magnets with organic and inorganic insulation layers. *Sens. Transduc. J.* 2008;3:3–13.
7. Waldschik, A. *Elektromagnetische Mikroaktoren: Konzepte, Herstellung, Charakterisierung und Anwendungen.* Aachen, Germany: Shaker Verlag; 2010. (In German).
8. Feldmann, M.; Büttgenbach, S. Novel versatile electro magnetic micro actuators with integrated polymer magnets: Concept, fabrication and test. In Proceedings 10th International Conference on New Actuators, Bremen, Germany, 14–16 June 2006, 709–712.

ULTRASONIC INSTRUMENTS

Ultrasonic instruments have been used in dentistry since the 1950s. Initially they were used to cut teeth but very quickly they became established with ultrasonic scalers which were used to remove deposits from the hard tissues of the tooth. This enabled the soft tissues around the tooth to return to health. The ultrasonic vibrations are generated in a thin metal probe, and it is the working tip that is the active component of the instrument. Scanning laser vibrometry has shown that there is much variability in their movement which is related to the shape and cross-sectional shape of the probe. The working instrument will also generate cavitations and microstreaming in the associated cooling water. This can be mapped out along the length of the instrument indicating the active areas. Ultrasonics has also found use for cleaning often inaccessible or different surfaces including root canal treatment and dental titanium implants. The use of ultrasonics to cut bone during different surgical techniques shows considerable promise. More research is needed to determine how to maximize the efficiency of such instruments so that they are more clinically effective.[1, 2]

The ultrasonic instruments used in dentistry work at frequencies of 25 to 40 kHz. They were first introduced as a drill but then adapted as a scaling instrument used to clean deposits from the teeth. Such deposits are comprised of bacterial biofilms, which may or not be calcified. The vibrations transferred to a steel probe are used to physically remove them from the tooth. Such action also has the potential to damage the tooth structure if the instrument is not used correctly. The instruments present as either a magnetostrictive or piezoelectric generator with a series of interchangeable probes fashioned in the form of a dental hand instrument. It is the working tip that is used to remove the deposits from the tooth. The shapes of the probes are often curved which allows the working tip to negotiate difficult-to-reach places around or inside the tooth.[3, 4]

Mechanical Action of the Ultrasonic Scaler

The ultrasonic scaler works mainly in a "chipping" action, mechanically removing the deposits from the teeth. This removal is due to the longitudinal chipping motion and rapid movement of the tip. This is seen as the primary method of action. During use a flow of cooling water is passed over the tip, which acts as an irrigant removing debris from the area. Within the water biophysical effects such as cavitation and acoustic microstreaming will arise which may prove useful in the cleaning process. Until recently most authorities claimed differences between magnetostrictive and piezoelectric generators led to differences in the movement of the scaling tips. Using scanning laser vibrometry, it has now been shown that the movement of such tips is elliptical in nature and this is seen whether the tips are loaded or unloaded. The magnitude of this movement may differ between classes of instruments, and it is the lack of standardization that has been highlighted. It is known that different tips powered by different power generators show variation in either the unloaded or loaded situation. It is also possible to measure the vibration in 3D where the vibration picture is built up with the use of the three scanning heads of scanning laser vibrometer (SLV). The elliptical motion of all ultrasonic scalers is an important concept for researchers and clinicians. For researchers it means a change in thinking about how in vitro root surface investigations are evaluated. During use the ultrasonic scaler will not only remove the deposits but also partially impact the tooth surface. Any defects produced are directly related to the shape and cross section of the tip. The elliptical motion of the tip will produce some damage which will be most pronounced if the tip of the instrument is allowed to dwell in one position. Clinicians should be made aware of the motion and at all times orientate the body of the probe parallel to the surface of the tooth to minimize damage. Ultrasonic scalers have their own irrigation mechanism, which is related to the associated water supply. This is primarily needed to cool the heat generated from the rapid movement of the tip. The flow of water removes loosely attached plaque and dead bacteria from the tooth surface. It also improves clinician visibility by flushing debris from the pocket, and contributes to the occurrence of cavitation and acoustic microstreaming in the water. There have been various chemical additives added to the water supply with the aim of increasing the effectiveness of ultrasonic scaling, but clinical trials have so far not shown any evidence that this provides any advantage.[5-7]

Ultrasonics is firmly established as a routine clinical procedure in dentistry. While the major use of the instrument relies on the metal probe–tooth contact to achieve the result of removing deposits off the tooth surface, there is a contribution from cavitation and acoustic microstreaming occurring in the water supply. There have also been new and exciting developments in other specialties in dentistry for cleaning difficult to access areas (root canal treatment) or new surfaces such as dental implants. The use of the instrument to cut bone also opens up new opportunities. One area of further research that shows merit is using the phenomena of cavitation and acoustic microstreaming to break up bacterial biofilms.

References

1. Walmsley, A.D.; Lea, S.C.; Landini, G.; Moses, A.J. Advances in power driven pocket / root instrumentation. *J. Clin. Periodontol.* 2008;35(8) Supplement:22–28.
2. Felver, B.; King, D.C.; Lea, S.C.; Price, G.J.; Walmsley, A.D. Cavitation occurrence around ultrasonic dental scalers. *Ultrason. Sonochem.* 2009;16:692–697.
3. Lea, S.C.; Landini, G.; Walmsley, A.D. The displacement amplitude of ultrasonic scaler inserts. *J. Clin. Perio.* 2003;30:505–510.
4. Lea, S.C.; Felver, B.; Landini, G.; Walmsley, A.D. Three dimensional ultrasonic scaler probe oscillations. *J. Clin. Periodontol.* 2009a;36:44–50.
5. Lea, S.C.; Felver, B.; Landini, G.; Walmsley, A.D. Ultrasonic scaler probe oscillations and tooth surface defects. *J. Dent. Res.* 2009b;88:229–234.
6. Lea, S.C.; Landini, G. Reconstruction of dental ultrasonic scaler 3D vibration patterns from phase-related data. *Med. Eng. Phys.* 2010;32:673–677.
7. Lea, S.C.; Walmsley, A.D.; Lumley, P.L. Analysing endosonic root canal file oscillations: an in vitro evaluation. *J. Endodont.* 2010;36:880–883.

LIGHT CURE UNIT

Since the birth of dentistry there has been a continuous attempt to formulate a material and technique which fulfill aesthetic requirements, besides having the expected physical, mechanical and biological properties to behave favorably in the oral environment. Visible light-cured resin-based composites are the predominant restorative materials for both anterior and posterior restorations. In 2000, 94% of US dentists used visible light curing units. Light-cured composites allow the dentist to actively initiate the polymerization step which is a significant advantage compared to auto cured composites. Furthermore, a meticulous layering technique was employed to reduce polymerization shrinkage for application even in larger stress-bearing cavities in re-dentistry. This enables the dentist to generate aesthetic and durable restorations such as pit and fissure sealants, direct and indirect resin composite restorations and the luting of ceramic restorations. Even resin-modified glass ionomer relies on photo polymerization. There have been three major evolutions in dental composite curing lights since 1991. The relatively simple guidelines for clinicians involve three variables: Light intensity, exposure duration and incremental layering of the composite material. Restorative dentists are instructed to routinely monitor their light's output to ensure that the intensity is above 300 mW/cm², to cure each increment for at least 40 seconds and to cure the composite in increments less than 2 mm in thickness. There are basically three types of visible light curing units: Countertop units, gun type units and fiber optic handpiece attachment units.[1-3]

Countertop Units

The countertop unit contains all the functional parts in one box. A fiber optic or fluid-filled cord carries the light from the box to the patient. Some of these units have a control switch at the end of the cord so the operator does not have to leave the operating field to activate the light source. The advantages of counter-top units are that the fan and working parts of the unit are outside of the operating field and that they are generally less expensive than other designs. The disadvantages are that many units lack a switch at the cord end and many models do not have wide diameter curing tips. In addition, many countertop units have fiber optic cords that need periodic replacement because of fiber optic bundle breakdown.[4, 5]

Different Types[7-12]

Gun Type Units

The second type of visible light curing unit has its light source in a gun handle. The light passes through a small fiber optic cord or glass rod that forms the barrel of the gun. Generally, these units are attached to an additional table-top or wall-mounted unit that contains the necessary transformers to operate the light. This type of unit is activated at the operator site. They typically have large diameters of cure with good intensity and are generally small and easily made portable. Gun type units have no fiber optic cords to be replaced since the gun barrels are usually inflexible. The disadvantages of gun type units are the fan in the handle, which can be noisy and become warm with extended use, the gun bulk and weight (more bulky than fiber optic cord ends) and higher cost.

Fiber Optic Handpiece Curing Attachments

The third type, the fiber optic handpiece curing attachment, is generally adapted to existing fiber optic handpiece light sources. Attachment units have curing tips that are usually smaller than but similar to those in countertop units. Some of these units generate considerable heat, owing to inefficient or missing blue light filters. These units are less expensive, especially if the fiber optic handpiece is already in place. They are small and require no additional counter space. Their drawbacks include, generally, a smaller diameter of cure, less intense light source, release of excessive heat (some units) and periodic need for the replacement of fiber optic cords.

Curing Lamps/Curing Units

There are four main types of light sources that have been developed for use in the polymerization of light-curable dental materials and that are listed below. Out of these, halogen lights and LED units are by far the most frequently used in daily clinical practice.

QTH Lamps
Quartz Tungsten Halogen (QTH) lamps have been the standard curing units for several years, despite a remarkably low efficiency compared to heat generation. Since QTH lamps emit a rather wide range of wavelengths, band-pass filters are required to limit the wavelength between 370 and 550 nm in order to fit the peak absorption of camphoroquinone. QTH lamps have a limited lifespan of 100 hours with subsequent degradation of the bulb, reflector and filter caused by high operating temperatures and the considerable quantity of heat being produced during operating cycles.

PAC Lamps
Plasma arc curing (PAC) lamps emit visible light at higher intensities and were primarily designed to save irradiation time as an economic factor. PAC units typically produce power density greater than

2000 mW/cm^2, and have been shown to polymerize composite in the least amount of time. The plasma arc lamps (short-arc xenon) used for pulse energy curing usually have a 5-mm spot size and a wide bandwidth covering 380 to 500 nm. They yield a power density up to 2500 mW/cm^2. This is a tremendously powerful light energy source that requires a wait time (minimum 10 seconds) after each use to allow the unit to recover.

Argon-IPN-Lasers

Dental lasers were introduced and recognized as a tool for better patient care in the early 1990s. The wavelength of the argon laser (between 450 and 500 nm) has been used effectively to polymerize composite resins because it enhances the physical properties of the restorative material compared with conventional visible light curing. Lasers produce little heat, because of limited infrared output. The argon laser is useful in class 2 composite restorations, not only because of the decreased curing time needed, but also because the small fiber size allows for easy access of the curing light to the interproximal box area and provides a highly satisfactory result for the completed restoration.

Light Emitting Diodes (LED) Curing Light

To overcome the shortcomings of halogen bulb visible light curing units, Mills proposed using a solid-state light emitting diode, or LED technology in 1995 to polymerize light activated dental materials. The spectral emittance of gallium nitride blue LEDs covers the absorption spectrum of camphoroquinone so that no filters are required in LED light curing units. Recent reports have revealed that blue LED lamps offer the highest photo polymerization efficiency. LEDs use junctions of doped semiconductors for generating light. LEDs have a lifetime of more than 10,000 hours and undergo little degradation of output over time. LEDs are resistant to shock and vibration and consume little power on operation. The newer gallium nitrides LEDs produce a narrow spectrum of light (400–500 nm) that falls closely within the absorption range of camphoroquinone and initiates the polymerization of resin monomers. Halogen-based lights have a much broader light spectrum in comparison. LEDs are more efficient converters of electrical power into visible blue light, and do not generate the large quantities of heat associated with halogen lamps. Much of the spectral radiant intensity of many blue LEDs lies in the 468 nm region peak absorption of the photo initiator, and therefore produces an almost ideal bandwidth of the light that is required. LEDs, unlike halogen lamps, lend themselves to being driven by a pulsed supply. Today, LED technology has considerably changed towards high-power LEDs capable of delivering a rather high output with one single diode inside the curing unit.

References

1. Rueggeberg, F.A. From vulcanite to vinyl, a history of resins in restorative dentistry. *J. Prosthet. Dent.* 2002;87(4):364–379.
2. Craig, R. Symposium on composite resins in dentistry. In: Horn H, editor. *The Dental Clinica of North America.*Philadelphia: Saunders; 1981, 219–239.
3. Craig, R.G. Denture materials and acrylic base materials. *Curr. Opin. Dent.* 1991;1(2):235–243.
4. Chen, Y.C.; Ferracane, J.L.; Prahl, S.A. Quantum yield of conversion of the photoinitiator camphorquinone. *Dent. Mater.* 2007;23(6):655–664.
5. Oliveira, D.C.; Rocha, M.G.; Correa, I.C.; Correr, A.B.; Ferracane, J.L.; Sinhoreti, M.A. The effect of combining photoinitiator systems on the color and curing profile of resin-based composites. *Dent. Mater.* 2016 Oct;32(10):1209–1217.
6. Neumann, M.G.; Schmitt, C.C.; Ferreira, G.C.; Corrêa, I.C. The initiating radical yields and the efficiency of polymerization for various dental photoinitiators excited by different light curing units. *Dent. Mater.* 2006;22(6):576–584.
7. Neumann, M.G.; Miranda, W.G. Jr, Schmitt, C.C.; Rueggeberg, F.A.; Correa, I.C. Molar extinction coefficients and the photon absorption efficiency of dental photoinitiators and light curing units. *J. Dent.* 2005 Jul;33(6):525–532.

8. Schneider, L.F.; Cavalcante, L.M.; Consani, S.; Ferracane, J.L. Effect of co-initiator ratio on the polymer properties of experimental resin composites formulated with camphorquinone and phenyl-propanedione. *Dent. Mater.* 2009;25(3):369–375.
9. Rueggeberg, F.A. State-of-the-art: Dental photocuring: A review. *Dent. Mater.* 2011;27(1):39–52.
10. Rueggeberg, F. Contemporary issues in photocuring. *Compend Contin Educ Dent.* 1999;25:S4–S15.
11. Friedman, J., inventor. Dental light curing lamp unit with interchangeable autofocus light guides. *United States patent US 4,948,215*; 1990.
12. Curtis, J.W. Jr, Rueggeberg, F.A., Lee, A.J. Curing efficiency of the Turbo Tip. *Gen Dent.* 1995;43(5):428–433.

ELECTRIC PULP TEST

The response to an electric pulp tester, as indicated before, has no qualitative aspect. In cases where there is no reaction to heat or cold, the reasonable presumption might be that the pulp is necrotic. This would be a valid conclusion if all the teeth tested provided comparable responses. Occasionally in a given dentition, heat and cold tests elicit little response on any of the teeth. The electric pulp test (EPT) can at least provide the information of response or no response that may help differentiate normal from necrotic pulps. During usage, a medium such as toothpaste or gel is used to ensure electrical contact between the tooth and the tip of the tester. Ideally the tip of the tester is placed at the incisal edge for the anterior teeth. On posterior teeth, the favored location for the placement of the tester is on the buccal cusp tip.[1]

The limitation of the EPT is the lack of response on teeth with immature root development; this can be particularly confusing. Such teeth commonly have open apices and periapical-type radiolucencies associated with the development of the dental papilla. In these cases, a widened apical periodontal ligament space is also typical and completely normal. If any diagnostic questions arise regarding pulpal pathosis in teeth with immature apical development, pulp testing will be unhelpful. It is appropriate to monitor such teeth over time for the emergence of periapical symptoms or lack of continued root development before making the diagnosis of pulpal pathosis.[2]

Traumatically injured teeth may also fail to respond reliably and predictably immediately following the traumatic event, but many teeth will regain sensibility within three to six months. Once again, long-term monitoring is in order. The development of periapical pathosis either clinically or radiographically would support endodontic intervention. The same is true for sensibility testing of teeth during orthodontic tooth movement, where responses may be highly unreliable.

The EPT delivers a graduated increase in electric current (alternating or direct) to excite a response from the Aδ nerve fibers within the viable pulp. Most modern pulp testers are monopolar, meaning there is only one probe. When used as a pulp tester, a pulsating stimulus is produced starting at a low value, which increases automatically. The pulse amplitude of the stimulus begins at 15 volts and rises to a maximum of 350 volts.[3]

Pulp Testing Technique

The test and control teeth should be dried and isolated with cotton wool or a rubber dam, the latter applied as small strips placed between the teeth. Contacts may also be isolated by inserting acetate strips between teeth. A conducting medium must be used – the one most readily available is toothpaste. The pulp tester is applied to the middle third of the tooth, avoiding contact with the soft tissues and any restorations. A lip electrode is placed over the patient's lip. If the pulp is vital the patient describes feeling a sensation which is variously described as tingling, vibration, pain or shock. Before testing the tooth in question, it is important to educate and acclimatize the patient to the sensation first on a control tooth. The patient is instructed that they should only respond to a sensation that matches the one elicited from the control tooth (assuming the pulp in this tooth is normal). Asking the patient to respond to *any* sensation will yield a false positive because if the potential difference is high enough, a sensation could be elicited from the periodontal ligament or adjacent teeth. A more user-friendly method is to ask the patient to hold the lip electrode. The plastic cable is held in one hand and the metal electrode between the forefinger and thumb of the other hand. This method allows the patient to have control by releasing their finger grip on the metal electrode when they feel the defined (not any) sensation; thus reducing the element of an anxiety-driven response. Electric pulp testers should be used with caution on patients who have a cardiac pacemaker; although modern pacemakers are shielded from electrical interference. Pulp testing of crowned teeth is possible provided a small area of dentine or enamel is available for electrical contact without touching the gingival tissue. The electric pulp tester cannot discriminate partial pulp necrosis, which happens in the root of a molar tooth.[4]

EPT works on the premise that electrical stimuli cause an ionic change across the neural membrane, thereby inducing an action potential with a rapid hopping action at the nodes of Ranvier in myelinated nerves. The pathway for the electric current is thought to be from the probe tip of the test device to the tooth, along the lines of the enamel prisms and dentine tubules, and then through the pulp tissue. The "circuit" is completed via the patient wearing a lip clip or by touching the probe handle with his/her hand; alternatively, the operator can have one "gloveless" hand that touches the patient's skin. A "tingling" sensation will be felt by the patient once the increasing voltage reaches the pain threshold, but this threshold level varies between patients and teeth, and is affected by factors such as individual age, pain perception, tooth surface conduction and resistance.[5]

The correct technique for using the electric pulp tester is also important for accurate responses. In order to ensure that the appropriate current pathway is followed, correct placement of the EPT probe tip flat against the contact area, and having a conducting medium such as toothpaste between the probe tip and the tooth surface are essential. Jacobson found, in an in vitro experiment involving incisors and premolars, that placing the probe tip labially within the incisal or occlusal two-thirds of the crown gave more consistent results.

Safety Concerns of EPT

In EPT operation manuals, warnings are given that the current produced by the testing device may cause danger to patients who have cardiac pacemakers, with the risk of precipitating cardiac arrhythmia via pacemaker interference. This concern is based on a sole animal study where EPT interfered with a pacemaker fitted in a dog. At the time of that study (the early 1970s), cardiac pacemakers were primitive, but as pacemakers have become equipped with better shielding, more recent studies have shown no interference from EPT or similar electrical dental devices.

Accuracy of EPT

Electric pulp tests are known to be unreliable in many instances, producing false results in healthy immature teeth with incompletely formed roots which may be erupting since these teeth may take up to five years before the maximum number of myelinated fibers reaches the pulp-dentine border at the plexus of Rashkow. This is also when apical root maturation occurs. Teeth with pulp canal calcification (PCC) and patients suffering from primary hyperthyroidism frequently have an increased sensory response threshold to EPT. In the case of PCC, the sensory response may be completely blocked, whereas hypercalcemia from hyperthyroidism may require twice as much current as that which is normally needed to elicit a response from a clinically normal pulp. False results are also possible in teeth with healthy pulps undergoing orthodontic treatment because the pulp's sensory elements may be disturbed for up to nine months. Similarly, recently traumatized teeth undergoing pulp repair may also have false results and thus may not respond to EPT.

Theories proposed by Öhman for this loss of pulp sensibility include pressure or tension on the nerve fibers, blood vessel rupture and ischemic injury. It is then assumed that these effects were reversible in the cases where the pulp sensation recovered. Pileggi et al. have shown in ferrets that

10–12 days are required for the sensory component of the pulp to start to respond to EPT again as damage from trauma heals. It has also been observed that hyperemia and/or transient nerve decompression may be responsible for temporary sensory loss. Inaccurate responses are known to occur with EPT when the current is conducted to adjacent teeth, for example, when two adjacent teeth have contacting proximal metallic restorations. Periodontal tissues, breakdown products from pulps undergoing necrosis and remnants of inflamed pulp tissues may also cause sensory stimulation leading to false responses.[5, 6]

References

1. Anderson, R.W.; Pantera, E.A. Jr. Influence of a barrier technique on electric pulp testing. *J Endodont.* 1988;14:179–180.
2. Bender, I.B.; Landau, M.A.; Fonsecca, S., Trowbridge, H.O. The optimum placement-site of the electrode in electric pulp testing of the 12 anterior teeth. *J Am Dent Assoc.* 1989;118:305–310.
3. Bhaskar, S.N.; Rappaport, H.M. Dental vitality tests and pulp status. *J Am Dent Assoc.* 1973;86:409–411.
4. Chambers, I.G. The role and methods of pulp testing in oral diagnosis: A review. *Int Endodont J.* 1982;15:1–15.
5. Civjan, S.; Barone, J.J.; Vaccaro, G.J. Electric pulp vitality testers. *J Dent Res.* 1973;52:120–126.
6. Cooley, R.L.; Stilley, J.; Lubow, R.M. Evaluation of a digital pulp tester. *Oral Surg Oral Med Oral Pathol.* 1984;58:437–442.

LASERS

Light has been used as a therapeutic agent for many centuries. In ancient Greece, the sun was used in heliotherapy, that is, exposure of the body to the sun for the restoration of health. During the early 20th century, the physical principles of laser began to be realized with the introduction of quantum theory of Neils Bohr (1913). At the turn of century, Albert Einstein developed theories essential for the laser, almost 60 years before the first laser was built, which showed weak flashes of red light. [1]

Laser is an acronym for light amplification by stimulated emission of radiation.[2] This acronym describes the lasing principle. Several decades ago a laser was considered to be like a death ray, the ultimate weapon of destruction, something you would find in a science fiction story. Dental procedures performed today with lasers are so effective that they should set a new standard of care. Laser instruments allow easy access to the anatomic site and are capable of the ablation of lesions in proximity to normal structures. Access is provided by a handpiece and delivery system using either a non-touch (free) or touch (contact tip) technique and a series of mirrors or the conduction of radiant energy through a flexible quartz fiber. Lesions in proximity to normal tissue can be managed with minimal destruction of adjacent normal cells, because the precision of lasers with extremely small focal spot sizes causes minimal penetration and cell death collateral to laser incision.[1–3]

Lasers are employed in various disciplines of dentistry including oral medicine and maxillofacial radiology, prosthetics, periodontics, pedodontics, endodontics, implantology, cosmetic and operative dentistry and oral and maxillofacial surgery. Lasers can be employed in the detection of caries, the removal of incipient caries, for curing composite resins and for enamel etching. Newer versions of lasers have been developed to cut enamel without endangering the pulp. Thus lasers may replace mechanical drills for cavity preparation in the near future. Lasers can also be used in periodontal, stage II implant, pre-prosthetic and endodontic surgeries, for the treatment of vascular lesions and in photodynamic therapy. In the management of premalignant lesions such as leukoplakia, lasers have proven to be the treatment of choice. Lasers have also been used for the resection of T1 and T2 squamous cell carcinoma with successful results and varied advantages over other modalities of treatment.

For some procedures in dentistry such as maxillary midline frenectomy, lasers are so clinically effective that they should become the state of the art, as they have in certain medical procedures. Regardless of the wavelength used, lasers in dentistry offer a variety of advantages. Because lasers seal blood vessels, they offer a dry operating field, excellent visibility and reduced operative time. In addition, lasers seal lymphatic vessels which yields minimum post-operative swelling. Lasers offer the ability to negotiate curves and folds in the oral cavity and can vaporize, cut and coagulate tissue. With the use of lasers pain is reduced probably due to the sealing of nerve fibers. The chances of mechanical trauma are reduced, scaring is minimal and sutures are rarely needed. They also cause a reduction in bacterial counts. Besides these advantages, the greatest advantage of lasers is a high rate of patient acceptance.[4–6]

A laser is a device that converts electrical or chemical energy into light energy. In contrast to ordinary light that is emitted spontaneously by excited atoms or molecules, the light emitted by a laser occurs when an atom or molecule retains excess energy until it is stimulated to emit it. All the radiation emitted by a laser including both visible and invisible light is most generally termed as electromagnetic radiation.[7]

Electromagnetic radiation is the movement of energy through space as a combination of electric and magnetic fields. It is generated when the velocity of an electrically charged particle is altered. Gamma rays, X-rays, ultraviolet rays, visible light, infrared radiation, microwaves and radio waves are all examples of electromagnetic radiation. The types of radiation in this spectrum are ionizing or non-ionizing depending on their energy. If sufficient energy is associated with the radiation to remove orbital electrons from atoms in the irradiated matter, the radiation is ionizing. All electromagnetic waves travel at the velocity of light (3×10^8 m/s) in a vacuum.[8]

A laser consists of a lasing medium contained within an optical cavity, with an external source to maintain population inversion so that the stimulated emission of a specific wavelength can occur, producing a monochromatic, collimated and coherent beam of light.[7, 8]

The word laser is an acronym for light amplification by stimulated emission of radiation. A brief description of each of those five words begins to explain the unique qualities of laser instruments and, in turn, becomes the foundation for further elaboration of the uses of lasers in dentistry.

Properties of Lasers[8–11]

The important properties of laser light that distinguish it from white light are monochromaticity, directionality, collimation and coherence.

Monochromaticity

Lasers emit light that is monochromatic or specifically has a single wavelength. Lasers of varying types emit a specific wavelength. Each type of tissue absorbs a given wavelength far better than others. This factor is based on the consistency of the tissue, its thickness and significant tissue chromophores such as hemoglobin and melanin.

Directionality

There is little divergence of the laser as it exits the laser device, and the beam can travel a considerable distance maintaining its parallelism. Most gas or solid-state lasers emit laser beams with a divergence angle of approximately a milli radian. This means they will spread out to one meter in diameter after traveling one kilometer. Because of this lasers are extremely hazardous.

Collimation

Collimation refers to the beam having specific spatial boundaries which ensures that there is a constant size and shape of beam emitted from the laser cavity. Thus, the laser produces a pencil beam of light that is very nearly parallel. If the parallel laser light is focused through a lens, it will focus down to a diffraction limited spot, the smallest possible focal spot. This property is especially useful in medicine. Thus a laser is able to focus the light to the minimum focal spot size with the highest energy density to ablate the tissue with light.

Coherence

Coherence is a property unique to lasers. The light waves produced by a laser are a specific form of electromagnetic energy. A laser produces light waves that are physically identical. They are all in phase with one another, that is, they have identical amplitude (all the peaks and valleys are the same size) and identical frequency.

High Power

The high energy density of lasers is useful in medicine as it allows surgeons to use lasers for ablation. It is the ability of lasers to focus the laser beam to a small point that achieves high power density (irradiance).

Components of Lasers

The basic components of lasers include:

- Housing tube/optical cavity
- Lasing/active medium
- Pump energy source/power supply
- Cooling system
- Delivery system
- Control panel

Housing Tube/Optical Cavity

The housing tube or optical cavity encapsulates the laser medium and functionally contains the process of absorption, spontaneous emission and stimulated emission. The tube material may consist of metal, ceramic or both. At both ends of the housing are mirrors, a fully reflecting mirror on one side and a partially reflecting mirror on the other side. They are precisely mounted so that they are exactly parallel to one another. This arrangement allows for the reflection of photons of light back and forth across the chamber, eventually resulting in the production of an intense photon resonance within the medium. The second mirror which is partially reflective allows some of the laser light to escape as the output device. Since the process is not 100% efficient and some energy is converted to heat, it is necessary to provide some cooling.[5, 12]

Lasing/Active Medium

A lasing medium is a material which is capable of absorbing the energy produced by an external extension source and subsequently gives off the excess energy as photons of light. This is usually achieved through the excitation of electrons to higher energy levels with photons of light being generated as these electrons drop to lower energy bands. Lasing media can be solid (crystal or semiconductor), liquid or gas. The composition and structure of the lasing medium determine the wavelength output and name of a particular laser.[13] The medium is located within the resonating chamber (laser tube).

Pump Energy/Power Supply

An energy source is used to excite or pump the atoms in the lasing medium to their higher energy levels that are necessary for the production of laser radiation. The pumping source can be electrical, chemical, thermal or optical energy. Energy from this primary source is absorbed by the active medium, resulting in the production of laser light. This process is very inefficient, with only some 3–10% of incident energy resulting in laser light, the rest being converted to heat energy. The dynamics of incident energy with time has a fundamental bearing on the emission mode characteristics of a given laser. A continuous-feed electrical discharge will result in a similar continuous feed of laser light emission.[2]

Cooling System

Heat production is a by-product of laser light propagation. It increases with the power output of the laser and hence, with heavy-duty tissue cutting lasers, the cooling system represents the bulkiest component. Co-axial coolant systems may be air- or water-assisted.[2]

Control Panel

This allows variation in power output with time which is defined by the pumping mechanism frequency. Other facilities may allow wavelength change (multi-laser instruments) and print-outs of delivered laser energy during clinical use.[2]

Types of Lasers[14, 15]

I. **According to physical construction of the laser**:
   1. Gas
      a. Argon
      b. Helium-neon
      c. Carbon dioxide
   2. Liquid
   3. Solid
      a. Potassium titanyl phosphate (KTP)
      b. Neodymium:Yttrium Aluminum Garnet (Nd:YAG)
      c. Erbium, Chromium:Yttrium-Scandium-Gallium-garnet (Er,Cr:YSG)
      d. Erbium:Yttrium Aluminium Garnet (Er:YAG)
   4. Semiconductor
      a. Diode
II. **According to potential hazards – American National Standards Institute (ANSI) and Occupational Safety & Health Administration (OHSA) standards**:
III. **Lasers are classified as hard and soft lasers**:
   a) Soft lasers
      These are a source of cold low energy emitted at wavelengths thought by some to stimulate cellular activity. These generally utilize semiconductor laser diodes. They are principally used for tissue generation, to relieve pain, to reduce inflammation and edema and to accelerate healing. The three main soft lasers are helium-neon (He-Ne), gallium-arsenide (Ga-As) and gallium-aluminum-arsenide lasers.
   b) Hard lasers
      Hard lasers have a longer wavelength and produce thermal effect which cut the tissue by coagulation, vaporization and carbonization. Three commonest types used in dentistry are argon, carbon dioxide and Nd:YAG.
IV. **According to type of medium which undergoes lasing**:
   1. Argon
   2. Diode
   3. Nd:YAG
   4. Holmium:YAG

5. Erbium family (Er,Cr:YSG, Er:YAG)
6. Carbon dioxide (CO_2)
7. KTP
8. Helium-neon (He-Ne)
9. Excimer laser
10. Ruby

Advantages[5, 15]

1. Precise delivery of energy to the diseased tissue via microscopes; thus there is minimal damage to surrounding tissues.
2. The laser beam exerts a hemostatic effect by sealing blood vessels rendering a bloodless surgery field. This allows excellent visibility and precision in tissue removal.
3. Precision in tissue destruction because of good visualization of tissue planes by means of an operating microscope provides precise control together with illumination and magnification of the operative field.
4. Reduction of post-operative inflammation and edema due to sealing of the lymphatic vessels; no serous or lymph leakage occurs into the tissue.
5. There is little post-operative scarring resulting in little induration or restriction in movements of soft tissue intraorally and the healed area is soft on palpation.
6. Reduced post-operative pain sensation due to the sealing of nerve endings and decreased releases of pain mediators.
7. Pressing or suturing is not required for wound closing.
8. Operating time is reduced, and immediate tissue destruction can be done.
9. Sterilization of the wound due to reduction in amount of micro-organisms exposed to laser radiation.
10. Relative absence of scarring and wound closure.
11. Malignant cells or immunologically active cell particles are destroyed during laser surgery and also blood vessels and lymphatics are sealed; thereby tumor seeding can be prevented.
12. Laser surgery requires minimal instrumentation and handling of surrounding tissue.
13. Any recurrence in the lesion can be easily treated.
14. Laser exposure to tooth enamel causes a reduction in demineralization or enamel permeability or morphological microscopic alteration which makes the enamel more acid resistant thereby decreasing the caries activity.
15. No ionizing radiation to cause cellular mutation as with X-rays or gamma rays.
16. Access to difficult-to-reach anatomical sites is easy.
17. It has the ability to coagulate, vaporize and incise tissue.
18. High patient acceptance.

Disadvantages[15]

1. Specialized didactic and clinically oriented instruction required for laser use by the surgeon and ancillary staff.
2. Laser equipment is expensive.
3. Specialized wiring and a plumbing connection are required.
4. The laser beam could injure the patient or operator by the direct beam or the reflected light causing retinal burn.

5. Laser exposure to the surface of the teeth, whether accidental or intentional, can cause irreversible pulpal damage.
6. General anesthesia is usually required for patients undergoing laser treatment in the mouth.
7. If the laser beam strikes a combustible anesthetic tube which is carrying anesthetic gases, it will ignite and can be fatal.
8. Delays in healing of wounds due to delays in epithelial regeneration.
9. Loss of tactile feedback while incising in the laser instrument.
10. Aqueous solutions may be used for preparation and tissues must be dried since fluid reduces laser efficiency.
11. The removal of soft tissue overlying the bone can damage the underlying bone and cause delayed healing and sequestration of devitalized bone fragments.
12. It is available only in hospitals.

References

1. Reinisch, L.; Ossof, R.H. Introduction-Laser applications in otolaryngology. *Otolaryngol Clin North Am.* 1996;29(6):891–914.
2. Parker, S. Introduction, history of laser and laser light production. *Br Dent J.* 2007;202:21–31.
3. Chionchio, F. The use of lasers in treatment of vascular and pigmented lesions. *Oral Maxillofac Surg Clin North Am.* 1998;10(1):141–154.
4. Pick, R.M. The use of the lasers for treatment of gingival diseases. *Oral Maxillofac Surg Clin North Am.* 1997;9(1):1–18.
5. Miserendino, L.M.; Pick, R.M., editors. *Lasers in Dentistry.* Quintessence Publishing; 1995.
6. Frame, J.W. Carbon dioxide laser surgery for benign oral lesions. *Br Denta J.* 1985;158:125–128.
7. Coluzzi, D.J. An overview of laser wavelength in dentistry. *Dent Clin North Am.* 2000;44(4):753–765.
8. Coluzzi, D.J. Fundamentals of dental lasers: Science and instruments. *Dent Clin North Am.* 2004;48(4):751–770.
9. White, S.; Pharoah, M. *Oral Radiology: Principles and Interpretation: 5th Edition.* Elsevier Publication; 2004.
10. Catone, G.A.; Alling, C.C., editors. *Laser application in Oral and Maxillofacial Surgery.* W.B. Saunders Company.
11. Reinisch, L. Laser physics and tissue interaction. *Otolaryngologic Clinics of North America* 1996;29(6):893–913.
12. Spivey, J.D. Lasers and implant dentistry. *Oral Maxillofac Surg Clin North Am.* 1996;8(3):347–359.
13. Cobb, C.M.; McCawley, T.K.; Killoy, W.J. A preliminary study on the effects of the Nd:YAG laser on root surfaces on subgingival microflora in vivo. *J Periodontol.* 1992;63:701–707.
14. Midda, M.; Renton-Harper, P. Lasers in dentistry. *Br Dent Surg.* 1991;11:343–346.
15. Walsh, L.J. The current status of laser application in dentistry. *Aust Dent J.* 2003;48(3):146–155.

DENTAL IMAGING DEVICES

The invention of X-ray was described by Wilhelm Conrad Roentgen on November 8, 1845, Wilhelm Conrad Roentgen discovered a new radiation which he named as X-rays. After his invention of X-ray, he said 'I didn't think, I experimented'. The potential for using X-ray pictures in medical and dental diagnosis was recognized at once and exploited almost immediately. Credit for the first dental radiograph is given to Dr. Otto Walkhoff. The first dental radiograph was taken on January 14, 1896, by Walkhoff exposing himself for 20 minutes.[1]

Roentgen was a German physicist working with vacuum tubes operating at high voltages. When an electric current passed between the positively and negatively charged points of a tube, in a dark room, excited a supply of platicocyanide which had been casually stored nearby, Roentgen concluded that the voltage moving through the vacuum tube must have emitted energy. He called this unknown energy

X-ray after a short time. The first dental radiograph in the United States was taken by Dr. William Herbert Rollins on a skull, and Dr. C. Edmond Kells, a well-known pioneer in dental radiography, took the first dental intraoral radiograph in the United States. He suffered a series of surgical attempts to remedy his radiation injuries, losing his left arm, eventually leading to his death from suicide. Dr. William Herbert Rollins recognized very early the potential hazards of X-radiation and made recommendations for protection. Dr. William Herbert Rollins is considered to be the father of modern radiation protection, and many of the ideas he advanced are now widely accepted as good radiation protection practices.[1]

Dental radiography is a double-edged sword, capable of the diagnosis of physical conditions that would otherwise be difficult to identify, and its judicious use is of considerable benefit to the patient. It is one of the most valuable tools used in modern dental health care. The use of X-rays requires the adoption of measures to limit the exposure of both the patient and the clinician.

Radiation protection in dental practice is focused on three basic principles: Justification, optimization and dose limitation. These principles imply the definition of selection criteria, methods to reduce radiation dose and education. Although widely accepted selection criteria are lacking, there is general agreement about the methods to reduce radiation dose. One of the basic beliefs of radiation safety is to ensure that all exposure to ionizing radiation is clinically justified. All radiation exposure must be kept "as low as reasonably achievable (ALARA principle)". This principle states that exposure to radiation which can be decreased without loss of critical diagnostic information and without too much expense or inconvenience should be done. This is achieved in three ways, the application of selection criteria when choosing whether or not to use a radiographic examination, using physical methods of minimizing dose (i.e. equipment and film factors) and finally by quality assurance programmers. In the latter, efforts are made to ensure the consistent production of high-quality radiographs, thereby avoiding repeat exposure and maximizing the benefit to the patient.[1, 2]

The application of intraoral radiography in dentistry plays a major role in the diagnosis and treatment of diseases which contributes directly to patient care and pathology; it provides a vital diagnostic backup to all the specialties. The biological effects of ionizing radiation have been well documented; therefore all dental exposure should involve a balance between benefits and risk for the patients and dental professionals. In many procedures, diagnostic radiographs are essential for the production of a treatment plan, and treatment may be contraindicated without them. Periapical radiographs ("peri" meaning "around" and apical meaning "apex" or end of tooth root) record images of the outlines to position a mesiodistal extent of the teeth and its surrounding tissues.[3]

In periapical radiographs it is essential to obtain the full length of the tooth and at least 2 mm of the periapical bone. The purpose of the intraoral periapical examination is to obtain a view of the entire tooth and its surrounding structures. Intraoral periapical radiography is a commonly used intraoral imaging technique in dental radiology and may be a component of intraoral periapical radiologic examination. Periapical radiographs provide important information about the teeth and surrounding bone. The film shows the entire crown and root of the teeth and surrounding alveolar bone which provides vital information to aid in the diagnosis of the most common dental diseases, specifically tooth decay, tooth abscesses and periodontal bone loss or gum disease. Additional important findings may be detected, including the condition of restorations, impacted teeth or broken tooth fragments and variations in tooth and bone anatomy.[3]

Technique for Periapical Radiography[3]

Two exposure techniques are used for periapical radiography. Prior to presenting the techniques, a clear understanding of the techniques must be established; although the bisecting angle technique is utilized by practitioners, the paralleling technique is the method of choice for intraoral radiography. The paralleling angle technique provides less distortion and reduces excess radiation to the patient.

Instruments

The film holder consists of three basic components:

The film holder holds the film packet parallel to the teeth and prevents the bending of the film. It has a bite block and beam aiming device, which may or may not prevent the collimation of the beam.

A number of commercial devices are available that will hold the film parallel and at varying distances from the teeth:

1. The extension cone paralleling (XCP) instruments.
2. The precision rectangular collimating instruments which restrict the beam size at the patient's face to the size of radiograph.
3. The stable disposable film holder.
4. The Snap-A-Ray intraoral film holder
5. A hemostat inserted through a flattened rubber bite bock.

The choice of holder is a matter of personal preference.

The introduction of digital computers in the early 1940s fueled a revolutionary chain of rapid developments in various fields of science, including the beginning steps in digital imaging for diagnostic applications. The computational power of digital computers, coupled with image- and signal-processing algorithms, provided a wide range of options for image enhancement and analysis. The early approach to digital radiography involved scanning (digitizing) film-based radiographs into a computer, followed by image processing and display. This two-step process, also known as indirect digital radiography, gained significant popularity in research activities but not much use in clinical procedures. Moreover, such an indirectly formed digital image had, at best, the same information content as the film-based radiograph along with its characteristics and artifacts. The introduction of electronic image receptors in the late 1960s and their rapid improvements not only made direct digital radiography possible, but also led to the introduction of computed diagnostic imaging methods, such as computed tomography (CT).[4]

The first technology is composed of a group of digital image receptors that can transfer the captured image electronically in real time to the computer system.

Charge-coupled device (CCD) technology is the first electronic receptor introduced in 1989 for dental application. Currently, CCD-based receptors are the most common electronic receptors and have gone through significant improvements since their introduction. A CCD image receptor is composed of an array of individual small sensors, configured in a uniform and rectangular form. Each small sensor collects the X-ray energy imparted. The collection of these sensed signals will be transferred to the computer via the ADC unit to form the digital radiographic image. An active pixel sensor (APS) image receptor has a structure similar to the CCD receptor, except it offers direct access to each individual location within the sensor. This allows operations such as reading a small region of interest (ROI) or location-dependent processing of images on the chip.[4]

Photostimulable storage phosphor (PSP) is the second category of imaging technology that has found some acceptance in dental radiography and caries diagnosis. PSP image receptors are fundamentally different from electronic receptors in terms of design and structure. PSP imaging requires a scanning step and does not provide an immediate image. Despite the differences, PSP shares many of the characteristics of the electronic image receptor which makes it an alternative approach for digital radiography.

Digital radiography refers to a method of capturing a radiographic image using a sensor, breaking it into electronic pieces and presenting and storing the image using a computer. Instead of having an analog radiographic image on a film, in digital imaging the sensor is used to receive the analog information and through an analog-to-digital converter (ADC) analog radiographic image on a film is converted into a digital image that is an array of picture elements called pixels, with discrete gray values for each one. Special software is used to store and manipulate the digital image in the computer. The image is displayed within seconds or minutes on the computer screen in front of the clinicians and the patient.[4, 5]

Another digital imaging technique, storage phosphor radiography, first introduced in medical radiography in 1981, became available for intraoral imaging in 1994 (Table 9.2).

Digital Radiographic Imaging[4–7]

Digital imaging is simply an image acquisition technique that generates an electronic image to be viewed and manipulated on a computer. The goal of radiography is not merely to capture an accurate image, but also to produce diagnostic information. Digital image processing can provide this information more effectively than can film-based imaging.

For a better understanding of the mechanism of image processing, it is good to know what a digital image actually is. Solid-state sensors and phosphor plate sensors principle are not different with respect to the end result of the image acquisition process. The sensor system measures the photon intensity of the X-ray beam after it has passed through the object (the patient). These measurements are done in a two-dimensional array of small regions of 20 to 30 mm², called pixels (the abbreviation of "picture element").

The photon intensity is measured electronically on a scale of 256 gray values (0–25). Zero on this scale means that the maximum radiation is measured, which corresponds to radiolucent (black) in the radiographic image, and 255 represents no radiation at all, or complete radiopacity (white). The measurements of the photon intensities for each pixel are sent to the computer and stored as an array of numbers representing the X and Y coordinates and the photon intensity of each pixel. In fact, the digital image can be conceived as a table with columns and rows. The columns represent the X coordinates of the pixels and the rows the Y coordinates. The values in each cell indicate the gray level of the pixel represented by that cell. The numerical information contained in the array subsequently is used to display the gray values on the monitor screen. Some systems use a more detailed gray value scale, one that can contain up to 64,000 values, to express the photon intensity for each pixel; however the image always is displayed on the monitor screen that uses only up to 256 gray values.[3] The table can also be used to perform image processing: A mathematical procedure is applied to the numerical representation of the digital image which results in a new set of pixel values. The resulting set of numbers then is used to display the processed image on the monitor screen.[8, 9]

The algorithm, for instance, reverses the order of the gray values, resulting in a negative of the original image. More advanced algorithms can be used for higher resolution, for instance, in a three-dimensional reconstruction of radiographic information or the automated recognition of image features. Currently, there are two types of digital radiography systems available without an analog precursor: Direct and semi-direct.[8–10]

Semi-direct Image Plate System

This image plate method involves the use of PSP. This plate stores energy after exposure to radiation and emits light when scanned by a laser. The scanner stimulates the phosphor plate and stores a record of the number of light photons detected.

Loading of the scanners generally only requires subdued lighting as the plates are slightly sensitive to visible light. Some products are more sensitive than others. The lasers used are centered around the 600-nm band and are usually of the helium-neon variety. Scanners, the size of a bread maker, can accommodate multiple image plates at any one time. The exact number varies between manufacturers. There is a delay while the image is developed before it appears on the monitor. Up to 8 bitewing radiographs take about 90 seconds, and a panoramic image can take approximately 3 minutes to be scanned. Although the plate can store energy for a number of days, information starts to be lost within minutes after exposure, and it is advised to scan the plate quite quickly to optimize the image recovered. To fully remove the latent image the plate should be exposed to high-intensity light.

Image plates are available in exactly the same size as conventional film and come with disposable plastic barriers. They have no wires attached and are reusable for thousands of exposures, but do need careful handling to avoid surface damage. Current systems have a spatial resolution of 6–8 LP/mm.[10, 11]

Direct Sensor System

The sensor for the radiation is usually a CCD. It consists of silicon crystals arranged in a lattice and converts light energy into an electronic signal. This technology is widely used in video cameras. The sensor cannot store information and must be connected via fiber optic wires to the monitor, which can make the sensor awkward to use.

Image Acquisition

There are two ways to acquire a digital image:

Indirect Acquisition

A digital image can be produced by scanning and a transparency adaptor, or by using a charged coupled device camera instead of the flatbed scanner. This image can then be manipulated using software packages or passed on to a second party via a modem.[4]

Direct Digital Imaging

There are two systems available, one produces the image immediately on the monitor post-exposure and is therefore called direct imaging. The second has an intermediate phase, whereby the image is produced on the monitor following scanning by laser. This is known as semi-direct imaging.[4]

Conventional versus Digital Radiography

Conventional radiography is based on the interaction of X-ray photons with electrons of silver bromide crystals in the film emulsion, production of a latent image and subsequently chemical processing that transforms the latent image into a visible one.

The film-based radiograph may have a continuous density distribution, limited only by the maximum and minimum values of density (black and white). Each optical density in between the maximum and minimum is related to the amount of light that can pass through the film at a certain site. Based on the continuous density scale film-based images are called analog images.

A digital image, on the other hand, consists of a matrix of cells having a range of various gray levels on the computer monitor.

The X-ray intensity is translated into discrete values, called gray levels. The number of gray levels normally used is 256, which is equivalent to 8 bits per pixel. This range of gray levels is called contrast resolution. The contrast resolution of the human eye is usually between 50 and 100 gray levels, so the 256 gray levels in a digital image are sufficient enough for the human visual system to simulate a continuous gray scale. In digital images gray values are found only at well-defined spatial positions, called pixels (picture elements). The number of pixels per inch or centimeter defines the so-called spatial resolution. The more pixels are arranged in a matrix, the better the quality of the image that is captured. The limited number of pixels that can be grouped together restricts the digital spatial image resolution in solid-state systems. In phosphor plate systems the accuracy of laser scanner and the scattering of laser light within the phosphor layer limit the spatial resolution. The smallest detectable object depends on the spatial resolution as well as the contrast resolution.[11, 12]

Different Types of Systems

Solid-State Systems

A solid-state system includes an electronic X-ray sensor, a digital interface card and a computer with a screen monitor and software. Current systems are mostly based on personal computer (PC) technology and require a Pentium III processor (or higher), sufficient internal memory (at least 128 MB), a super video graphics array (SVGA) graphics card and a high-resolution monitor (1024 × 768 pixels).

Solid-state sensors are either a CCD or a complementary metal oxide semiconductor active pixel sensor (CMOS-APS).

A CCD is made up of arrays of X-ray sensitive or light-sensitive pixels. The size of one pixel is approximately 40 μm × 40 μm; in some CCDs a pixel is even as small as 20 μm × 20 μm. The pixels, in fact photoelectric cells, generate voltage in proportion to the amount of X-rays or light striking them. This charge is transferred (coupled) to a readout amplifier for an image display. Intraoral CCD sensors fall into two categories: Fiber optically coupled sensors and directly exposed sensors. Fiber optically coupled sensors use a scintillation (intensifying) screen coupled to a CCD. Light photons, that are the result of the interaction of X-rays with the screen, are transmitted by the fibers to the CCD. The directly exposed CCDs capture the image directly without the intermediate scintillation layer.

In contrast to CCD sensors CMOS-APS sensors use an active pixel technology. The technology provides design integration which makes the sensor less expensive to manufacture and may improve the reliability and the lifespan of the sensor. However, CMOS-APS sensors have more fixed pattern noise and a smaller active area for image acquisition.[13, 14]

The physical performance of different sensor systems: It was found that gray level values in images from solid-state systems decrease faster with increasing exposure than in images from phosphor plate systems, resulting in darker images and deterioration of the image caused by blooming effects; solid-state systems have better resolving power due to higher contrast and smaller pixel sizes than phosphor plate systems.

Phosphor Plate Systems

Storage phosphor plate systems (SPP), also called photostimulable phosphor systems (PSP), temporarily store the radiation energy of the latent X-ray image on a sensitive plate.

By stimulating the phosphor on the plate with a laser beam in a readout scanner, the energy stored on the plate is emitted as light. The intensity of the light in a given area is linearly proportional to the amount of X-ray energy that has been absorbed. The scanner measures the emitted light. The measurements are displayed on the monitor as a digital image.

The phosphor plate is able to store the X-ray energy for many days; however, it is best to read it as soon as possible. In one day an exposed imaging plate, stored in a dark environment and enclosed in a protective bag, loses half of its stored energy. After readout, flooding the plate with bright light erases any residual energy. The phosphor plates are reusable, and therefore should be enclosed in an infection control barrier before placement in the mouth of the patient. The image plates cannot be sterilized. The image size and the fact that the plates are cordless, in contrast to solid-state systems, make phosphor systems and conventional film very similar with respect to the manipulation of the plates in the mouth of the patient. The pixel size of phosphor plate systems is dependent on the focal spot of the laser beam and the accuracy of the movement of the plate or laser beam in the scanner. The pixel size of the first Soredex Digoraphosphor plate system (Soredex-Orion Co., Helsinki, Finland) (white plates) is 70 μm. The new version, the DigoraFmx system, produces an image of 628 × 466 pixels for the same active area, resulting in a pixel size of 64 μm.

The development of digital radiographic systems is still going on. Especially for solid-state systems this development is rapid. In the last two years, many manufacturers have developed high-resolution sensors that are producing 12 bit data output, giving 1024 gray levels.

Direct digital imaging was introduced into oral radiology at the end of the 1980s. Since then, a range of digital systems based on different receptors, CCD, PSP and APS, have been developed. Vuchich et al suggested the use of a more pragmatic approach to the evaluation of image quality, namely subjective evaluation of the degree to which predefined anatomical landmarks are clearly visualized. It is assumed that such an analysis combines the overall effect of those physical parameters which influence the diagnostically important aspects of image quality.

Kundel suggested a similar approach to defining image quality. He noted that the role of observer performance in the evaluation of diagnostic image quality has been underemphasized compared with the technical aspects.

A number of studies have compared the image quality of solid-state and PSP systems with conventional film. For instance Borg and Grondahl found that PSP images scored similar to film but over a larger exposure range, while solid-state images were rated lower and over a considerably smaller range. Kashima also found that PSP images of normal structures were comparable with, slightly better than, the conventional images while Lim et al. found that they were consistently scored as diagnostically acceptable throughout a wider exposure range. Knowledge of the performance of newer digital systems is scarce, and comparisons of the efficacy of the different sensor technologies almost non-existent. There are no studies comparing the performance of different digital systems under similar conditions to determine the radiation dose required to produce optimal images. The Digora, manufactured by Soredex-Orion Corporation, Helsinki, Finland, was the first digital intraoral radiographic system based on PSP technology. Its clinical imaging characteristics and performance have been described by a number of authors. The Digora system has been modified since then. The dose response of the system has been described recently. A reason for the limited information on the physical properties of the Digora may be due to the fact that there is no obvious relationship between exposure and gray levels in the final radiograph. In order to produce radiographs with an optimum dynamic range, the Digora system is calibrated to the maximum exposure that will be used clinically. Careful selection of the calibration exposure is essential since exceeding the exposure range will result in inferior image quality. The useful exposure range is between 10 and 100% of the calibration exposure. During calibration a high voltage (HV) value is set on the photomultiplier tube (PMT) of the reading device which is subsequently used in scanning the PSPs.[8–11]

When assessing the physical properties of any digital radiographic system quantitatively, the relationship between actual exposure and gray levels stored in the image file must be known. In the Digora this can be achieved if the internal HV value and the PMT and the gain set at the pre-scanning stage are known. These values cannot be read by the commercial Digora software.

The Digora system has properties that make it suitable for intraoral digital radiography. The pixel size is relatively large compared with intraoral digital systems and the pre-sampling MTF approaches zero at a Nyquist frequency which is as low as about 7 cycles/mm. On the other hand, the MTF exhibits typical properties in the frequency range up to about 3 cycles/mm where most diagnostic information is likely to be represented, and object details characterized by spatial frequencies approaching the Nyquist frequency, for example small objects or relatively distinct edges, are still perceptible in Digora radiographs. Noise in Digora radiographs is relatively low and, consequently, the DQE is relatively high compared with CCD sensors. It is an advantage that the Digora system compensates for underexposure and displays radiographs with suitable gray level range. However, the Digora system also compensates for overexposure which, from a radiation protection point of view, may be a drawback. When the calibration exposure is not exceeded, the user has no absolute indication that an overexposure has been made.[12]

The Digora system for intraoral radiography, developed by Soredex-Orion Corporation, Helsinki, Finland, is based upon PSP plates.

On exposure to an X-ray field, high-energy electrons are created in the phosphor material which produces secondary ionization events resulting in a significant number of electron hole pairs. In conventional intensifying screens such pairs immediately recombine and emit light that exposes the film. In storage phosphors less than half of the electron hole pairs recombine. Some electrons are trapped for a considerable period of time, and the number of such trapped electrons is proportional to the number of X-ray photons absorbed by the phosphor material. The distribution of stored electrons forms the latent radiograph. The electrons will be trapped until liberated by stimulation with a laser beam of a specific wavelength whereupon they travel to the holes, recombine and emit light with a wavelength of about 390 nm. The emitted light is conducted via fiber optics to a photomultiplier tube which produces a voltage proportional to the light intensity. This voltage is amplified with a gain determined during pre-scanning. The gain is chosen in order to optimize the range of voltages presented to the AD converter and therefore, the range of gray levels present in the final radiograph.[11, 12]

The Digora system is calibrated by exposing an imaging plate to a uniform exposure. The exposure is selected to represent the maximum exposure that will be used with a particular X-ray unit. During calibration, the device reads the plate and sets the high voltage on the photomultiplier tube by an iterative process. Once the calibration is complete, a new gain is selected each time a plate is exposed and read in an attempt to optimize the gray scale. The useful range within which the Digora system compensates adequately for exposure differences is between 10 and 100% of the calibration exposure. As a result of this arrangement there is no obvious relationship between gray levels in a radiograph and exposure. Consequently, a dose response function for the Digora system can only be obtained from knowledge of factors set at the calibration and the pre-scanning of each individual radiograph.

Another digital radiographic system, DenOptix, unlike CCD-based systems, uses a film-like sensor to capture and store the radiographic image. Instead of film, this system uses storage phosphor imaging plates, which are thin and flexible like film and can be produced in the same sizes as film. For this reason, the DenOptix system enables both intraoral digital radiography, and digital panoramic and cephalometric imaging, too. Storage phosphor-based imaging technology has been used in medicine for many years but the high cost of scanning devices has prevented the use of the technology in dentistry. These medical systems, which cost several hundred thousand dollars, are typically hospital based and used for chest X-rays and large format studies. The key to the DenOptix system has been the development of an affordable scanner that produces extremely high-quality images captured on imaging plates.[12, 13]

The intraoral imaging plates, which are housed in disposable sanitary barriers, are exposed just like traditional film with one important exception: With storage phosphor technology the exposure settings on the X-ray machine can be reduced. These storage plates are thin and flexible and do not have wires attached. The imaging plates can be bent to fit the palate and are indistinguishable to the patient from film. For each patient, all necessary images can be taken in sequence (just like film) and the imaging plates set aside until the session is complete.[12, 13]

The combo DenOptix digital imaging system includes accessories needed to generate digital images in all common formats from #0 intraoral through panoramic. The new ceph version will also be able to work with ceph sizes (8 ×10 inch or 18 × 24 cm) (Table 9.3) (Table 9.4).

References

1. Forrai, J. History of X-ray in dentistry. *Rev Clin Pesq Odontol* 2007;3(3):205–211.
2. VaDer Stelt, P.F. Filmless imaging. *JADA.* 2005;136:1379–1387.
3. Mulligan, T.W.; Aller, M.S.; Williams, C.A. Intraoral imaging techniques. *Atlas Canine Feline Dent Radiol.* Trenton, NJ: Veterinary Learning Systems; 1998, 27–44.
4. Brennan, J. An introduction to digital radiography in dentistry. *J Orthodont.* 2002;29:166–169.
5. van der Selt, P.F. Principles of digital imaging. *Dent Clin North Am* 2000;44:237–246.
6. Christensen, G.J. Digital radiography sensors: Which is best? *Clin Rep.* 2011 Sept;4(9):1–2.
7. Versteeg, C.H.; Sanderink, G.C.; van der Stelt, P.F. Efficacy of digital intra-oral radiography in clinical dentistry. *J Dent.* 1997;25:215–224.

8. Karjodkar, F.R. *Digital Radiography. Textbook of Dental and Maxillofacial Radiology*, 2nd ed., 339–346.
9. Brennan. An introduction to digital radiography. *J Orthodont.* 2002;29:66–69.
10. Parks, E.T.; Gali, F.; Willamson. Digital radiography: An overview. *J Contemp Dent Pract.* 2015;3(4):23–39.
11. Abesim, F.; Mirshekar, A.; Moudi, E.; Seyedmajidi, M.; Haghanifar, S.; Haghighat, N.; Bijani, A. Diagnostic accuracy of digital and conventional radiography in the detection of non-cavitated approximal dental caries. *Iran J Radiol.* 2012;9(1):17–21.
12. Williamson, G.F. *Best Practices in Intraoral Digital Radiography.* ADA CERP; 2010, 1–11.
13. Mouyen, F.; Benz, C.; Sonnabend, E.; Lodter, J.P. Presentation and physical evaluation of RadioVisioGraphy. *Oral Surg Oral Med Oral Pathol.* 1989;68:238–242.

INTRAORAL RADIOGRAPHY

Intraoral periapical (IOPA) Machine

Working of an IOPA Machine[1–14]

The components of an X-ray machine:
Head: Tube and accessories
Timers: Manual and automatic

X-Ray Tube

- Design introduced by W. C. Coolidge in 1913.
- Also called Coolidge's tube or self-rectification tube or shock-proof tube or Crookes-Hittorf's tube.
- The X-ray tube is composed of an anode and cathode.

Cathode

The cathode is the negative electrode of the tube, which serves as the source of electrons.
It consists of:

a) The filament
b) A focusing cup

Anode

- The anode is the positive electrode of the tube.
- It consists of target and a copper block.

Line Focus Principle

- Benson line focus principle: Use of an anode with target angulated such that the effective focal spot is smaller than the actual focal spot size.
- Target is inclined about 17°–20° to the central ray of the X-ray beam.
- The projection of a focal spot perpendicular to the X-ray beam is the effective focal spot.
- The actual focal spot is projected perpendicular from target.
- Actual focal spot = 1× 3 mm; effective focal spot = 1× 1 mm.

Heel Effect

- Variation in beam intensity along the longitudinal axis.
- Cathode intensity is greater than anode intensity due to absorption of the beam by the anode.
- Increases as anode angle decreases.

Power Supply

Functions:

a) Provide a low-voltage current to heat the X-ray tube filament by use of a step-down transformer.
b) Generates a high-potential difference between the anode and cathode by use of a high-voltage transformer.

The transformers and X-ray tube lie within the head of the X-ray machine, an electrically grounded metal housing.

- 60–70 KVp usually used in dental radiography

Electrical Circuit of the X-Ray Unit

- Electric current
- Direct current
- Alternating current
- Voltage

Timer

- Is built into high-voltage circuit to control the duration of X-ray exposure
- 0.1 to 3 sec is usually the time range used in dental radiography

Intraoral Radiography

- Intraoral radiographic techniques are used in routine dental practice.
- They are divided into three categories.

Periapical Radiograph – Radiographic technique of oral structure taken by placing film in the oral cavity with an X-ray source outside the oral cavity.

Indications

- Apical lesion, cyst and apical surgery
- Dental caries
- Pulp pathology
- Periodontal status
- Trauma
- Unerupted tooth
- Endodontic treatment and implant prosthesis

Technique

Angulation of Tube Head

- Horizontal angulation: 0°
- Vertical angulation depending on the tooth of interest

Bitewing Radiography

- Bitewing radiography is also called interproximal radiography.
- This includes the crowns of the maxillary and mandibular teeth and alveolar crest on the same film.

Principle

- The film is placed in the mouth parallel to the crowns of both the upper and lower teeth.
- The film is stabilized when the patient bites on the bitewing tab of the bitewing holder.
- The central ray of the X-ray beam is directed through the contacts of the teeth, using a +10 vertical angulation.

Clinical Indications

- Detection of interproximal caries.
- Monitoring the progression of dental caries.
- Detection of secondary caries below restorations.
- Evaluating periodontal conditions.
- Useful for evaluating alveolar bone crest, and changes in bone height can be assessed by comparison with the adjacent teeth.

Film Holder

- The film holder is used to stabilize the film.
- Those used for bitewing radiographs are Rinn XCP.
- Reproducible film packet holder and bite tab.

Occlusal Radiograph

- Synonym: Sandwich radiography.
- Used to examine large areas of the upper and lower jaw.
- The palate and floor may also be examined.

This is a supplementary radiographic technique that is usually used in conjunction with periapical or bitewing radiographs.

Indications

- To locate retained roots of extracted teeth.
- To locate supernumerary, unerupted or impacted (canine/third molar) teeth.
- To locate foreign bodies in either jaw.

- To locate salivary stones in Wharton's duct at the floor of mouth.
- To locate and evaluate the extent of lesions (e.g. cyst, tumor, tori, etc.) in the maxilla and mandible.
- To evaluate boundaries of the maxillary sinus.
- To evaluate fractures of maxilla and mandible (location, extent and displacement).
- To aid in the examination of a patient who is unable to open the mouth fully or in adults and children who are unable to tolerate periapical films.
- To examine the area of a cleft palate.
- To measure changes in the size and shape of the maxilla and mandible.
- As a middle view, when using the parallax method for determining the buccal/palatal position of unerupted/impacted canines.

Principle

- Film is positioned with white side facing the arch, i.e. being exposed.
- Film is placed between the occlusal surfaces of the maxillary and mandibular teeth.
- Film is stabilized when the patient bites on the surface of the film.
- For maxillary occlusal films the patient's head must be positioned so that the upper arch is parallel to the floor and mid-sagittal plane is perpendicular to the floor.
- For mandibular occlusal films the patient's head must be reclined and positioned so that the occlusal plane is perpendicular to the floor (Table 9.6).

References

1. MacDonald, D. Basics of radiological diagnosis. *Oral and Maxiillofacial Radiology: A Diagnostic Approach.* Chichester, UK: Wiley-Blackwell; 2011, 5–36.
2. Pharoah, W.S.C. *M.J. Oral Radiology: Principles and Interpretation*, 7th ed. St Louis: Mosby; 2014.
3. Langland, O.E.; Langlais, R.P. Early pioneers of oral and maxillofacial radiology. *Oral Surg Oral Med Oral Pathol Oral Radiol Endod.* 1995;80:496–511.
4. Frederiksen, N.L. Health physics. In: Pharoah, M.J.; White, S.C., editors. *Oral Radiology: Principles and Interpretation*, 4th ed. St. Louis: Mosby; 2001, 49.
5. Niemiec, B.A.; Sabitino, D.; Gilbert, T. Equipment and basic geometry of dental radiography. *J Vet Dent.* 2004;21:48–52.
6. Mulligan TW, Aller MS, Williams CA. Intraoral imaging techniques. *Atlas Canine Feline Dent Radiol.* Trenton, NJ: Veterinary Learning Systems; 1998, 27–44.
7. Button, T.M.; Moore, W.C.; Goren, A.D. Causes of excessive bite-wing exposure: Results of a survey regarding radiographic equipment in New York. *Oral Surg Oral Med Oral Pathol Oral Radiol Endod.* 1999;87(4):513–517.
8. Naitoh, M., et al. Observer agreement in the detection of proximal caries with direct digital intraoral radiography. *Oral Surg Oral Med Oral Pathol Oral Radiol Endod.* 1998;85:107–112.
9. Williamson, G.F. *Digital Radiography in Dentistry: Moving from Film-based to Digital Imaging.* American Dental Assistants Association Continuing Education Course.
10. Goren, A.D., et al. Updated quality assurance self-assessment exercise in intraoral and panoramic radiography. *Oral Surg Oral Med Oral Pathol Oral Radiol Endod.* 2000;89:369–374.
11. Stuart, C. White, Edward, W. Helop, et al. Parameters of radiologic care: An official report of the american academy of oral and maxillofacial radiology. *Oral Surg Oral Med Oral Pathol Oral Radiol Endod.* 2001;91:498–511.
12. Sikorski, P.A.; Taylor, K.W. The effectiveness of the thyroid shield in dental radiology. *Oral Surg.* 1984;58:225–236.
13. White, S.C.; Heslop, E.W., et al. Parameters of radiologic care: An official report of the American Academy of Oral and Maxillofacial Radiology. *Oral Surg Oral Med Oral Pathol Oral Radiol Endod.* 2001;91(5):498–511.
14. Razmus, T.F. The biological effects and safe use of radiation. In: Razmus, T.F.; Williamson, G.F., editors. *Current Oral and Maxillofacial Imaging.* Philadelphia: WB Saunders;1996.

EXTRAORAL RADIOGRAPHY

Digital Orthopantogram/Panoramic Radiography[1–7]

- *"Panorama"* means an unobstructed view of a region in any direction.
- Panoramic radiography is a technique for producing a single image of the facial structures that includes both maxillary and mandibular dental arches and their supporting structures.
- Also called *pantomography or rotational radiography.*
- Orthopantomography (OPG) is a curvilinear variant of conventional tomography which is based on the principle of reciprocal movement of the film and the source around the central plane called the image layer. This is called the focal trough which is a 3D curved zone located within the object whose image is seen clearly on the radiograph.
- Panoramic radiography, also called panoramic X-ray, is a two-dimensional (2D) dental X-ray examination that captures the entire mouth in a single image, including the teeth, upper and lower jaws, surrounding structure and tissue that cannot be seen with a simple oral exam, such as permanent teeth, pathological cyst and fractured jaws.

Cephalogram AP/Lateral View

A cephalogram, also called cephalometric, is an X-ray image of the structures of the head. It can also mean a radiograph of the head, including the mandible, in full lateral view, that is used for making cranial measurements.

Features

- Fully automatic mode operation.
- Aesthetic look and compact design.
- Soft press key (soft press control pad) for simple and faster operations.
- Three positioning laser beams to ensure precise position.
- Head auxiliary fixing device for keeping patient's head stable.
- Dual speed vertical movement for adjusting scan frame smoothly.
- Convex positioning mirror allowing operator to position the patient's face accurately and quickly.
- Four modes: PAN, HALF PAN L, HALF PAN R, TJM (TJM 1 and TJM 2).
- Ceph with different patient size – small, medium, large.
- Low investment, lower running cost, more profits.
- Double stage voltage regulation.
- Automatic exposure termination at end of travel.
- Test mode without exposure.
- Automatic audible and visible error alarm.
- No installation hazards.
- Quick after-sales service with ready availability of spares.
- 0.4 mm focus dedicated OPG X-ray tube.
- Full wave rectification.
- Microcontroller-based system.
- Control panel with LCD display and soft keypad.
- Anatomical selection for different ages/modes.
- Remote control operations.

The Principal Advantages of Panoramic Images/OPGs

- Low patient radiation dose
- Convenience of examination for the patient
- Ability to be used in patients who are restricted in opening their mouth
- Short time required for producing the image
- Useful visual aid in patient education and case presentation

Principles

- *Tomo* (Greek): Section.
- *Tomography* is a radiographic technique that allows radiographing in one plane of an object while blurring or eliminating images of structures in other planes.
- Focal plane or focal trough.
- Requires controlled and accurate movement of the X-ray tube head and film.

Procedure

- Ask the patient to remove jewelry, eyeglasses and any metal objects that may obscure the images.
- The patient will be asked to stand with their face resting on a small shelf and to bite gently on a sterile mouth piece to steady their head.
- It is important that the patient stays very still while the X-ray is taken.

Indications

1) When intraoral radiography is not possible due to gagging or trismus.
2) When large anatomic coverage is required, e.g. cysts, benign or malignant tumors, osteomyelitis, fibro-osseous lesions, multiple lesions, generalized periodontitis.
3) To study growth and development and its disorders.
4) To detect and study extent and nature of oral and maxillofacial trauma.
5) Pre-operative, intra-operative and post-operative assessment in implantology.
6) To study Temporomandibular joint (TMJ) and its disorders.
7) To study maxillary sinus.
8) To detect and assess involvement of jaws by metastatic lesions.
9) As a part of FMRS.

Exposure Parameters

- Tube voltage – 60–100 kVp
- Tube current – 8–12 mA
- Exposure time – 14–20 sec
- Target to image receptor – 14 inches
- Size – 6 × 12 or 6 × 14 inches
- Type of film – screen

Advantages

- The entire jaws (maxilla and mandible) can be studied in one film.
- It is a relatively easy procedure.
- Minimum patient co-operation is required.

- The entire procedure requires less than five minutes as compared to full mouth radiographic interpretation.
- Better for patient education.
- Radiation dose is less as compared to full mouth radiographic interpretation.

Disadvantages

- Image quality is inferior as compared to IOPA view because of magnification, geometric distortion and unsharpness.
- *Overlapping*: Panoramic units have a tendency to produce overlapping images especially in the premolar area.
- *Image quality*:
  - Inadequate sharpness and detail due to rotational movement.
  - Other factors that tend to degrade the image as compared with intraoral films are:
    - (a) External placement of film with resultant increased object-film distance
    - (b) Use of intensifying screen
    - (c) Faster film
- *Focal trough*: Only structures that lie within the focal trough are visualized clearly.
- Exposure to radiation of other structures (vertebral column).
- High initial cost.

References

1. Langland, A.N.D., Langlais, R.P.; Morris, C. R. *Principles and Practice of Panoramic Radiology*. 1st ed., ch. 1. Philadelphia: W. B. Saunders; 1982.
2. Mcdavid, W. D., Welander, U.; Tronje, G. Preliminary evaluation of a digital system for rotational panoramic radiography. *Oral Surg. Oral Med. Oral Pathol.* 73 (1992), 623.
3. Paatero, Y. V. Radiography of the temporo-mandibular joint. A new method. *Ann. Chir. Gynaecol. Fenn.* 42 (19S3), 259.
4. Welander, U. Layer formation in narrow beam rotation radiography. *Acta Radiol.* 16 (1975), 529.
5. Welander, U.; Mcdavid, W. D.; Tronje, G.; Morris C. R. A method of increasing the anterior layer thickness in rotational panoramic radiography. *Dentomaxillofac. Radiol.* 12 (1983), 133. 33.
6. Welander U., Tronje G. & Mcdavid W. D. Layer thickness in rotational panoramic radiography. Some specific aspects. *Dentomaxillofac. Radiol.* 18 (1989), 119.
7. Molander B. Molander B. Panoramic radiography in dental diagnostics. *Swed Dent J* 1996;119:1–26.

GENERAL RADIOGRAPHY[1–10]

Introduction

General radiographic imaging dates to the discovery of X-rays by Conrad Roentgen in 1895. Radiographic imaging includes all plain film radiographic imaging of the body. Radiographic imaging is also used in veterinary and industrial radiography.

Important Principles

Radiographic imaging involves the complex combination of various types of specialized equipment and processes. The process used for chest radiography is not satisfactory for mammographic imaging, nor is it suitable for radiographs of the pelvis and abdomen. Dental radiography is included in this area of imaging and has specialized equipment for general dental imaging, cephalometric applications and panoramic imaging.

Image quality is dependent upon the X-ray tube voltage, tube current and exposure time, size of the X-ray tube focal spot, focal spot to image distance and scatter reducing grids (used to increase image contrast). Although patient dose is important, image quality is the essential element in general radiographic imaging. An X-ray, or general radiology, is a painless, non-invasive procedure that creates images of a patient's internal organs or bones to aid in diagnosis and treatment. It's the oldest and most commonly used type of medical imaging.

X-ray exams help doctors identify and treat a broad range of conditions, including:

- Broken bones
- Arthritis
- Joint injuries
- Pneumonia

Digital X-ray provides several important benefits to both patients and physicians:

- Faster than analog X-ray
- Reduces repeat exposures
- Maximizes image quality
- Can highlight or magnify areas of interest
- Can electronically view images and reports, expediting patient care

Extraoral radiographs (outside the mouth) are taken when large areas of the skull or jaw must be examined or when patients are unable to open their mouths for film placement.

- Extraoral radiographs are very useful for evaluating large areas of the skull and jaws but are not adequate for the detection of subtle changes such as the early stages of dental caries or periodontal disease.
- There are many types of extraoral radiographs. Some types are used to view the entire skull, whereas other types focus on the maxilla and mandible.

Definitions of Some Extraoral Landmarks Used for Patient Positioning

- *The median plane of the head* (*mid-sagittal plane*) line that is coincident with the sagittal suture between the upper margins of the parietal bones, running from the top of the skull backwards.
- *The infraorbital line*: This line runs across the face from one infraorbital margin to the other.
- *The orbitomeatal line* (*canthomeatal line*): This is an imaginary line from the outer canthus of the eye to the tragus of the ear.

Canthomeatal line is known as the radiological base line and joins the upper edge of the auditory meatus with the outer canthus of the eye.

Most Commonly Used Views for Maxillofacial Imaging

A. *Radiography of Sinuses*
  1. Posteroanterior projection (also known as occipitofrontal projection of nasal sinuses)
       There are two methods for obtaining this projection.
       a. Posterior anterior (*Granger projection*)
       b. Modified method, inclined posterior anterior (*Caldwell projection*)
  2. Standard occipitomental (OM) projection (0° OM)
  3. Modified method (30° occipitomental projection)

    4. Bregma Menton
    5. Posteroanterior (PA) Waters
B. **Radiography of the Mandible**
    1. PA mandible
    2. Rotated PA mandible
    3. Lateral oblique
      – Anterior body of mandible
      – Posterior body of mandible
      – Ramus of mandible
C. **Radiography of Base of the Skull**
    Submento vertex projection
D. **Radiography of the Zygomatic Arches**
    Jug handle view (a modification of submento vertex view)
E. **Radiography of the Temporomandibular Joint**
    1. Transcranial projection
    2. Transpharyngeal projection
    3. Transorbital projection
    4. Reverse Towne's projection
    5. Dental panoramic tomograph (including specific TMJ field limitation techniques)
    6. Tomography, both linear and spiral
F. **Radiography of the Skull**
    1. Lateral cephalogram
    2. True lateral
    3. PA cephalogram
    4. PA skull
    5. Towne's projection

Radiography of the Paranasal Sinuses

- This is used to study the relationship of the sinuses to each other and to the surrounding structures.

Posteroanterior Projection (Also Known as the Occipitofrontal Projection of the Nasal Sinuses)

There are two methods for obtaining this projection:
    A. Posteroanterior (Granger) projection
    B. Modified method, inclined posteroanterior (Caldwell) projection

Radiography of the Maxillary Sinuses

Standard Occipitomental Projection (0° OM)

This projection shows the facial skeleton and maxillary antra, and avoids superimposition of the dense bones of the base of the skull.

Indications

- For investigating maxillary antrum

- Detecting the following middle third facial fractures (*using Campbell lines*):
  - LeFort I
  - Le Fort II
  - Le Fort III
  - Zygomatic complex
  - Naso-ethmoidal complex
  - Orbital blow-out
  - Coronoid process fractures
  - Investigation of the frontal and ethmoidal sinuses
  - Investigation of the sphenoidal sinus (projection needs to be taken with the patient's mouth open)
- Examining the 0° OM using an approach based broadly on that suggested originally by McGrigor and Campbell (1950), often referred to as Campbell's lines

Modified Method (30° Occipitomental Projection)

This method also shows the facial skeleton, but from a different angle from the 0° OM, enabling certain bony displacements to be detected.

Main Indications

The main clinical indications include:

- Detecting the following middle third of facial fractures:
  - LeFortI
  - Le Fort II
  - Le Fort III
- Coronoid process fractures

PA Waters

Structures Seen

- Maxillary sinus, frontal and ethmoidal sinuses.
- The sphenoidal sinuses can be seen if the patient is asked to open his mouth, whereby the sphenoidal sinuses are projected on the palate.

The orbit, frontozygomatic suture, nasal cavity, coronoid process of the mandible and the zygomatic arch are also seen.

Angulation

The central ray passes through a point 2 inches above external occipital protuberances.

Tube film distance (TFD) – 3 feet
kVp – 80
mAS – 15

Radiography of the Mandible

PA Mandible

- A posteroanterior projection of the mandibular body and the ramus.
- The symphysis region is not well seen because of the superimposition of the spine.

Indications

- Used to study fractures of the posterior third of the body of the mandible, angles, rami and lower condylar neck
- Medio-lateral expansion of the posterior third of the body or rami in case of tumor or cystic lesions, maxillofacial deformities and mandibular hypoplasia and hyperplasia

Rotated PA Mandible

This is used to show the tissues of one side of the face and used to investigate the parotid gland and the ramus of the mandible.

Indications

- Stones/calculi in the parotid glands.
- Lesions such as cysts or tumors in the ramus to note any medio-lateral expansion.
- Submasseteric infection – to note new bone formation.

Anterior Body of the Mandible

- In anterior body of the mandible, position of the teeth is seen.

Indications

- To evaluate impacted teeth
- Fractures
- Lesions located in the anterior portion of the mandible

Posterior Body of the Mandible

Structures Seen

- In posterior body of the mandible, position of the teeth is seen. Also shows angle and ramus of the mandible
- same area, ramus of the mandible, angle of the
- mandible

Indications

- To evaluate impacted teeth
- Fractures
- Lesions located in the posterior border of the mandible

Ramus of Mandible

Structures Seen

- A view of the ramus from the angle of the mandible to the condyles

Indications

- To evaluate impacted third molars
- Large lesions
- Fractures that extend into the ramus of the mandible

Radiography of the Base of the Skull

Submento Vertex Projection

Structures Seen

- The base of the skull sphenoidal sinuses facial skeleton from below.

Indications

- Destructive/expansive lesions affecting the palate, pterygoid region or base of the skull
- Investigation of the sphenoidal sinus
- Assessment of the thickness (medio-lateral) of the posterior part of the mandible before osteotomy
- Fracture of the zygomatic arches – to show these thin bones the Sub Mento Vertex (SMV) is taken with reduced exposure factors

Angulations
The central ray passes through a point 1.5 inches below the symphysis menti through the Median Sagittal Plane (MSP).

TFD – 3 feet
kVp – 80
mAS – 15

Radiography of the Zygomatic Arches

Jug Handle View (a Modification of the Submentovertex View)

Structures Seen

- A symmetrical axial view of the zygomatic arches.

Radiography of the Temporomandibular Joints

Transcranial

Structures Seen

- Lateral aspect of glenoid fossa:
- Articular eminence
- Joint space
- Condylar head

Indications

- TMJ pain dysfunction syndrome.
- Internal derangements of the joint producing pain, clicking and limitation in opening.
- To investigate the size and position of the disc.
- This can only be inferred indirectly from the relative positions of the bony elements of the joints.
- To investigate the range of movement in the joints.

Diagnostic Information
Open Mouth

- The range and type of movement of the condyle
- A comparison of the degree of movement on both sides

Closed Mouth

- The size of the *joint space*
- The position of the head of the condyle within the fossa
- The shape and condition of the glenoid fossa and articular eminence (on the lateral aspect only)
- The shape of the head of the condyle and the condition of the articular surface (on the lateral aspect only)
- A comparison of both sides

Transpharyngeal (Infracranial or McQueen Dell Technique)

Structures Seen

- Lateral view of condylar head and neck:
- Articular surface

Indications

- TMJ pain dysfunction syndrome
- To investigate the presence of joint disease, particularly osteoarthritis and rheumatoid arthritis
- To investigate pathological conditions affecting the condylar head, including cysts or tumors
- Fractures of the neck and head of the condyle

Transorbital (Zimmer Projection)

- Conventional frontal TM joint projection.

Structures Seen

- The anterior view of the temporomandibular joint.
- Medial displacement of fractured condyle.
- Fractures of neck of condyle are clearly seen in this view.

Reverse Towne's

Structures Seen
Posterior view of both condylar heads and necks

Indications

- To investigate the articular surface of the condyles and disease within the joint
- Fractures of the condylar heads and necks
- Condylar hypo/hyperplasia

Skull Projection

Lateral Cephalogram

Indications

- Orthodontics
- Initial diagnosis – confirmation of the underlying skeletal and/or soft tissue abnormalities
- Treatment planning
- Monitoring treatment progress
- Appraisal of treatment results, e.g. one or two months before the completion of active treatment to ensure that treatment targets have been met and to allow planning of retention
- Orthognathic surgery
- Pre-operative evaluation of skeletal and soft tissue patterns
- To assist in treatment planning
- Post-operative appraisal of the results of surgery and long-term follow-up studies

True Lateral

Structures Seen

- Shows the skull vault and facial skeleton from the lateral aspect

Indications

- Fractures of the cranium and the cranial base
- Middle third facial fractures, to show possible downward and backward displacement of the maxillae
- Investigation of the frontal, sphenoidal and maxillary sinuses

- Conditions affecting the skull vault, particularly:
  - Paget's disease
  - Multiple myeloma
  - Hyperparathyroidism
- Conditions affecting the sella turcica, such as:
  - Tumor of the pituitary gland in acromegaly

PA Cephalogram

This projection is identical to the PA view of the jaws, except that it is standardized and reproducible. This makes it suitable for the assessment of facial asymmetries and for pre-operative and post-operative comparisons in orthognathic surgery involving the mandible.

Indications

- Used for the assessment of facial asymmetries
- Pre-operative and post-operative comparisons in orthognathic surgeries involving the mandible

PA Skull

- Structures seen in the skull vault, primarily the frontal bones and the jaws

Indications

- Fractures of the skull vault
- Investigation of the frontal sinuses
- Conditions affecting the cranium, particularly:
  - Paget's disease
  - Multiple myeloma
  - Hyperparathyroidism
- Intracranial calcification

Towne's Projection

Structures Seen

- Occipital area of the skull
- Neck of the condylar process

References

1. Oldnall Tameside, N.J. *Radiography of the Skull.* NJO / SKULL ISO PENDO TECHNIQUE; 1998. doc 1996:1-35.
2. Torsten, B.; Reif, M. *Pocket Atlas of Radiographic Positioning.* Thieme; 2009, 1–392.
3. Koong, B. The basic principles of radiological interpretation *Aust Dent J.* 2012;57(1) Supplement 1:33–139.
4. Bernaerts, A.; Vanhoenacker, F.M.; Geenen, L.; Quisquater, G.; Parizel, P.M.; Bernaerts, A., et al. Conventional dental radiology: What the general radiologist needs to know. *JBR-BTR.* 2006;89(1):23–32.
5. MacDonald, D. Basics of radiological diagnosis. In *Oral and Maxiillofacial Radiology: A Diagnostic Approach.* Chichester, UK: Wiley-Blackwell; 2011: 5–36.

6. Pharoah, W.S.C. *M.J. Oral Radiology: Principles and Interpretation*. 7th ed. St Louis: Mosby; 2014.
7. Timmenga, N.; Stegenga, B.; Raghoebar, G.; van Hoogstraten, J.; van Weissenbruch, R.; Vissink, A.; Timmenga, N., et al. The value of Waters' projection for assessing maxillary sinus inflammatory disease. *Oral Surg Oral Med Oral Pathol Oral Radiol Endod*. 2002;93(1):103–109.
8. De Sutter, A.; Spee, R.; Peersman, W.; De Meyere, M.; Van Cauwenberge, P.; Verstraete, K.; De Maeseneer, J.; De Sutter, A., et al. Study on the reproducibility of the Waters' views of the maxillary sinuses. *Rhinology*. 2005;43(1):55–60.
9. Young, J.; Young, J. The value of a Waters' projection. *Oral Surg Oral Med Oral Pathol Oral Radiol Endod*. 2003 May;95(5):512–513.
10. Uysal, T.; Malkoc, S. Submentovertex cephalometric norms in Turkish adults. *Am J Orthodont Dentofac Orthoped*. 2005;128(6):724–730.

COMPUTED TOMOGRAPHY

The term "computed" in computed tomography (CT) refers to calculated or reconstructed, and the term "tomography" is a composite word comprising the term "tomo" (which means to "cut" or "section" in Greek) and "graphy" (which means "to describe" in Greek).[1] CT uses X-rays for the production of images. It was invented in 1972 by British engineer Godfrey N. Hounsfield using image reconstruction mathematics developed by Allan M. Cormack, an American physicist, in the early 1960s. Hounsfield jointly shared the Nobel Prize in Physiology and Medicine with Allan M. Cormack for the development of CT in 1979.[1, 2] The projection data is acquired in approximately 5 minutes, and the tomographic image reconstructed in approximately 20 minutes.[3] The first commercially available X-ray CT scanner was built and designed by the Electric and Musical Industries (EMI) Company and was developed in collaboration with the UK Department of Health and London's Atkinson Morley Hospital.[4, 5] In an EMI CT scanner, translate-rotate geometry was used to create EMI CT images, but, within a couple of years, there were eight manufacturers using different scanning methods to image the head and body.[5]

Components of a CT Scanner

A basic CT scanner generally consists of a gantry, a patient table, a control console and a computer. The gantry contains the X-ray source, X-ray detectors and the data-acquisition system (DAS). The X-ray source and detector are situated on opposite ends of the patient, mounted on a rotational gantry that spins the imaging chain at very high speeds.[6, 7]

X-Ray System

The X-ray system consists of the X-ray source, detectors and a DAS.

- X-Ray Source
  Except for the fifth-generation system, all CT scanners use bremsstrahlung X-ray tubes as the source of radiation. These tubes produce X-rays by accelerating a beam of electrons onto a target anode. Most systems have two possible focal spot sizes, approximately 0.5×1.5 mm and 1.0×2.5 mm. A collimator assembly is used to control the width of the beam between 1.0 and 10 mm, which in turn controls the slice thickness. Machine is operated at 120–140 kilovolts peak (kVp) and 200–800 milliamperes (mA). Most of the power used by the tubes results in heating of the anode; thus, a heat exchanger on the rotating gantry is used to cool the tube.[2, 3]

- X-Ray Detectors

  Detectors used in CT scanners must (1) have a high overall effectiveness to minimize the patient radiation dose, (2) have stability with time and (3) be insensitive to temperature changes within the gantry. Three factors that contribute to the detector efficiency are geometric efficiency, quantum (also called *capture*) efficiency and conversion efficiency. *Geometric efficiency* is the area of the detectors sensitive to radiation as a fraction of total area exposed. *Quantum or capture efficiency* is the fraction of incident X-rays that are absorbed on the detector and contribute to the measured signal. *Conversion efficiency* is the ability to accurately convert the absorbed signal into an electrical signal. *Overall efficiency* is the product of the three that ranges between 0.45 and 0.85. A value less than 1 indicates a non-ideal detector system and requires an increase in the patient radiation dose to maintain the image quality.[3, 5, 6]

Modern scanners use either of the two types of detectors, namely, solid-state detectors or gas-filled detectors.[2, 3, 5, 7]

Solid-state detectors: These consist of an array of scintillating crystals and photodiodes. Scintillators are either cadmium tungstate (CdWO4) or a ceramic material made of rare earth oxides. These detectors have very high quantum and conversion efficiencies and a large dynamic range.

Gas ionization detectors: These consist of an array of chambers which contain compressed gas (usually xenon at 30 atm pressure). These detectors have high stability and a large dynamic range but, in general, they have lower quantum efficiency when compared to that of solid-state detectors.

- Data-Acquisition System

  It converts the electrical signal produced by the detector to a digital value for the computer.[3] The basic requirements of data acquisition include that one tomographic image is reconstructed from X-ray projection data of the object obtained at different angles for 360° (or 180°) rotations and during the scan, object must be included in every projection data set, and the object should be still.[1, 2]

Data-Acquisition Geometries

Projection data is obtained based on the configuration, scanning motions and detector arrangement.[1, 3] The evolution of these geometries is termed "generations."[3]

First Generation: Parallel-Beam Geometry
Parallel beam geometry is the simplest one and technically it's easy to understand the principles of CT. Multiple measurements of data are obtained using a single highly collimated X-ray pencil beam and detector providing excellent rejection of the scattered radiation in the patient, but the complex scanning motion results in long scan times. This was used by Hounsfield in his original experiments (Hounsfield, 1980) but is not in use in modern scanners.

Second Generation: Fan Beam, Multiple Detectors
These scanners use a fan beam of X-rays and a linear detector array due to which scan times are reduced to approximately 30 s. But the reconstruction algorithms are slightly more complicated than those of first-generation algorithms as they need to handle fan-beam projection data.

Third Generation: Fan Beam, Rotating Detectors
These were introduced in 1976; in these detectors a fan beam of X-rays is rotated 360 degrees around the isocenter.

Fourth Generation: Fan Beam, Fixed Detectors
In a fourth-generation scanner, the X-ray source and fan beam rotate about the isocenter, while the detector array remains stationary consisting of 600 to 4800 independent detectors in a circle which completely surrounds the patient. Scan times are similar to those of third-generation scanners.

Fifth Generation: Scanning Electron Beam

These are unique in that the X-ray source becomes an integral part of the system design. The detector array remains stationary, while a high-energy electron beam is electronically swept along a semicircular tungsten strip anode. Projection data can be obtained in approximately 50 ms, which is fast enough to image the beating heart without any significant motion artifacts.

Image Reconstruction

Image reconstruction is a mathematical calculation which calculates the 2D cross-sectional attenuation distribution function from a series of one-dimensional projections obtained as the line integrals at different angles around the 3D object.[1] Hounsfield divided a slice into a matrix of 3D rectangular boxes, called voxels.[2, 8] Each square of the matrix is called a pixel, and images typically consist of 512×512 or 1024×1024 pixels. The sizes of the pixels in the image matrix need not be necessarily the same as those in the reconstruction matrix but rather can be interpolated from the reconstruction matrix to meet the requirements of the computer.[2, 3, 8] To reconstruct an image, the row of voxels through which a particular ray passes during data collection is considered and the linear attenuation coefficients of each box are computed simultaneously. But this method of image reconstruction is not practical for 512^2 or 1024^2 pixels, so filtered back projection algorithms are used involving Fourier transformations. A modification of these methods called Feldkamp reconstruction is used in multidetector helical CT (MDCT).[2, 8]

CT Image[2, 3, 8]

Each pixel in a CT image is given a CT number which represents its tissue density. These CT numbers are also called Hounsfield units (HU) and range from −1000 to +1000.

Advantages[1, 2, 9]

1. High-contrast resolution differentiates tissues with even 1% difference in the density.
2. Multiple images in all three planes – axial, coronal and sagittal.
3. Prevents superimposition of structures outside the area of interest.

Limitations[9]

1. Metallic objects create artifacts across the image.
2. Expensive.
3. Since the pixels represent discrete subdivisions, blurring is greater compared to conventional radiographs.

Advancements

Advances in CT can be categorized into helical/spiral data acquisition, multi-slice CT, wide-cone CT, DSCT and spectral CT.[9, 10]

Spiral or Helical CT

In 1990, CT scanners with continuous rotation of the gantry using slip-ring technology and continuous transport of the patient during data acquisition were introduced. For the first time, volume data became available where whole body organs could be covered in a single-breath-hold without missing anatomical details and overlapping images could be reconstructed at arbitrary positions. This was a big development compared to previous step-and-shoot data-acquisition techniques that provided only a few slices for the organ of interest. Volume data has become the very basis for applications such as CT angiography, which has revolutionized the assessment of vascular disease. The ability to acquire volume data also led the way for the use of 3D image processing techniques such as multiplanar reformations, maximum intensity projections, surface shaded displays and volume rendering techniques (VRT) in CT.[10]

Multi-Slice CT

This is similar to spiral or helical CT except there is more than one detector ring. It has increased speed of volume coverage allowing large volumes to be scanned in minimal time. A two-row scanner was introduced in 1992 (Elscint CT Twin); multi-slice scanners that significantly impacted clinical practice were introduced in 1998. For MDCT, reconstruction algorithms are very complex as compared to those of single-slice CT.[9, 10]

Wide-Cone CT

The introduction of multi-slice CT enabled organ coverage with an isotropic spatial resolution. For temporally sensitive clinical applications, such as coronary CT angiography (CCTA), the ability to capture the whole organ in a single rotation is important. These technical challenges have been overcome by wide-cone CT systems.[10]

Cone Beam CT

This uses a round or rectangular cone-shaped X-ray sensor that scans 360° around a patient's head.[1, 2, 9, 10]

SPECT/CT and PET/CT

Single photon emission CT (SPECT/CT) and positron emission CT (PET/CT) use nuclear medicine with CT imaging. These techniques have the advantage of functional assessment along with anatomical assessment.[2, 10]

The understanding of CT will provide successful and precise patient care in the fields of diagnostics and radiotherapy, and lead to the improvement of image quality and optimization of the exposed doses.

References

1. Jung, H. Basic physical principles and clinical applications of computed tomography. *Prog Med Phys.* 2021 Mar;32(1):1–17.
2. White, S.C.; Pharoah, M.J. *Oral Radiology: Principles and Interpretation*, 6th ed, 2011; 207–210.
3. Cunningham, I.A.; Judy, P.F. *Computed Tomography.* CRC Press Release LLC; 2000.
4. Webb, S. A brief history of tomography and CT. *RPI: Radiography.* 1995:429–430, Volume 273.
5. Rubin, G.D. Computed tomography: Revolutionizing the practice of medicine for 40 years. *Radiology.* 2014 Nov;273(2 Suppl):S45–S74. radiology.rsna.org.
6. Ginat, D.T.; Gupta, R. Advances in computed tomography imaging technology. *Annu Rev Biomed Eng.* 2014;16:431–453.
7. Pelc, N.J. Recent and future directions in CT imaging. *Ann Biomed Eng.* 2014 Feb; 42(2):260–268.
8. Goldman, L.W. Principles of CT and CT technology. *J Nucl Med Technol.* 2007;35:115–128.
9. Karjodkar, F.R. *Textbook of Dental and Maxillofacial Radiology*, 2nd ed., 2009, 270, 283, 284.
10. Hsieha, J.; Flohr, T. Computed tomography recent history and future perspectives. *J Med Imag.* 2021; 8(5):1–24.

CONE BEAM COMPUTED TOMOGRAPHY

Cone beam computed tomography (CBCT) is a three-dimensional imaging technology that was developed for angiography in 1982 and later used in maxillofacial imaging.[1, 2] It is used to overcome the limitations of conventional radiographic techniques.[1]

The term "cone beam" refers to the conical shape of the beam which scans the patient in a circular path around the vertical axis of the head, in contrast to the fan-shaped beam and more complex scanning movement of multidetector computed tomography (MDCT) used in medical imaging.[3, 4] Two factors contributed to the rapid application of CBCT technology in dentistry, the first of which was the availability of improved, fast and cost-effective computer technology and the second was the ability to develop software programs that can be used for multiple dental imaging applications for CBCT with broad diagnostic capability.[3, 5]

History of CBCT

Though the first clinical CBCT scanner was made for angiographic application in 1982, the availability of commercial CBCT scanners was delayed for more than a decade.[6] In 1998, CBCT was introduced for dentoalveolar imaging.[4] In one of the very first commercially available cone beam machines, the NewTom 9000 (QR srl, Verona, Italy), had a large unit that scanned the patient in a supine position. It was subsequently followed by the NewTom 3G. Eventually, smaller, sit-down chair units and stand-up units were developed. These smaller units with good quality images more readily fit into dental office space.[3, 6]

Principles of CBCT

A CBCT machine uses a cone-shaped beam and a reciprocating solid-state flat-panel detector that rotates once around the patient, 180–360 degrees, covering the defined anatomical volume rather than slice-by-slice imaging as seen with conventional CT.[5]

Image Acquisition

As with any radiographic imaging system, CBCT also requires X-ray production, X-ray attenuation by an object, signal detection, image processing and image display. Multiple exposures referred to as a basis image are taken at fixed intervals/angles of the rotation during a rotational scan.[2, 3, 6] Once the rotation is finished, the complete set of basis images is referred to as the "projection data."[2, 3] The total number of basis images ranges from 100 to 600 per scan. The greater the number of basis images, the longer the scan time, the greater the radiation dose and the better the quality of the constructed images.[3]

X-Ray Generation

- X-Ray Generator

In CBCT, exposure time is dependent on the number of basis images and the degree of spatial resolution requested in the voxel size. The smaller the voxel size and the greater the number of basis images, the longer is the exposure, leading to continuous radiation exposure to the patient.[2, 3] Hence, exposure is pulsed at intervals and the X-ray tube does not generate X-rays for the entire rotational cycle thereby reducing patient exposure during the time interval that the detector is not ready to receive X-rays. These intervals also reduce heat buildup during an exposure cycle.[2, 3, 5, 6] The time for the acquirement of basis images is known as the frame rate.[3] A higher frame rate increases the signal-to-noise ratio resulting in images with less noise. Further, it reduces metallic artifacts. But the disadvantage is that the higher the frame rate, the longer the scan time and hence patient dose.[2]

The "as low as reasonably achievable" (ALARA) principle should be followed. As per the International Commission on Radiation Protection, the effective dose ranges from 52 to 1025 microsieverts for CBCT.[5]

• Scan Volume or Field of View (FOV)

The size of the scanned object volume is called the field of view (FOV) or scan volume. The FOV for CBCT units with a flat-panel detector is cylindrical or spherical in the middle of the scanner between the detector and the X-ray source. The FOV depends on the size and shape of the detector, beam projection geometry and collimation of the beam.[2, 3] The size of the FOV largely influenced the evolution of the CBCT scanner. Early CBCT units were restricted to a single-size FOV that was either large or small, which limited its use. As a general rule, the larger the FOV, the greater is the cost of the scanner.[3]

Image Detectors

Based on the type of detector CBCT units can be divided into image-intensifier tube/charge-coupled device combinations or amorphous silicone flat-panel imagers.[2, 3] Early CBCT units were mostly constructed with large, heavy image-intensifier detectors. Later CBCT scanners have nearly all transitioned to the smaller, flat-panel linear array detectors.[3]

The image-intensifier detectors are larger, sensitive and susceptible to distortion from magnetic fields; also images displayed from these detectors demonstrate greater distortion of the grid dimensions while moving away from the center of the detector which reduces the measurement accuracy of the reconstructed images. On the other hand, being smaller and less bulky, the flat panels have minimal distortion at the periphery of an image display; hence, these units are considered to produce better data sets.[3, 6]

Another important factor of the image detector is the bit depth, an exponential expressing the total number of gray shades the detector is able to distinguish. If a 14-bit detector (i.e. 2^{14}) is used it can display 16,384 shades of gray. The bit depth of commercially available CBCT units ranges between 12 and 16 bits indicating the wide range of contrast distinguishing capability.[2, 3, 6]

Image Reconstruction

Once the basis images are obtained, they have to be processed to create a volumetric data set called primary reconstruction.[2] Primary image reconstruction of the object is displayed in the three anatomic planes of imaging: The axial, sagittal and coronal planes referred to typically as the multiplane or multiplanar images.[3, 5] This volumetric data set can also be used to construct multiple secondary reconstructions. Reconstruction occurs in two stages. Acquisition stage: Once the multiplanar (MPR) images are acquired these are corrected by inherent pixel imperfections and uneven exposure. Reconstruction stage: Corrected images are then converted to sinogram, a composite image of a row of pixels from each projection. This process is referred to as random transformation which is then reconstructed with a filtered-back-projection algorithm called a Feldkamp algorithm.[2, 5]

Image Artifacts
An artifact is a distortion or error in the image that is not related to the subject being studied. This affects the CBCT image quality and limits adequate visualization of the structures in the dento-alveolar region.[2, 5–7]

Noise
The irradiation of large volumes during CBCT scanning resulting in heavy interactions with tissues produces scattered radiation, which in turn leads to nonlinear attenuation by the detectors. This additional detection of X-rays is called noise and contributes to image distortion.[5, 7]

Scatter and Beam-Hardening Artifact
Scatter and beam-hardening artifacts occur where image reconstructions of a data set are needed for review of the data volume. Dense metal structures in the FOV present metal artifacts on CBCT reconstructions. These artifacts present as light or dark streaks, or as a dark periphery next to metallic

borders. Scatter artifacts are seen as radiopaque lines and patterns of metallic density that "scatter" on image reconstructions. The main type of beam hardening is the dark streaks or dark bands that show up in the image reconstructions often simulating disease such as recurrent caries or fractures in endodontically treated teeth. The light streaks often overlap with regular anatomy and significantly degrade image quality.[2, 3, 5, 7]

Aliasing Artifacts

Undersampling and divergence of the cone beam cause aliasing. Undersampling occurs when too few basis images are provided for the image reconstruction leading to misregistration, sharp edges and noisier images. Aliasing appears as fine striations in the image called moire patterns.

Ring Artifacts

These are seen as concentric rings centered on the location of the axis of rotation. They are most prominent when homogeneous media are imaged. They result from imperfections in scanner detection or poor calibration.[2, 7]

Motion Artifacts – Misalignment Artifacts

These two types of errors are closely related in that a misalignment of any of the three components, i.e. source, object and detector, causes inconsistencies in the back projection process. Motion artifacts present as double contours. Proper fixation of the patient's head during the scan process will help to limit the movement of the patient.[2, 3, 7] Misalignment also occurs for minute deviations, e.g. deviations from a truly planar circular source and detector trajectory.[7]

Applications of CBCT in Dentistry

CBCT produces 3D images that are useful for many oral and maxillofacial situations which can guide in the diagnosis and assessment of disease severity, planning and delivery of treatment and follow-up.[2, 4, 5]

Advantages[1, 2, 5]

- Lower radiation than traditional CT scan
- Aids in the diagnostics, treatment plan and procedure
- High-speed scanning (<30 seconds)
- Submillimeter resolution
- Can analyze position of surrounding structures (sinuses, roots and nerves)
- Cost effective
- Safe for patients of all ages

Disadvantages[1, 2, 5]

- Poor soft tissue contrast
- Noise
- Streaking and motion artifacts are possible

CBCT produces accurate, submillimeter resolution images in a short scan time and at low cost. It overcomes the limitations of 2D imaging and incorporates advantages of 3D imaging.

References

1. Dr. Fathima, S. Dr. Manikandan. Cbct in dentistry: An overview. *Eur J Mol Clin Med.* 2020;7(5):1403–8.
2. White, S.C.; Pharoah, M.J. *Oral Radiology: Principles and Interpretation*, 6th ed., 2011, 225–242.

3. Abramovitch, K.; Rice, D.D. Basic principles of cone beam computed tomography. *Dent Clin N Am.* 2014; 58:463–484.
4. Alamri, H.M.; Sadrameli, M. et al. Applications of CBCT in dental practice: A review of the literature. *Gen Dentist.* 2012;www.agd.org:390–402.
5. Venkatesh, E.; Elluru, S.V. Cone beam computed tomography: basics and applications in dentistry. *J Istanbul Univ Fac Dent.* 2017; 51(3 Suppl 1):S102–S121.
6. Miracle, A.C.; Mukherji, S.K. Conebeam CT of the head and neck, part 1: physical principles. *AJNR Am J Neuroradiol.* 2009;30(6):1088–1095.
7. Schulze, R; Heil, U. et al. Artefacts in CBCT: A review. *Dentomaxillofac. Radiol.* 2011;40:265–273.

MAGNETIC RESONANCE IMAGING

Magnetic resonance imaging (MRI) is an imaging modality that uses a magnetic field and radiofrequency pulses to obtain images of the internal structures of the body. Tissue contrast with MRI is the best among all the current imaging techniques. It is non-invasive, non-ionizing and doesn't cause any significant harm to tissues.[1]

History

The history of nuclear magnetic resonance (NMR) dates back to studies performed in 1938 by Isidor Isaac Rabi where a beam of molecules was sent through a magnetic field and demonstrated that they could emit radio waves at specific frequencies. In 1944, he was awarded the Nobel Prize in Physics for his work. Subsequently, Felix Bloch and Edward Mills Purcell extended this work to solids and liquids, for which they were jointly awarded the 1952 Nobel Prize in Physics. Anticipating medical applications, in 1971 Raymond Damadian suggested that magnetic resonance (MR) relaxation times could be used to differentiate cancer from healthy tissue. In 1973, Paul Lauterbur demonstrated the usage of nuclear MR to obtain an image. The 2003 Nobel Prize in Physiology or Medicine was jointly awarded to Lauterbur and Sir Peter Mansfield in recognition of their pioneering efforts. But the first human MR images were published in 1977, six years after the first human CT images. The first human MR imaging study took nearly five hours to acquire and is based on the field focused nuclear MR (or FONAR) voxel-imaging technique.[2]

Equipment

The MR system consists of two main groups of equipment. First, a control center, where the operator sits, that houses the "host" computer, its associated electronics and power amplifiers situated in an adjacent room connected to the second equipment group. The second group of equipment is housed within the machine where the patient lies. It has parts that produce and receive the MR signal and also has a set of main magnet coils, three gradient coils, shim coils and a radiofrequency (RF) transmitter coil.

The patient is positioned within the bore of the machine surrounded by coils lying concentric to each other in the order: Main magnet coils, gradient coils and radiofrequency (RF) coils.

Due to use of RF electromagnetic waves or radio waves, the room containing this second set of equipment needs to keep potential sources of electromagnetic noise out and its own RF in. This is accomplished by enclosing the magnet and its coils in a special, copper-lined examination room, forming something called a Faraday shield.[3]

Magnets

Magnets with higher field strength are needed to increase the strength of the emitted signal.[4] [(KJ)] Hence, superconducting magnets are typically used in clinical MR systems. The main magnet coils are made of a superconducting metal-alloy that generates a strong, constant magnetic field (B_0) throughout the exposure. The strength of the magnetic field is measured in units of tesla (T). Approximately, 1 Tesla is equivalent to 20,000 times the magnetic field of Earth. Most clinical MR systems operate at 1.5 T or 3 T.[3]

Gradient Coils

Gradient coils represent the three orthogonal directions (x, y and z) lying concentric to each other within the main magnet that operate relatively close to room temperature. Each gradient coil has the capability of generating a magnetic field in the same direction as B_0, but the strength changes with position along the x, y or z directions, depending on which gradient coil is being used.[3] It is the use of these gradient coils that differentiates MR scanners from conventional NMR systems. Practically, gradient coils are constructed by winding them on a cylindrical coil form that surrounds the patient.[4]

Radiofrequency (RF) Coils

RF coils receive and/or transmit the RF signal. They transmit RF energy to the tissue of interest and receive the induced RF signal back from the tissue of interest.[1, 3, 4] The RF field is also referred to as the B_1 field. When it is turned on, the B_1 field combines with B_0 to produce MR signals creating an MRI. The output signal picked up by the receiver coil is digitized and then sent to a reconstruction computer processor where the image is generated after a complex mathematical calculation.[3]

Shim Coils

Localization of the MR signal needs homogeneity within the local magnetic field. Nevertheless, the placement of an object in the main B_0 field generates local susceptibility effects reducing the homogeneity. Shimming is adjustments made to the magnet to improve its homogeneity. It can be passive or active. Passive shimming is done during magnet installation by placing sheets or small coins of metal at certain places at the edge of the magnet bore, close to where the RF and gradient coils lie. Active shimming provides additional field correction of an object of interest by using shim coils.[3, 4]

MR Signals

To generate almost all clinical images, MR signals come from hydrogen nuclei. A hydrogen nucleus consists of a single proton that carries a positive electrical charge.[3] The proton constantly spins and creates a tiny magnetic field. As a result, protons have their own magnetic fields and behave like little bar magnets.[4]

The magnetic field of each proton is called a *magnetic moment*. Magnetic moments are randomly oriented when there is no external magnetic field. But, when an external magnetic field (B_0) is applied, they align either parallel or anti-parallel to the external field. Generally, they prefer to align in the direction that requires the least energy, that is, parallel to B_0 represented as the z-axis.[3-5]

Precession

When in an external static magnetic field, in addition to aligning either parallel or anti-parallel to B_0 the magnetic moments of protons also precess or wobble about the external field.[6] This motion is called *precession*. Precession can be compared to the movement of a spinning top that wobbles when spun but does not fall over and the axes over the top circles form a cone shape.

The frequency of precession is called the *Larmor frequency* (ω_0) *or resonance frequency* and is defined by the Larmor equation:

$$\omega_0 = \gamma B_0$$

γ is a constant for a particular nucleus and is termed the gyromagnetic ratio. For a proton it is 42.6 MHz/T. The Larmor equation represents that precession frequency is proportional to the strength of the magnetic field.[3–6]

Longitudinal Magnetization

Protons which are precessing parallel to B_0 begin to cancel each other out in all directions. The net result is a sum magnetic field or sum magnetization (M), with the value M_0 which is shown as a vector. Since this sum magnetization parallels the external magnetic field it is also referred to as *longitudinal magnetization*.

Longitudinal magnetization. Here, protons are vector (A). The magnetic moments of protons precessing in the external magnetic field begin to cancel each other out. Opposing protons A and A_0 and B and B_0 "neutralize" each other leaving a net number of protons parallel to B_0. Protons precessing parallel to B_0 cancel each other out. C on the left and C_0 on the right oppose and neutralize each other. This happens in all the directions bar one: The direction of the z-axis, along B_0. The result is a sum of magnetic field that is typically depicted as a vector (B).

RF Pulses and Transverse Magnetization

Patient in the magnet while processing longitudinal magnetization, RF pulses are switched on and off to disturb the protons resulting in them being out of alignment with B_0. This happens because of the transfer of energy from the RF pulse to the protons. This can happen only when the RF pulse is the same as the precessional frequency of the protons, a phenomenon called *resonance*. RF pulses are set accordingly at the Larmor frequency. Due to the activation of an RF pulse some of the protons gain energy and move to the higher energy state, i.e. anti-parallel to B_0. Subsequently, those parallel and anti-parallel to B_0 cancel each other out, resulting in overall reduction of longitudinal magnetization. Also, the RF pulse will result in the protons moving in phase (i.e. in the same direction, at the same time). The resultant magnetization vector is transverse magnetization in the x–y plane which moves in line with the precessing protons at the Larmor frequency.[3–5]

The transverse magnetization vector is a moving magnetic field, so, if a conductive receiver coil is placed closed to it, an alternating voltage will be induced across it which in turn generates an electrical current that can be picked up in the form of an *MR signal*.[3] The magnitude of this signal is proportional to the overall concentration of hydrogen nuclei in the tissue. Tightly bound hydrogen atoms like those in bone do not align themselves with the external magnetic field and produce a weak signal. Loosely bound hydrogen atoms produce a detectable signal at the end of the RF pulse. The concentration of available loosely bound hydrogen atoms to create the signal is called the proton density or spin density of a tissue.[4] When the RF pulse is switched off the protons start to fall out of phase and return to a lower energy state, called *relaxation*.[3, 4]

T1 Relaxation

T1 relaxation is a process where protons transfer energy to their surroundings to return to their low energy state causing the return of longitudinal magnetization.[1–3] The time required for 63% of net magnetization to return to equilibrium is called the *T1 relaxation time or spin-lattice relaxation time*.[3, 4] The T1 relaxation time varies for different tissues and reflects the tissue's ability to transfer its excess energy to surrounding molecules.[4]

T2 Relaxation

At the end of the RF pulse, the magnetic moments of neighboring hydrogen nuclei start to interfere with each other resulting in the dephasing of nuclei, which further leads to loss of transverse magnetization. The time constant that describes this loss is called the *T2 relaxation time or spin-spin relaxation time*. T2 is a constant describing the time taken for transverse magnetization to decay about 37% of its initial value.

(A) T1 curve: In plotting the recovery of longitudinal magnetization, over time, following the switching off of an RF pulse results in a T1 curve.
(B) T2 curve: A 180° refocusing pulse acts to "combat" the effects of external magnetic field inhomogeneity by rephasing the protons. This results in a temporary gain in signal intensity at echo time (TE) termed spin echo. A sequence of 180° pulses results in a chain of spin echoes. Each subsequent echo will be of lower intensity due to T2 effects. The c curve connecting the spin echo intensities is the T2 curve.
(C) T2* curve: This curve results when 180° refocusing pulses are not used. The signal decays much faster due to T2* effects.

TR - repetition time is the amount of time between successive pulse sequences applied to the same slice.

Free Induction Decay (FID)

When the RF pulse is switched off, T1 and T2 relaxation occur simultaneously and also independently. Protons continue to precess and the net magnetization vector follows a spiral path where its magnitude and direction constantly change resulting in an electrical signal in a suitable receiver coil. The MR signal thus generated from the spiraling net magnetization vector is called FID. FID is subjected to further dephasing by the magnetic field gradients used to localize and encode the MR signal. As a result the signal generated by FID is not usually measured in MRI. Instead, it is measured in the form of an echo: Typically, a spin echo (SE) or a gradient echo (GRE).[3-5]

Free Induction Decay

Transverse magnetization is at its greatest following an initial 90° excitatory RF pulse. Its amplitude along with signal intensity then decreases as the protons begin to lose phase coherence. The resultant decay signal is termed free induction decay.

Tissue Contrast

Contrast between tissues allows them to be differentiated from one another and they are further determined by the signal intensities governed by the T1 and T2 relaxation times of tissues within an image.[3, 4] An image in which the difference of signal intensity is predominantly due to differences in tissue T1 relaxation time is called a *T1-weighted image*. T1 weighted images are generated mostly by manipulating the time between two RF excitation pulses, i.e. repetition time (TR).[3, 5] Tissues with fast T1 times like fat appear bright whereas tissues with long T1 times like water and cerebrospinal fluid (CSF) appear dark. T1-weighted images are usually used to demonstrate anatomy.[3-5]

An image in which the difference of signal intensity is predominantly due to differences in tissue T2 relaxation time is called a *T2-weighted image*. T2 images are generated by using long TR times and long echo times (TE). TE is the time after the application of the RF pulse when MR signal is read.[4, 5]

Contrast Agents

Signal intensity emitted by a tissue can be altered using contrast agents. These agents change the signal intensity by altering the T1 or T2 relaxation times. Contrast enhancement is predominantly determined by the vascularity and the interstitial vascular space of the tissue involved.[6]

MR contrast agents are classified into ferromagnetic, paramagnetic and super magnetic. The paramagnetic type is the most popularly used and has the greatest relaxation as protons in water molecules. A paramagnetic agent, lanthanide also known as gadolinium diethylene thiamine pantothenic acid (Gd-DTPA), shortens T1 and T2 relaxation times.[4, 6]

Advantages[1, 3, 4, 6]

- Differentiation among various types of normal and abnormal tissues due to greater tissue contrast, with clarity that is supreme to any other imaging technique.
- Non-ionizing radiation and relative lack of side effects. High patient acceptability.
- The absence of artifacts due to bone or air.
- Direct multiplanar imaging without changing the orientation of the patient.

Disadvantages[1, 3, 4, 6]

- Relatively long imaging times.
- Potential hazard caused by the presence of ferromagnetic metals in close proximity to imaging magnet.
- Excessive noise and potential to hearing loss.
- RF pulses can cause local tissue heating through the dissipation of energy. Typically this is negligible (<1°C) but is potentially a risk in patients with implantable devices.

References

1. Patralekh, M.K.; Kalra, M. Basics of magnetic resonance imaging. https://www.researchgate.net/publication/294088588 2012.
2. Edelman, R.R. The history of MR imaging as seen through the pages of radiology. *Radiology*. 2014 Nov;273(2 Suppl):S181–S200.
3. Currie, S.; Hoggard, N.; Craven, I.J; Hadjivassiliou, M.; Wilkinson, I.D. Understanding MRI: Basic MR physics for physicians. *Postgrad Med J.* 2013;89:209–223.
4. White, S.C.; Pharoah, M.J. *Oral Radiology: Principles and Interpretation*, 6th ed., 2011, 212–217, Mosby Elseiver.
5. Brown, M.A.; Richard, C.S. *MRI Basic Principles And Applications*, 3rd ed., 2003, 1–8, 11, 24, 27, John Wiley & Sons, Inc.
6. Dr. Tekale, P.D.; Dr. Mhaske, A.R.; Dr. Chitko, S.S.; Dr. Parhad, S.M.; Dr. Bhandari, A.P.; Dr. Patil, H.A. MRI and dentistry: A contemporary review. *Eur J Biomedi Pharmaceut Sci.* 2014;1(3):490–503.

Index